SYSTEMIC THERAPY FOR GENITOURINARY CANCERS

Systemic Therapy for Genitourinary Cancers

DOUGLAS E. JOHNSON, M.D.

W.A. "Tex" and Deborah Moncrief, Jr., Chair in Urology
Professor of Urology
The University of Texas M. D. Anderson Cancer Center
Houston, Texas

CHRISTOPHER J. LOGOTHETIS, M.D.

Chief, Section of Genitourinary Oncology
Associate Professor of Medicine
The University of Texas M. D. Anderson Cancer Center
Houston, Texas

ANDREW C. VON ESCHENBACH, M.D.

Chairman, Department of Urology
Professor of Urology
The University of Texas M. D. Anderson Cancer Center
Houston, Texas

YEAR BOOK MEDICAL PUBLISHERS, INC.
CHICAGO • LONDON • BOCA RATON

1 2 3 4 5 6 7 8 9 0 PR 93 92 91 90 89

Library of Congress Cataloging-in-Publication Data
Systemic therapy for genitourinary cancers / [edited by] Douglas E.
    Johnson, Christopher J. Logothetis, Andrew C. von Eschenbach.
        p.   cm.
    Includes bibliographies and index.
    ISBN 0-8151-4935-2
    1. Genitourinary organs—Cancer—Chemotherapy.   2. Genitourinary
organs—Cancer—Immunotherapy.   I. Johnson, Douglas E., 1934–
II. Logothetis, Christopher J., 1950– III. von Eschenbach, Andrew C.,
1941–
        [DNLM: 1. Carcinoma.   2. Genital Neoplasms, Male—therapy.
3. Sarcoma.   4. Urologic Neoplasms—therapy.   WJ 700 S995]
RC280.G4S985   1989
616.99'46061--dc19   88-38639
DNLM/DLC   CIP
for Library of Congress

Sponsoring Editor: David K. Marshall
Associate Managing Editor, Manuscript Services: Deborah Thorp
Production Project Manager: Gayle Paprocki
Proofroom Manager: Shirley E. Taylor

Dedicated to
Melvin L. Samuels, M.D.
physician, oncologist, teacher, and friend.
His uncompromising commitment to providing the best patient care
possible made all of us who worked with him better and more caring physicians.

CONTRIBUTORS

RICHARD ABBOTT, M.B.B.S.,
F.R.A.C.P.
Visiting Physician in Oncology
Royal Adelaide Hospital
Adelaide, Australia

ALBERTO G. AYALA, M.D.
Professor of Pathology
Deputy Chairman, Department of
  Pathology
Director, Section of Surgical Pathology
The University of Texas M. D. Anderson
  Cancer Center
Houston, Texas

R. JOSEPH BABAIAN, M.D.
Associate Professor of Urology
University of Texas M. D. Anderson
  Cancer Center
Houston, Texas

NEIL BANDER, M.D.
Assistant Professor of Surgery (Urology)
Cornell University Medical Center
Assistant Attending Surgeon (Urologist)
New York Hospital
New York, New York

ROBERT S. BENJAMIN, M.D.
Professor of Medicine
Chief, Section of Melanoma/Sarcoma
Department of Medical Oncology
The University of Texas M. D. Anderson
  Cancer Center
Houston, Texas

RALPH C. BENSON, JR., M.D.
Professor of Urology
Mayo Medical School
Rochester, Minnesota
Consultant, Section of Urology
Mayo Clinic Jacksonville
Jacksonville, Florida

PETER BILENKIJ, M.B.B.S.,
F.R.A.C.S.
Urologist
The Orange Base Hospital
Orange, Australia

JAMES BISHOP, M.B.B.S.,
F.R.A.C.P., F.R.C.P.A.
Department of Cancer Medicine
University of Melbourne
Peter MacCallum Cancer Institute
Melbourne, Australia

GEORGE J. BOSL, M.D.
Associate Professor of Medicine
Cornell University Medical College
Associate Attending Physician
Memorial Sloan-Kettering Cancer Center
New York, New York

JOHN BOULAS, M.B.B.S., F.R.A.C.S.
University of Sydney
Royal Prince Alfred Hospital
Sydney, Australia

ISADORE BRODSKY, M.D., PH.D.
Professor and Chairman
Department of Neoplastic Diseases
Hahnemann University Hospital
Philadelphia, Pennsylvania

RONALD M. BUKOWSKI, M.D.
Staff Physician
Hematology/Oncology and Cancer
*   Immunology*
Cleveland Clinic Foundation
Cleveland, Ohio

W. IVON BURNS, M.B.B.S.,
F.R.A.C.P.
Senior Associate
Department of Medicine
University of Melbourne
Director Medical Oncology
St. Vincent's Hospital
Melbourne, Australia

MICHAEL BYRNE, M.B.B.S.,
F.R.A.C.P.
Head, Department of Medical Oncology
Medical School, University of Western
*   Australia*
Sir Charles Gairdner Hospital
Nedlands, Australia

WILLIAM A. CARTER, M.D.
Department of Neoplastic Diseases
Fred Kroll Chemotherapy Testing Center
Hahnemann University of Health Sciences
Philadelphia, Pennsylvania

CLAYTON D.K. CHONG, M.D.
Assistant Professor of Medicine
Section of Genitourinary Oncology
Department of Medical Oncology
The University of Texas M. D. Anderson
*   Cancer Center*
Houston, Texas

GLEN J. COOREY, M.B.B.S.,
F.R.C.S., F.R.A.C.S.
Lecturer in Surgery
University of Sydney
Chairman and Visiting Urologist
Royal Prince Alfred Hospital
Sydney, Australia

D. DAVID DERSHAW, M.D.
Assistant Professor of Radiology
Cornell University Medical College
Memorial Sloan–Kettering Cancer Center
New York, New York

WILLIAM D. DEWYS, M.D.
Department of Medicine
Capital Area Permanente Medical Group
Attending Physician
Fairfax Hospital
Falls Church, Virginia

FRANCISCO DEXEUS, M.D.
Assistant Professor of Medicine
Section of Genitourinary Oncology
Department of Medical Oncology
The University of Texas M. D. Anderson
*   Cancer Center*
Houston, Texas

PETER DUVAL, M.B.B.S., F.R.C.R.,
F.R.A.C.R.
Acting Head
Department of Radiation Oncology
The Orange Base Hospital
Orange, Australia
Royal Alexander Hospital for Children
Sydney, Australia

WILLIAM R. FAIR, M.D.
Professor of Surgery
Cornell University Medical College
Chief, Urology Service
Memorial Sloan-Kettering Cancer Center
New York, New York

TRENT DOUGLAS FAREBROTHER,
PH.C., M.B.B.S., F.R.A.C.S.
Master, University of New Castle
Visiting Urologist
Gosford Hospital
Gosford, Australia

ISAIAH J. FIDLER, D.V.M., PH.D.
R. E. "Bob" Smith Chair in Cell Biology
Professor and Chairman
Department of Cell Biology
The University of Texas M. D. Anderson
*   Cancer Center*
Houston, Texas

LAURY FINN, R.T.
Coordinator—Research Data
Section of Genitourinary Oncology
Department of Medical Oncology
The University of Texas M. D. Anderson
*   Cancer Center*
Houston, Texas

RICHARD FOX, M.B.B.S., PH.D.,
F.R.A.C.P.
Professor and Director
Department of Haematology and Medical
Oncology
University of McAconne
The Royal Melbourne Hospital
Melbourne, Australia

FUAD S. FREIHA, M.D.
Associate Professor and Chief
Urologic Oncology
Stanford University School of Medicine
Stanford, California

RAM GANAPATHI, PH.D.
Staff Scientist
Research Institute
Cleveland Clinic Foundation
Cleveland, Ohio

MARC B. GARNICK, M.D.
Associate Professor of Medicine
Harvard Medical School
Dana-Farber Cancer Institute
Boston, Massachusetts

MICHAEL A. GEISINGER, M.D.
Department of Hospital Radiology
Cleveland Clinic Foundation
Cleveland, Ohio

NANCY L. GELLER, PH.D.
Associate Member
Memorial Sloan-Kettering Cancer Center
Associate Attending Biostatistician
Memorial Hospital
New York, New York

DONALD F. GLEASON, M.D., PH.D.
Associate Professor (Retired)
Laboratory Medicine and Pathology
University of Minnesota
Minneapolis, Minnesota

VERNON HARVEY, M.D., M.R.C.P.,
F.R.A.C.P.
Consultant, Medical Oncologist
Auckland Hospital
Auckland, New Zealand

HARRY W. HERR, M.D.
Associate Professor of Surgery
Cornell University Medical College
Associate Attending Surgeon
Memorial Sloan-Kettering Cancer Center
New York Hospital
New York, New York

DANIEL C. IHDE, M.D.
Professor of Medicine
Uniformed Services University of the
Health Sciences
Deputy Chief, NCI-Navy Medical
Oncology Branch
Naval Hospital
Bethesda, Maryland

NORMAN JAFFE, M.D., D.SC.
Professor of Pediatrics
Chief, Section of Solid Tumors
Division of Pediatrics
The University of Texas M. D. Anderson
Cancer Center
Houston, Texas

DOUGLAS E. JOHNSON, M.D.
W.A. "Tex" and Deborah Moncrief, Jr.,
Chair in Urology
Professor of Urology
The University of Texas M. D. Anderson
Cancer Center
Houston, Texas

ZOLTAN KERESTES, B.SC., PH.D.
(PHYSICS)
Computer Scientist
Royal North Shore Hospital
Sydney, Australia

MARIAN LEE, M.D.
Department of Hematology/Medical
Oncology
Cleveland Clinic Foundation
Cleveland, Ohio

JOHN LEVI, M.B.B.S., F.R.A.C.P.
University of Sydney
Director, Department of Clinical
Oncology
Royal North Shore Hospital
Sydney, Australia

W. MARSTON LINEHAN, M.D.
Head, Urologic Oncology Section
Surgery Branch
National Cancer Institute
Bethesda, Maryland

RICHARD K. LO, M.D.
Assistant Professor of Surgery (Urology)
Stanford University School of Medicine
Chief, Section of Urology
Palo Alto Veterans Administration Medical
*   Center*
Palo Alto, California

CHRISTOPHER J. LOGOTHETIS, M.D.
Chief, Section of Genitourinary Oncology
Associate Professor of Medicine
Department of Medical Oncology
The University of Texas M. D. Anderson
*   Cancer Center*
Houston, Texas

BERT LUM, PHARM. D.
Stanford University Medical Center
Stanford, California

HEDY MAMEGHAN, B.M., B.CH.
(OXON), F.R.C.R., F.R.A.C.R.
Radiation Oncologist
University of New South Wales
Prince of Wales Hospital
Sydney, Australia

DEVORAH T. MAX, M.D.
Abbott Laboratories
Abbott Park
North Chicago, Illinois

JAMES E. MONTIE, M.D.
Department of Urology
Cleveland Clinic Florida
Ft. Lauderdale, Florida

MICHAEL J. MORSE, M.D.
Department of Surgery (Urology)
Memorial Sloan-Kettering Cancer Center
New York, New York

SEIJI NAITO, M.D.
Visiting Assistant Professor
Departments of Cell Biology and Urology
The University of Texas M. D. Anderson
*   Cancer Center*
Houston, Texas

JEROME NISSELBAUM, PH.D.
Associate Professor
Cornell University
Associate Attending
Memorial Sloan-Kettering Cancer Center
New York, New York

SHERYL OGDEN, B.S.N.
Supervisor, Research
Section of Genitourinary Oncology
Department of Medical Oncology
The University of Texas M. D. Anderson
*   Cancer Center*
Houston, Texas

ROBERT F. OZOLS, M.D., PH.D.
Head, Experimental Therapeutics Section
Medicine Branch
National Cancer Institute
Bethesda, Maryland

NICHOLAS E.J. PAPADOPOULOS, M.D.
Assistant Professor of Medicine
Section of Melanoma/Sarcoma
Department of Medical Oncology
The University of Texas M. D. Anderson
*   Cancer Center*
Houston, Texas

BRUCE SAMUEL PEARSON, M.B.B.S.,
F.R.C.S., F.R.A.C.S.
Lecturer in Urology
University of Sydney
VMO Royal Prince Alfred Hospital
Sydney, Australia

CHARLES E. PIPPENGER, PH.D.
Head, Section of Applied Clinical
*   Pharmacology*
Cleveland Clinic Foundation
Cleveland, Ohio

J. EDSON PONTES, M.D.
Head, Section of Urologic Oncology
Cleveland Clinic Foundation
Cleveland, Ohio

JORGE R. QUESADA, M.D.
Department of Clinical Immunology and
*   Biological Therapy*
The University of Texas M. D. Anderson
*   Cancer Center*
Houston, Texas

DEREK RAGHAVAN, M.B.B.S., PH.D.,
F.R.A.C.P.
Department of Clinical Oncology
Royal Prince Alfred Hospital
Sydney, Australia

A. KEVIN RAYMOND, M.D.
Associate Professor of Pathology
The University of Texas M. D. Anderson
*   Cancer Center*
Houston, Texas

VICTOR REUTER, M.D.
Assistant Attending Pathologist
Memorial Sloan Kettering Cancer Center
New York, New York

BARBARA RISIUS, M.D.
Department of Radiology
Cleveland Clinic Foundation
Cleveland, Ohio

JOHN ROGERS, M.B.B.S., F.R.C.S.,
F.R.A.C.S.
Lecturer, University of Sydney
Visiting Urologist
Royal Prince Alfred Hospital
Sydney, Australia

JAE Y. RO, M.D., PH.D.
Assistant Professor of Pathology
The University of Texas M. D. Anderson
*   Cancer Center*
Houston, Texas

I. M. ROSEN, M.B.B.S., F.R.C.S.,
F.R.A.C.S.
Urologist, Illawarra Urology Unit
Consultant Urologist
Illawarra Area Health Service Hospitals
Figtree, Australia

THOMAS F. SANDEMAN, M.B., CH.B.,
D.M.R.T., F.R.C.R., F.R.A.C.R.
Consultant, Radiation Oncologist
Peter MacCallum Cancer Institute
Melbourne, Australia

HOWARD I. SCHER, M.D.
Assistant Professor of Medicine
Cornell University Medical College
Assistant Attending Physician
Solid Tumor Service
Department of Medicine
Memorial Sloan-Kettering Cancer Center
New York, New York

MORTON SCHWARTZ, PH.D.
Professor of Biochemistry
Cornell University Medical College
Chairman, Department of Clinical
*   Chemistry*
Memorial Sloan-Kettering Cancer Center
New York, New York

AVISHAY SELLA, M.D.
Assistant Professor of Medicine
Section of Genitourinary Oncology
Department of Medical Oncology
The University of Texas M. D. Anderson
*   Cancer Center*
Houston, Texas

SABRI E. SEN, M.D.
Resident in Urology
Mayo Graduate School of Medicine
Rochester, Minnesota

HIKMET SIPAHI, M.D.
Department of Medical Oncology
The University of Texas M. D. Anderson
*   Cancer Center*
Houston, Texas

TRACY SMART-CURLEY, R.N.
Department of Medicine
Memorial Sloan-Kettering Cancer Center
New York, New York

PRAMOD C. SOGANI, M.D., F.R.C.S.,
F.A.C.S.
Assistant Professor of Surgery
Cornell University Medical College
Associate Attending Surgeon
Memorial Sloan-Kettering Cancer Center
New York, New York

MARK S. SOLOWAY, M.D.
Professor, Department of Urology
Chief, Urologic Oncology
University of Tennessee at Memphis
Attending Physician
Baptist Memorial Hospital
Memphis, Tennessee

ROXANNE E. STEINLE, M.D.
Department of Biochemistry
Cleveland Clinic Foundation
Cleveland, Ohio

CORA N. STERNBERG, M.D.
Clinical Instructor in Medicine
Cornell University Medical College
Clinical Assistant Attending
Memorial Sloan-Kettering Cancer Center
New York, New York

DAVID R. STRAYER, M.D.
Professor, Department of Neoplastic
*   Diseases*
Hahnemann University
Philadelphia, Pennsylvania

DAVID A. SWANSON, M.D.
Associate Professor of Urology
Deputy Chairman, Department of Urology
The University of Texas M. D. Anderson
*   Cancer Center*
Houston, Texas

LINDA J. SWANSON, PH.D.
Senior Clinical Research Associate
Abbott Laboratories
North Chicago, Illinois

MARTIN H.N. TATTERSALL, M.D.,
F.R.C.P., F.R.A.C.P.
Royal Prince Alfred Hospital
Sydney, Australia

DENISE M. TENNEY, R.N., B.S.
Research Nurse
Department of Urology
The University of Texas M. D. Anderson
*   Cancer Center*
Houston, Texas

NORY TERIANA, B.S. HYGIENE
Data Manager
Urological Cancer Research Unit
Royal Prince Alfred Hospital
Sydney, Australia

GILLIAN M. THOMAS, M.D.
Assistant Professor of Radiology
University of Toronto
Staff Radiation Oncologist
Toronto Bayview Regional Cancer Center
Toronto, Ontario, Canada

DAMIEN THOMSON, M.B.B.S.,
F.R.A.C.P.
Clinical Lecturer
University of Queensland
Staff Medical Oncologist
Princess Alexandra Hospital
Brisbane, Australia

CARLO TONDINI, M.D.
Fellow, Division of Medical Oncology
Dana Farber Cancer Institute
Harvard Medical School
Boston, Massachusetts

FRANK M. TORTI, M.D.
Associate Professor of Medicine
Stanford University School of Medicine
Chief, Oncology Section
Veterans Administration Center
Palo Alto, California

E. DARRACOTT VAUGHAN, JR., M.D.
James J. Colt Professor of Urology
Director, Division of Urology
Cornell University Medical Center
Attending Urologist-in-Chief
The New York Hospital
New York, New York

ANDREW C. VON ESCHENBACH, M.D.
Chairman, Department of Urology
Professor of Urology
The University of Texas M. D. Anderson
*   Cancer Center*
Houston, Texas

ROBIN C. WATSON, M.D.
Professor of Radiology
Cornell University Medical College
Attending, Memorial Hospital
New York Hospital
New York, New York

W. HUNTER WATT, M.B.B.S.,
F.R.A.C.S.
Urologist, Illawarra Urology Unit
Consultant Urologist
Illawarra Area Health Service Hospitals
Wollongong, Australia

WILLET F. WHITMORE, JR., M.D.
Professor of Surgery (Urology)
Cornell University Medical Center
Memorial Sloan-Kettering Cancer Center
New York, New York

KENNETH I. WISHNOW, M.D.
Assistant Professor of Urology
The University of Texas M. D. Anderson
  Cancer Center
Houston, Texas

ALAN YAGODA, M.D.
Professor of Clinical Medicine
Cornell University Medical Center
Attending Physician
Memorial Sloan-Kettering Cancer Center
New York, New York

ROBERT C. YOUNG, M.D.
Associate Director
Centers and Community Oncology
  Program
National Cancer Institute
Bethesda, Maryland

GUNAR K. ZAGARS, M.D.
Associate Professor of Radiotherapy
The University of Texas M. D. Anderson
  Cancer Center
Houston, Texas

MARGARET ZELCH, M.D.
Head, Section of Vascular and
  Interventional Radiology
Department of Diagnostic Radiology
Cleveland Clinic Foundation
Cleveland, Ohio

HORST ZINCKE, M.D.
Professor of Urology
Mayo Medical School
Consultant, Department of Urology and
  Surgery
Mayo Clinic and Mayo Foundation
Rochester, Minnesota

PREFACE

Cancers of the urinary system and male genital tract account for 16% of all malignant disease. Although the overall incidence of cancer has decreased slightly in the past quarter-century, the number of new cases of genitourinary tumors has continued to rise. Efforts by numerous medical organizations and lay societies have done much to encourage earlier diagnosis, but unfortunately the majority of patients who have genitourinary tumors either have metastatic disease present at the time the primary tumor is diagnosed or will subsequently develop cancer at distant sites.

Over the past decade, major technologic advances—computed scans, magnetic resonance imaging, biochemical and radioimmunoassays for a wide range of tumor antigens (beta human chorionic gonadotropins, alpha-fetoprotein, carcinoembryonic antigens, prostatic-specific antigen, prostatic acid phosphatase, squamous cell antigen), flow cytometric studies for DNA content, and the emerging use of monoclonal antibodies—have significantly increased our ability to detect metastases or identify patients who are at risk for metastatic spread. During the same period a relatively large number of new active agents has been introduced—cisplatin, bleomycin, Adriamycin, epipodophylotoxin derivatives (VP-16, VM-26), vindesine, and ifosfamide. These drugs, when variously combined with older established agents such as mitomycin, vinblastine, vincristine, cyclophosphamide, and methotrexate, are providing effective treatment. Cures of germ cell tumors have become routine, and several combination chemotherapy programs have recently demonstrated their ability to eradicate metastatic urothelial tumors. These successes have given us cause to investigate ways of reducing drug toxicity and concomitant morbidity while simultaneously maintaining or increasing drug activity. In addition, the ready availability of these active chemotherapy programs combined with the increasing ability to identify patients who have or will develop metastasis has caused major changes in our approach to the treatment of patients who have early-stage genitourinary tumors.

New treatment strategies are especially evident for patients with testicular and bladder malignancies. Surveillance, rather than immediate retroperitoneal lymphadenectomy with its inherent risks, has become the standard approach at many centers for early-stage nonseminomatous germ cell tumors of the testis. In selected cases of regional lymph node spread, chemotherapy has eliminated the need for surgical intervention. Similarly, chemotherapy has reduced the employment of radiotherapy for patients with advanced testicular seminoma or invasive bladder carcinoma. The integrated programs of the 1970s, which used preoperative radiotherapy followed by radical cystectomy for patients with invasive bladder carcinoma, have given way today to neoadjuvant and adjuvant chemotherapy programs. Their effectiveness has led some clinicians to consider chemotherapy as the primary treatment for selected patients. At the same time immunotherapy, particularly using bacille Calmette-Guérin (BCG), has recently offered new promise for improving the control of superficial bladder cancer and lessening the need for radical cystectomy.

Prostatic carcinoma is less responsive to cytotoxic drugs than either testicular or urothelial tumors. Difficulties in assessing response together with problems arising from the advanced age of many of the patients have delayed advances in systemic therapy for this neoplasm. However, new agents have been introduced to treat prostatic carcinoma, including luteinizing hormone-releasing hormone (LH-RH) agonists, ketoconazole, and megestrol acetate. These hormonal agents have toxicities different from those of the cytotoxic agents and provide new therapeutic options for patients with metastatic prostate cancer. In addition, combination chemotherapy programs are playing an increasing role in helping palliate patients who suffer with hormonally refractory disease.

Although few drugs have proved to be effective in treating metastatic renal cell carcinoma, refinements in chemotherapy-sensitivity testing in vitro are making possible the rapid screening of a large number of potential agents. Interferons have demonstrated modest action against metastatic renal cell carcinoma, and encouraging results, admittedly preliminary, have been reported for lymphokine-activated killer cells activated with interleukin 2 (IL-2-activated LAK cells).

The wide range of therapeutic options currently employed for advanced genitourinary tumors is evidenced in the myriad recent publications detailing their use. Consequently, we have tried to synthesize the important developments and to provide the clinician—the primary care physician, internist, medical oncologist, urologist, or radiotherapist—with a ready resource detailing the treatment programs currently used to manage advanced genitourinary tumors.

Each of the four major sections contains three different types of chapters, an overview, a series of specific and sometimes controversial chapters, and a commentary. The overview is purposely written jointly with a pathologist and highlights what we consider to be the major clinically relevant advances made in the diagnosis, staging, and therapeutic approaches to each of these malignancies. The subsequent chapters comprise recent methods of therapy developed at leading cancer centers by experienced investigators in the United States, Canada, and Australia who treat patients with advanced genitourinary tumors. These chapters allow the clinician to examine and evaluate the complications and results that are to be expected with the varying treatment programs and, we hope, provide the information necessary for choosing the therapeutic approach that is best suited for his or her patient. We are privileged that these experts in the field have been so willing to share their experience in treating these patients. The final commentaries represent the joint conclusions of the editors. They review and highlight the preceding chapters, address existing controversies, and present our conclusions about the best ways of managing these difficult situations.

We hope, therefore, that this book will provide a thorough overview of the field and also serve as an immediate reference for the clinician needing to advise a patient of the treatment options available for his disease.

Douglas E. Johnson, M.D.
Christopher J. Logothetis, M.D.
Andrew C. von Eschenbach, M.D.

ACKNOWLEDGMENTS

This book represents a compilation of the diaries from hundreds of unselfish cancer patients willing to enter investigative studies with the hope of advancing the treatment of genitourinary tumors. They have provided the experience and given meaning to our work; to each, we give our thanks.

We wish, also, to express our deep appreciation to the contributors for sharing their experience and for completing their manuscripts within the confines of a rigid schedule.

To Lonna Sager we extend special thanks for her tireless, cheerful work in seeing the manuscript through all its various stages and endless revisions; without her secretarial skills *extraordinaire* we would never have met our deadline.

Finally, no amount of thanks can adequately acknowledge our appreciation to Barbara Reschke, our medical editor. She has been an integral part of the "team" from the beginning—coaxing authors into completing their manuscripts early, giving advice and counsel where needed, and sustaining our interests when work became drudgery. Without her untiring efforts in taking the diverse manuscripts and polishing and blending them into a unified array, this project could not have been completed in its allotted time.

Douglas E. Johnson, M.D.
Christopher J. Logothetis, M.D.
Andrew C. von Eschenbach, M.D.

CONTENTS

PART II GENITAL TUMORS 159

Prostatic Carcinoma

Penile, Scrotal, and Urothelial Carcinoma

Genitourinary Sarcoma

Germ Cell Tumors

TESTICULAR SEMINOMA

NONSEMINOMATOUS TESTICULAR TUMORS

LOCOREGIONAL DISEASE

ADVANCED DISEASE

PART I

Urinary Tract Tumors

Chapter 1

Bladder Cancer: Clinically Relevant Advances

Douglas E. Johnson, M.D.

Alberto G. Ayala, M.D.

Every 13 minutes in the United States, a new case of bladder carcinoma is diagnosed, resulting in 40,000 cases annually. In 80% of the cases the lesion is superficial, confined either to the mucosa or lamina propria. Although two out of three of these patients remain at risk for recurrent disease, their malignancy never becomes invasive and poses a problem only in local management. Unfortunately, however, in the remaining patients either the lesion is invasive at the time of the initial diagnosis or subsequent tumors become invasive as time passes. It is in these latter situations that distant metastases, which resulted in a high mortality until the recent availability of active chemotherapeutic programs, most frequently occur.

If we, as clinicians, are to have a major impact on the natural history of this disease, it is imperative that we (1) establish the diagnosis early, (2) stratify patients correctly into superficial and invasive disease categories, (3) identify those patients with superficial disease who are at high risk for recurrences or for developing invasive disease, (4) recognize those patients with invasive disease who are most likely to have or to develop metastasis, and (5) learn how best to integrate available therapies to maximize tumor responses and minimize patient morbidity. It behooves us, therefore, to be cognizant of the recent advances that have been made in these areas.

DIAGNOSIS

No simple, inexpensive, and reliable screening procedures for diagnosing bladder cancer are currently available. The development of symptoms is what most often leads to the initial diagnosis. The predominant symptom is hematuria, which is both painless and macroscopic in 75% to 80% of the patients. Symptoms of vesical irritability, including increased urinary frequency, dysuria, and pain on urination, have been recorded in over one fourth of the patients who present with bladder cancer. About 20% have no specific symptoms, however, and the malignancy is discovered during an evaluation for conditions such as occult hematuria or pyuria.

Although urinary cytology and flow cytometry, used either alone or in combination, are proving helpful in monitoring patients with a history of bladder cancer, these examinations are not reliable as single tests for establishing a diagnosis of previously undiagnosed cases (Badalament et al. 1987a,b; Cowan et al. 1987). Hemstreet and associates (1986) have recently introduced acridine orange staining and slide photometry image analysis to detect bladder cancer by quantitating absolute nuclear fluorescence intensity, but too few patients have been examined to confirm the reliability of this test. Consequently, the initial diagnosis of a bladder tumor is usually a three-step procedure: first, excretory urography; second, cysto-urethroscopy; and third, histopathologic confirmation.

Although in recent years debates have increased regarding the cost-effectiveness of excretory urography (intravenous pyelogram [IVP]) in screening patients with various urologic disorders, the first step in establishing the diagnosis of a bladder tumor in the majority of patients is still an IVP. This procedure helps to eliminate the upper urinary tracts (renal parenchyma, ureter, renal pelvis, and calyces) as sources of the patient's symptoms. Occasionally, however, the procedure demonstrates other associated urothelial tumors in addition to bladder carcinoma. The excretory cystogram, which is an integral part of the IVP, frequently raises the suspicion of a bladder tumor by demonstrating an irregular filling defect.

The second step in diagnosing a bladder tumor, careful cystourethroscopy, identifies the lesion(s), but their malignant nature can be confirmed only by histopathologic evaluation of *adequate* biopsy specimens. Even though today government and third-party payers apply increasing pressures to perform surgery in an outpatient setting, it is imperative, nevertheless, that the urologist carry out a careful, methodical inspection of the bladder and urethral urothelium and remove an adequate amount of tissue from the primary lesion and any suspicious-appearing areas. Ideally, tissue from the base of the tumor, including muscle, should be included with the specimen. In addition, biopsies of the primary tumor(s) should include adjacent normal-appearing epithelium. This usually requires regional or general anesthesia and a several-day hospitalization. *Inadequate biopsies can severely jeopardize proper treatment and adversely affect the patient's prognosis!*

The vast majority of bladder tumors (98%) are epithelial in origin. The World Health Organization (WHO) recommends classifying them according to four primary histologic types: transitional, squamous, adenocarcinomatous, and undifferentiated (Mostofi et al. 1973). Transitional cell carcinomas (TCC) constitute about 92%, squamous carcinoma 6% to 7%, and adenocarcinoma 1% to 2%; undifferentiated tumors account for less than 1%. When a tumor contains a mixture of primary types, the different components should be listed in decreasing order of magnitude. In the past, all epithelial tumors could be grouped together for treatment purposes, and treatment was determined by the stage of the disease (Johnson 1974). Today, however, therapy differs according to these primary histologic types. Moreover, transitional forms usually signal a poorer prognosis, and recognizing them may require altering therapy.

In addition to the histologic appearance of the tumor, other histopathologic features that need to be sought—since they are important in selecting and evaluating therapy—include the depth of tumor penetration, the presence of vascular or lymphatic invasion, and the extent of urothelial involvement (distal ureter, prostatic ducts, etc.).

SUPERFICIAL DISEASE

Stratification of patients into either superficial (stage O/A) or invasive (stage B/C) disease categories rests solely on the histologic examination of the biopsy specimen. Invasion of muscle by the malignancy has been the sine qua non for making this determination. Non-

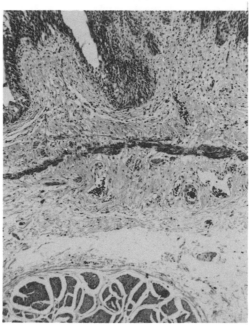

FIG 1–1.
Muscularis mucosa. This low-power illustration shows a band of smooth-muscle fibers running parallel to the mucosa, typical of the muscularis mucosa. A few large bundles of smooth muscle seen at the bottom of the picture represent the muscularis propria. (×60)

invasive (superficial) tumors of the bladder are defined as those without evidence of extension into the muscularis. Recently, however, Ro et al. (1987) have described the presence of a "muscularis mucosa," consisting of smooth muscle bundles located in the upper third of the lamina propria and forming a band that runs parallel to the overlying mucosa. In examining 100 consecutive cystectomy specimens, they found a complete muscularis mucosa (Fig 1–1) in 3; a discontinuant or interrupted layer in 20; and scattered, thin bundles of smooth-muscle fibers that did not form an obvious layer in 71. In only six cases were no muscle fibers evident in the lamina propria of the sections examined. Tumor invading the lamina propria may involve these muscle bundles without ever extending into the true muscularis; an unwary pathologist could, therefore, make an erroneous interpretation of muscle invasion (stage B). Although there is no diagnostic rule of thumb, when tumor invades only thin muscle bundles, the pathologist should suspect muscularis mucosa invasion. The presence of large blood vessels along with the thin muscle bundles should further raise the suspicion of muscularis mucosa. A histologic diagnosis of deep muscularis invasion should be restricted to those situations where tumor is found to surround or invade thick bundles of smooth muscle fiber. Whenever the pathologist is in doubt as to the actual depth of tumor penetration, he or she should encourage additional biopsies for clarification.

Another important histologic finding in patients with superficial disease that has not received proper emphasis concerns malignant changes occurring in von Brunn's nests. Frequently, as a result of proliferative changes in the bladder, the mucosa is thrown into folds, and cords of epithelium can become isolated below the surface epithelium, forming a von Brunn's nest. These epithelial nests may later undergo the full spectrum of changes, ranging from atypia to mild or moderate dysplasia and finally to carcinoma in situ (T_{is}) (Fig 1–2). It is unlikely that any currently employed intracavitary agent, such as thiotepa, doxorubicin (Adriamycin), mitomycin, or bacillus Calmette-Guérin (BCG), will penetrate deeply enough and in sufficient concentration to influence favorably this rather ominous development. Consequently, we usually favor radical surgery as treatment of patients in whom this change is evident.

Once superficial disease has been diagnosed, it becomes important to identify further those patients at risk for developing recurrent disease. Tumor recurrence and progression have been shown to relate to stage, grade, number, and size of tumors, duration of disease, positive or negative cytologic results, aneuploidy, and associated mucosal abnormalities (Herr 1987). The prognostic factor most significant for recurrence is the number of tumors present at diagnosis. Solitary superficial tumors recur in 46% of patients, whereas the recurrence rate for multifocal tumors is 73%. Lutzeyer et al. (1982) reported recurrences in only 29% of patients who presented with a solitary papillary grade 1 tumor, as contrasted to 94% of patients with multiple papillary grade 1 tumors. Similarly, the 50% recurrence rate for patients with solitary papillary grade 2 lesions rose to 100% when the lesions were grade 3. When the influence of grade on recurrence rate was examined as an independent variable, however, its effect was seen to be only slight: recurrence rates were 63%, 67%, and 71%, respectively, for grades 1, 2, and 3 tumors.

The prognostic factor second most significant for recurrence is chronology. A patient with a first tumor has a 45% risk of developing another lesion, but the patient who has developed a second tumor has an 84% risk of developing a third (Lutzeyer et al. 1982). The third most important predictor for recurrence is the simultaneous presence of dysplasia or T_{is} elsewhere in the bladder of a patient presenting with superficial bladder carcinoma. Smith et al. (1983) reported a recurrence rate of 42% when preselected quadrant biopsies failed to show epithelial abnormalities, but it increased to 73% when either dysplasia (25/34 patients) or T_{is} (2/3 patients)

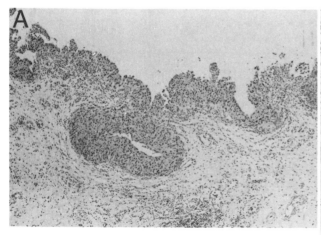
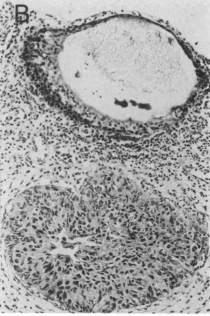

FIG 1–2.
A, T_{is} involving a von Brunn's nest. The surface mucosa shows marked nuclear atypia that extends down into a von Brunn's nest. **B**, a cystic structure (cystitis cystica) lined by slightly atypical cells is present right beneath the surface. Lower down, there is a von Brunn's nest completely replaced by transitional cell carcinoma in situ. (×150)

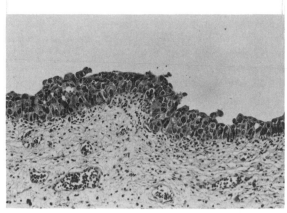

FIG 1–3.
Transitional cell carcinoma in situ. The full thickness of the mucosa is replaced by malignant cells. ($\times$ 150)

was documented. Other factors such as tumor size and location, positive or negative cytologic results, and aneuploidy have affected recurrence rates to a minor and conflicting extent.

Although most patients with superficial bladder tumors experience recurrences only of a similarly low stage and grade, as many as 30% go on to develop muscle-invasive disease. Factors associated with a higher risk for invasion parallel those associated with higher recurrence rates, namely, size, grade, and stage. Heney and associates (1983a) reported that progression to muscle invasion occurred in 35% of patients with superficial tumors larger than 5 cm as compared to 9% of patients with smaller tumors. They also found that invasive disease eventually occurred in 42% of patients whose tumors extended into the lamina propria but in only 28% of those with papillary tumors confined to the mucosa. Tumor grade also correlated with subsequent invasion: 2% of grade 1, 11% of grade 2, and 45% of grade 3 tumors ultimately became invasive.

Carcinoma in situ found concomitantly in a patient with superficial bladder tumors not only warns the clinician of the possibility of recurrent disease but also serves as a strong predictor for subsequent invasive disease. Prout and associates (1987) recently reported that of 16 patients presenting with concomitant T_{is} and papillary superficial tumor prior to the era of BCG therapy, 7 developed muscle invasions, 6 developed metastasis, and 6 died from their disease. This group had reported previously (Althausen et al. 1976) that when T_{is} is present in a bladder that also has superficial tumors, the risk of invasion may rise to as high as 83%. Carcinoma in situ remains a heterogeneous disorder that is difficult to characterize clinically; histologically, its diagnosis should be restricted to cases in which the entire thickness of the mucosa has undergone a malignant change (Fig 1–3).

A major reason why investigators have attempted to find pathologic criteria that can identify patients destined to develop invasive disease is to enable them to modify therapy from the beginning to prevent metastasis. Numerous studies have suggested that patients whose tumors contained abnormal chromosomes or failed to express either ABO(H) cell-surface or normal T (Thomsen-Friedenreich) antigens were more likely to develop invasive disease (Decenzo et al. 1975; Limas et al. 1979; Coon and Weinstein 1981; Limas and Lange 1982; Weinstein et al. 1984; Juhl et al. 1986). Initial studies, which employed the specific red cell adherence test (SRCA), were difficult to perform and often lacked reproducibility. Immunoperoxidase staining techniques were a major improvement, but because the test failed to predict invasion accurately in 20% to 30% of the patients tested, it was impossible to select definitively those patients who required more aggressive therapy. Similar problems have occurred when tumor chromosomes and T antigens were used.

Finally, the clinician monitoring and treating patients with superficial bladder carcinoma needs to be aware of the possibility that other urothelial areas, such as prostatic ducts or distal ureters, may develop similar surface changes. The usual scenario is a positive cytologic report for a patient whose cystoscopic studies are normal. In addition to employing tests such as excretory urograms, retrograde ureteral pyelograms, and ureteroscopy to exclude the upper urinary tracts as a source of the malignant cells, the physician must include transurethral prostatic biopsies to search for disease in this area. The incidence of prostatic ductal carcinoma (Fig 1–4) in patients who have bladder T_{is} has been reported to range from 26% to 43% (Farrow et al. 1976; Mahadevia et al. 1986; Wishnow and Ro, 1988). Prostatic ductal carcinoma is frequently silent and may escape notice by the inexperienced endoscopist. Its importance is highlighted by our recent finding that all patients in whom the disease invaded through the ducts into the prostatic stroma (Fig 1–5) developed metastatic disease despite radical surgery.

INVASIVE DISEASE

Treatment for patients with invasive bladder carcinoma has evolved through three readily distinguishable phases: surgery, radiotherapy, and integrated therapy consisting of preoperative radiotherapy followed by radical surgery. Early experience with either total or radical cystectomy yielded only a 13% to 18% 5-year survival rate for patients presenting with deeply invasive tumors (stage B_2) or extravesical extension (stage C) (Whitmore and Marshall 1962; Jewett et al. 1964; Marshall and McCarron 1977; Morabito et al. 1979). When supervoltage radiotherapy became available during the 1950s, urologists became interested in using it for patients with invasive bladder carcinoma. However, the early results were disappointing, as 5-year survival rates continued to be in the range of 20% (Miller and Johnson 1973). Consequently, a number of centers began exploring the use of preoperative radiation followed by radical cystectomy. Early results of this combination were encouraging, and after a decade, 5-year survival rates were generally reported in the neighborhood of 50% (Miller and Johnson 1973; van der Werf-Messing 1975; Whitmore et al. 1977). An analysis of 216 patients with invasive bladder cancer treated with integrated therapy at The University of Texas M. D.

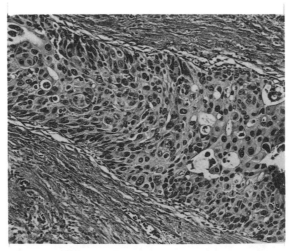

FIG 1–4.
Transitional cell carcinoma in situ involving a prostatic duct. (× 150)

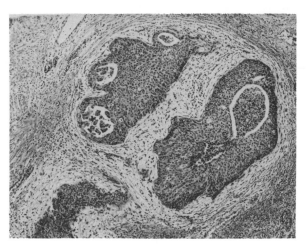

FIG 1–5.
Transitional cell carcinoma involving prostatic stroma. Desmoplastic resection manifested by myxoid fibrous proliferation around the nests of carcinoma indicate stromal invasion. (×150)

Anderson Cancer Center between 1969 and 1979 and monitored for a minimum of 5 years demonstrated that 44% of the patients remained alive and disease-free; 16%, however, died during the 5 years, but without evidence of recurrent malignant disease; and 40% died as a direct result of their bladder malignancy (Johnson, unpublished data). The disappointing realization that 40% of patients were dying of pelvic and visceral disease has led us to reappraise the treatment for patients with invasive bladder carcinoma.

Reassessment of the results of radical surgery when used alone in patients with invasive bladder carcinoma suggested in 1980 that improvements in surgical techniques and a concomitant reduction in operative mortality had increased survival rates to where they were comparable to the results that had been achieved during the previous decade with integrated therapy (Mathur et al. 1981; Montie et al. 1984). Consequently, as active drugs for treating metastatic bladder cancer began to become available, attention was focused on integrating chemotherapy with surgery (Samuels et al. 1979; Harker et al. 1985; Sternberg et al. 1985).

Past experience in treating patients with invasive bladder cancer has shown that those who are at high risk for developing pelvic recurrences, metastatic disease, or both after cystectomy have one or more of the following pathologic conditions: (1) tumor demonstrated to be outside the bladder (involving the perivesical fat) in the cystectomy specimen; (2) lymphatic or blood vessel involvement; (3) invasion of contiguous organs (prostate, vagina, etc.); and (4) regional lymph node involvement. The poor prognosis for patients whose cystectomy specimen documents perivesical extension has been emphasized by Mathur et al. (1981), who noted that only 33% of their patients were alive at 5 years following radical cystectomy. Similarly, in the era of integrated therapy we noted that, although survival rates among patients whose disease was confined to the bladder, whether it be P_0, P_{is}, P_1, P_2, or P_{3a}, did not differ significantly, a markedly significant reduction in survival occurred among patients whose disease was demonstrated by the pathologist to be outside the bladder wall (P_{3c}) (Johnson, unpublished data).

The presence of tumor cells within vessels (lymphatic, blood, or both), regardless of the stage of the disease, is likewise an ominous sign. Anderstrom and associates (1980) reported that all 10 patients with bladder tumor involving the lamina propria were dead within 6 years—7 of them from metastatic disease. Similarly, Heney et al. (1983b) reported that, when vessels were involved, 70% of their patients had succumbed to metastatic disease within 5 years.

The prognosis for patients whose disease has spread to the regional lymph nodes is also poor. Smith and Whitmore (1981) reported only a 7% 5-year survival rate for 134 patients who underwent radical cystectomy and bilateral pelvic lymph node dissection. Similar reports have been recorded by other investigators (Dretler et al. 1973; LaPlante and Brice 1973; Heney et al. 1983b). Although Skinner (1982) recently reported that 36% of his patients with involved lymph nodes who underwent radical surgery survived 5 years, the fact remains that regional lymph node involvement heralds a poor prognosis when surgery is the only treatment.

Consequently, adjuvant programs were developed to reduce our surgical failures in these situations, and a number of recent reports attest to their success (see Chapters 6, 7, and 9 in this book). However, the issues remaining still need to be addressed: Is chemotherapy best given in an adjuvant or neoadjuvant setting? How many courses need to be given and over what period of time? What is best for the patient who achieves a complete response with the bladder in situ—surveillance or cystectomy?

CONCLUSION

An increased appreciation of subtle histopathologic changes, such as dysplasia or T_{is} involving von Brunn's nests or the prostatic ducts, existence of a muscularis mucosa, and the ominous implication of prostatic stromal invasion and vessel involvement, is providing both urologic and medical oncologists with new information affecting patients with bladder malignancy who, heretofore, may have received inappropriate therapy. As clinicians increasingly garner knowledge of those factors that place patients at high risk for tumor recurrence, local invasion, and distant spread, they are able to tailor therapy to meet individual situations, thereby reducing its morbidity and increasing its effectiveness.

The subsequent chapters emphasize results of current chemotherapy regimens, either applied topically or administered systemically. We hope that the information presented in this chapter has provided the reader with a better basis for assessing these results and a better appreciation of those situations to which therapy should be directed in the future.

REFERENCES

1. Althausen AF, Prout GR Jr, Daly JJ. 1976. Noninvasive papillary carcinoma of the bladder associated with carcinoma in situ. *J Urol* 116:575–580.
2. Anderstrom C, Johansson S, Nilsson S. 1980. The significance of lamina propria invasion on the prognosis of patients with bladder tumors. *J Urol* 124:23–26.
3. Badalament RA, Gay H, Cibas ES, et al. 1987a. Monitoring endoscopic treatment of superficial bladder carcinoma by postoperative urinary cytology. *J Urol* 138:760–762.
4. Badalament RA, Gay H, Cibas ES, et al. 1987b. Monitoring intravesical bacillus Calmette-Guerin treatment of superficial bladder carcinoma by postoperative urinary cytology. *J Urol* 138:763–765.
5. Coon JS, Weinstein RS. 1981. Detection of ABH tissue isoantigens by immunoperoxidase methods in normal and neoplastic epithelium: Comparison with the erythrocyte adherence method. *Am J Clin Pathol* 76:163–171.
6. Cowan DF, Wu B, Young G, et al. 1987. Correlation of histopathological, cytological and flow cytometric findings in neoplastic and nonneoplastic lesions of the bladder. *J Urol* 138:753–757.
7. Decenzo JM, Howard P, Irish CE. 1975. Antigen detection and prognosis of patients with stage A transitional cell bladder carcinoma. *J Urol* 114:874–878.
8. Dretler SP, Ragsdale BD, Leadbetter WF. 1973. The value of pelvic lymphadenectomy in the surgical treatment of bladder cancer. *J Urol* 109:413–416.

9. Farrow GM, Utz DC, Rife CC. 1976. Morphological and clinical observations of patients with early bladder cancer treated with total cystectomy. *Cancer* 36:2495–2499.
10. Harker WG, Meyers FJ, Freiba FS, et al. 1985. Cisplatin, methotrexate, and vinblastine (CMV): An effective chemotherapy regimen for metastatic transitional cell carcinoma of the urinary tract. A Northern California Oncology Group study. *J Clin Oncol* 3:1463–1470.
11. Hemstreet GP III, West SS, Cook MS. 1986. Improved nuclear fluorescence screening technique. *J Occup Med* 28:1004–1010.
12. Heney NM, Ahmed S, Flanagan MJ, et al. 1983a. Superficial bladder cancer: Progression and recurrence. *J Urol* 130:1083–1086.
13. Heney NM, Proppe K, Prout GR Jr, et al. 1983b. Invasive bladder cancer: Tumor configuration, lymphatic invasion and survival. *J Urol* 130:895–897.
14. Herr HW. 1987. Intravesical therapy: A clinical review. *Urol Clin North Am* 14:399–404.
15. Jewett HJ, King LR, Shelley WM. 1964. A study of 365 cases of infiltrating bladder cancer: Relation of certain pathological characteristics after extirpation. *J Urol* 92:668–678.
16. Johnson DE. 1974. Surgery for carcinoma of the urinary bladder. *Cancer Treat Rev* 1:271–283.
17. Juhl BR, Hartzen SH, Hainau B. 1986. A, B, H antigen expression in transitional cell carcinomas of the urinary bladder. *Cancer* 57:1768–1775.
18. LaPlante M, Brice M II. 1973. The upper limits of hopeful application of radical cystectomy for vesical carcinoma: Does nodal metastasis always indicate incurability? *J Urol* 109:261–264.
19. Limas C, Lange P. 1982. A, B, H antigen detectability in normal and neoplastic urothelium: Influence of methodologic factors. *Cancer* 49:2476–2484.
20. Limas C, Lange P, Fraley EE, et al. 1979. A, B, H antigens in transitional cell tumors of the urinary bladder: Correlation with clinical course. *Cancer* 44:2099–2107.
21. Lutzeyer W, Rubben H, Dahm H. 1982. Prognostic parameters in superficial bladder cancer: An analysis of 315 cases. *J Urol* 127:250–252.
22. Mahadevia PS, Koss LG, Tar IJ. 1986. Prostatic involvement in bladder cancer: Prostate mapping in 20 cystoprostatectomy specimens. *Cancer* 58:2096–2102.
23. Marshall VF, McCarron JP. 1977. The curability of vesical cancer: Greater now or then? *Cancer Res* 37:2753–2755.
24. Mathur VK, Krahn HP, Ramsey EW. 1981. Total cystectomy for bladder cancer. *J Urol* 125:784–786.
25. Miller LS, Johnson DE. 1973. Megavoltage irradiation for bladder cancer: Alone, postoperative, or preoperative, in *Proceedings of the National Cancer Conference,* vol 7. Philadelphia, JB Lippincott Co, pp 771–782.
26. Montie JE, Straffon RA, Stewart BH. 1984. Radical cystectomy without radiation therapy for carcinoma of the bladder. *J Urol* 131:477–482.
27. Morabito RA, Kanzari SJ, Milam DF. 1979. Invasive bladder carcinoma treated by radical cystectomy. *Urology* 14:478–481.
28. Mostofi FK, Sobin LH, Torlini H. 1973. *Histological Typing of Urinary Bladder Tumours. International Histological Classification of Tumours, No. 10.* Geneva, World Health Organization.
29. Prout CR, Griffin PP, Daly JJ. 1987. The outcome of conservative treatment of carcinoma in situ of the bladder. *J Urol* 138:766–770.
30. Ro JY, Ayala AG, El-Naggar A. 1987. Muscularis mucosa of urinary bladder: Importance for staging and treatment. *Am J Surg Pathol* 11:688–673.
31. Samuels ML, Moran ME, Johnson DE, et al. 1979. CISCA combination chemotherapy for metastatic carcinoma of the bladder, in Johnson DE, Samuels ML (eds): *Cancer of the Genitourinary Tract.* New York, Raven Press, pp 101–106.
32. Skinner DG. 1982. Management of invasive bladder cancer: A meticulous pelvic node dissection can make a difference. *J Urol* 128:34–36.
33. Smith G, Elton RA, Beynon LL, et al. 1983. Prognostic significance of biopsy results of normal-looking mucosa in cases of superficial bladder cancer. *Br J Urol* 55:665–669.
34. Smith JA, Whitmore WF. 1981. Regional lymph node metastasis from bladder cancer. *J Urol* 126:591–595.
35. Sternberg CN, Yagoda A, Scher HI, et al. 1985. Preliminary results of M-VAC (methotrexate, vinblastine, doxorubicin and cisplatin) for transitional cell carcinoma of the urothelium. *J Urol* 133:403–407.

36. van der Werf-Messing B. 1975. Carcinoma of the bladder $T_3N_x M_0$ treated by preoperative irradiation followed by cystectomy (Third report of the Rotterdam Radio-Therapy Institute). *Cancer* 36:718–722.
37. Weinstein RS, Miller AW, Coon JS. 1984. Tissue blood group ABH and Thomsen-Friedenreich antigens in human urinary bladder carcinoma, in Kurth KH, Debruyne FMJ, Schroeder FH, et al. (eds): *Progress and Controversies in Oncological Urology.* New York, Alan R. Liss, pp 249–260.
38. Whitmore WF Jr, Marshall VF. 1962. Radical total cystectomy for cancer of the bladder: 230 consecutive cases five years later. *J Urol* 87:853–868.
39. Whitmore WF Jr, Batata MA, Ghoneim MA, et al. 1977. Radical cystectomy with or without prior irradiation in the treatment of bladder cancer. *J Urol* 118:184–189.
40. Wishnow KI, Ro JY. 1988. Importance of early treatment of transitional cell carcinoma of the prostatic ducts. *Urology* 32:11–13.

Chapter 2

Intravesical Mitomycin C Therapy*

Mark S. Soloway, M.D.

If the clinician feels certain that all tumor is confined to the urothelium (T_a or T_{is}) or lamina propria (T_1), a trial of an effective intravesical therapeutic agent is indicated. Drugs that have demonstrated activity include thiotepa, mitomycin C, doxorubicin (Adriamycin), and bacillus Calmette-Guérin (BCG). It is not my intent to review the effectiveness of all intravesical therapeutic agents in this chapter, however, but rather to emphasize the value of mitomycin C for treating transitional cell tumors in general and, more particularly, T_{is}.[†] To better appreciate the effectiveness of mitomycin C, I discuss my results in light of recent experiences with BCG.

When intravesical therapy is discussed, it is important to distinguish between those patients receiving intravesical agents as *treatment* of existing tumor and those receiving intravesical agents as *prophylaxis* following complete removal of all evident tumor. In the first instance, tumor remains in the bladder when therapy begins. Its presence may be documented by only a positive cytologic evaluation or, when visible, by a bladder diagram or endoscopic photograph. Although it is preferable, when possible, to resect all tumor before an intravesical agent is instilled, in instances of multifocal carcinoma this is often not possible.

PATIENT POPULATION

Eighty consecutive patients who had transitional cell carcinoma stages T_a (41 patients), T_1 (18 patients), or T_{is} (21 patients) have now been *treated* with eight weekly doses of mitomycin C. A diagnosis of T_{is} was restricted to those cases wherein the urothelium contained a high-grade (grade 3) flat carcinoma that did not extend beyond the basement membrane (Friedell et al. 1986). Mitomycin C was instilled in a dose of 40 mg in 40 ml sterile water and remained in the bladder for 2 hours. Patients were requested to limit their fluid intake for 8 hours before therapy. They were instructed to void spontaneously after the 2-hour instillation and to wash their hands and genitalia after the initial instillation and the first several voidings. This has reduced the incidence of mitomycin C-associated rashes on the genitalia and hands. A diffuse rash, believed to be a systemic allergic phenomenon, has been extremely uncommon in our experience.

*This research was supported in part by the Lillian and Morrie Moss Urologic Oncology Research Fund.

[†]The reader interested in reviewing the entire concept of intravesical therapy is encouraged to read Soloway (1984, 1987) and Torti and Lum (1984).

Among the 80 patients were 59 men and 21 women ranging in age from 48 to 82 years (mean, 65 years). All patients entering this treatment program had multifocal tumor, almost all had a history of bladder tumors, and in none had all of the tumor been resected before mitomycin C therapy. The mean follow-up of the entire 80 patients has been 40 months; the mean follow-up for those with only T_{is} has been 33 months. Fifty-four patients (67.5%) have been monitored for a minimum of 3 years, and 27 (34%) have been monitored at least 5 years. Follow-up for these durations provides meaningful data.

Forty-one patients received mitomycin C as first-line therapy, but the remainder had received at least one previous 3-month course of intravesical thiotepa. The majority of patients who received thiotepa had developed a subsequent tumor during treatment, i.e., were thiotepa failures.

The initial endoscopic evaluation was accompanied by a bimanual examination of the patient under anesthesia and a bladder washing for cytology. A bladder diagram was made showing the site and size of all areas of tumor. Endoscopic photographs also documented the lesion(s) in most patients. At least one tumor from each patient was biopsied or resected to determine the grade and stage. In most instances all easily resected tumor was removed, but in all cases some tumor remained. A patient whose tumor extended beyond the lamina propria was not considered suitable for treatment with intravesical mitomycin C.

Before beginning mitomycin C therapy, patients were required to have a white blood cell count greater than 3,500/ml and a platelet count greater than 100,000/ml.

EVALUATION OF RESPONSE

Response was initially evaluated at 12 weeks, or 4 weeks after the last of the 8 weekly mitomycin C instillations. Every patient with an initial diagnosis of T_{is} was evaluated by selected-site and random mucosal biopsies. A complete response required that the patient have no visible or histologic evidence of bladder cancer and that the urine cytology (bladder washing) specimen contain no tumor cells. In our earlier reports we used the partial-response category (Soloway et al. 1981; Soloway 1987). Most patients in this category had no endoscopic evidence of tumor but had positive bladder washings; the remainder had a greater than 50% reduction in the estimated tumor volume. We determined, however, that the prognosis for these patients was similar to that of patients who had failed treatment, and therefore we have eliminated the partial-response category and now group the partial responders with the failures (Soloway 1985).

All patients who had a complete response, and occasionally those with only a positive bladder washing, continued a monthly maintenance schedule of 40 mg mitomycin C in 40 ml sterile water for 9 to 12 months. Endoscopic evaluation and bladder washing cytology were performed every 3 months for the first 12 months and every 3 to 6 months subsequently.

RESULTS

Eighty patients completed the 8-week treatment course of mitomycin C. Among the 21 who had only T_{is}, 7 (33%) had a complete response (Table 2–1). In 10 of the others with T_{is} (48%), cytology was positive, but no abnormality was endoscopically visible at the first 12-week evaluation; biopsies from random and selected sites showed only dysplasia. Biopsies from four patients (19%) still had evidence of T_{is}. The complete-response rate for those with an initial T_a lesion was 37% (15/41), and for those with a T_1 tumor, 44% (8/18).

TABLE 2–1.
Carcinoma In Situ: Outcome vs. Initial Response to Mitomycin C*

| Response at 12 wk | Patients | | Outcome | | | | | |
| | | | Cystectomy | | T_{2+} | | Death From TCC | |
	No.	%	No.	%	No.	%	No.	%
CR	7	33	1	14	1	14	1	14
PR/F	14	67	8	51	2	14	0	
Total	21		9	43	3	14	1	5

*T_{2+} = $\geq T_2$; TCC = transitional cell carcinoma; CR = complete response; PR/F = partial response and failure.

Nine of the 21 patients (43%) with T_{is} eventually had a cystectomy; however, only 1 of the 7 who had a complete response at 3 months required a cystectomy. The indication for cystectomy in 3 patients was persistence of T_{is} despite mitomycin C therapy and a subsequent 6-week course of BCG. Transitional cell carcinoma in the prostatic urethra prompted the decision to perform a cystectomy in two. Only 3 (14%) of the 21 patients with initially only T_{is} developed a tumor that invaded the muscle. One of these (5%) died of bladder cancer.

The likelihood of cystectomy for those whose initial tumor was T_a was 20% (8/41, Table 2–2). The likelihood was lower if they had an initial complete response than if they failed, 13% (2/15) vs. 23% (6/26). The incidence of subsequent invasion into the muscle was twice as likely for those who failed as for the complete responders, 15% vs. 7%. The three deaths (7%) in the T_a group occurred among those who failed.

The results for those with an initial T_1 tumor were not very different from results in the T_a group. Only 1 of the 8 complete responders (13%) at 3 months eventually had a cystectomy (Table 2–3). Once again, those who failed at 3 months were more likely to have a cystectomy or to develop a more deeply invasive lesion ($\geq T_2$).

An analysis of the entire group of 80 patients treated for superficial bladder cancer provides prognostic information beyond the initial treatment interval, since the average follow-up has been 40 months (Table 2–4). Fifty-four (67.5%) have been monitored for at least 3 years or have had a cystectomy or have died of bladder cancer. Only seven patients (9%) died of bladder cancer, 3% of the initial complete responders and 12% of those who had a partial response or failed. Twenty-one patients (26%) eventually had a cystectomy, 13% of the complete responders and 34% of those who did not have a complete response after the initial 8-week course of mitomycin C.

The number of patients who developed a tumor that invaded the muscle ($\geq T_2$) was low

TABLE 2–2.
T_a Tumor: Outcome vs. Initial Response to Mitomycin C*

| Response at 12 wk | Patients | | Outcome | | | | | |
| | | | Cystectomy | | T_{2+} | | Death From TCC | |
	No.	%	No.	%	No.	%	No.	%
CR	15	37	2	13	1	7	0	
PR/F	26	63	6	23	4	15	3	11
Total	41		8	20	5	12	3	7

*T_{2+} = $\geq T_2$; TCC = transitional cell carcinoma; CR = complete response; PR/F = partial response and failure.

TABLE 2–3.

T$_1$ Tumor: Outcome vs. Initial Response to Mitomycin C*

| Response at 12 wk | Patients | | Outcome | | | | | |
| | | | Cystectomy | | T$_{2+}$ | | Death From TCC | |
	No.	%	No.	%	No.	%	No.	%
CR	8	44	1	13 or 12.5	1	13 or 12.5	0	
PR/F	10	56	3	30	3	30	3	30
Total	18		4	22	4	22	3	17

*T$_{2+}$ = ≥T$_2$; TCC = transitional cell carcinoma; CR = complete response; PR/F = partial response and failure.

in all groups: 3 of 30 (10%) complete responders and 9 of 50 (18%) who had evidence of tumor at 3 months (the partial-response/failure group).

Toxicity with intravesical mitomycin C has been minimal. Three men developed a penile rash, one of whom discontinued therapy as a result. Five patients developed palmar erythema, dermatitis, or both. Bladder irritative symptoms were intermittent and mild, in no case severe enough to discontinue therapy. We have not seen bladder contracture related to intravesical mitomycin C. Myelosuppression did not occur.

DISCUSSION

Mitomycin C has been used as treatment and prophylaxis for superficial bladder tumors for several years. One of the advantages of mitomycin C is its relatively high molecular weight (329), which accounts for its low level of absorption. Leukopenia and thrombocytopenia rarely, if ever, occur, and therefore I do not monitor blood counts.

The majority of published studies were designed to evaluate *treatment*, i.e., to determine whether mitomycin C was capable of eradicating existing superficial bladder tumors. The weekly dose varied from 20 to 60 mg, but most urologists have used 30 to 40 mg in an equal volume of solution weekly for 8 weeks. When the drug is used to *prevent* subsequent tumor following endoscopic resection, 20 mg in 20 ml solution delivered every other week has been a recent standard regimen.

In 1987, Koontz et al. (unpublished data) reported the results of the National Bladder Cancer Group trial that evaluated mitomycin C as treatment of residual tumor following

TABLE 2–4.

Prognosis vs. Initial Response to Mitomycin C: 80 Patients*

| Response at 12 wk | Patients | | Outcome | | | | | |
| | | | Cystectomy | | T$_{2+}$ | | Death From TCC | |
	No.	%	No.	%	No.	%	No.	%
CR	30	38	4	13	3	10	1	3
PR/F	50	63	17	34	9	18	6	12
Total	80		21	26	12	15	7	9

*T$_{2+}$ = ≥T$_2$; TCC = transitional cell carcinoma; CR = complete response; PR/F = partial response and failure.

biopsy or partial transurethral resection of stages T_a, T_1, and T_{is} bladder cancer. The dose was 40 mg in 40 ml solution delivered weekly for 8 weeks. All of the patients treated had failed intravesical thiotepa therapy. Six of the 17 patients (35%) with T_{is} had a complete response; 38 patients had an initial T_a lesion, 26% of whom had a complete response; and 12 had an initial T_1 lesion, none of whom had a complete response. Thus, 26% of those with superficial transitional cell carcinoma had a complete response. An additional 23% had a partial response; all tumor initially seen endoscopically was absent at the first 3-month evaluation, but cytologic studies remained positive.

Somerville et al. (1985) provided 1- and 2-year follow-up reviews of 23 patients treated intravesically with mitomycin C for superficial bladder cancer. Patients selected for treatment were those whose disease had become difficult to control endoscopically because of frequent recurrences or multiple tumors or, in six patients, because T_{is} was present. Dosage was 20 mg in 20 ml of solution three times per week for 7 weeks. No tumors were resected until the 12-week interval.

The initial results indicated that tumor had disappeared completely in 17 patients (74%) at the initial 5-week evaluation. The six patients with T_{is}, all of whom were symptomatic, became symptom-free after receiving mitomycin C; five had a complete response. At 1 year, five of the total group (22%) had progressed to invasive cancer after completing treatment. By 24 months, three patients had died of bladder cancer, and disease in six (26%) had progressed to invasive cancer.

These results from Somerville et al. differ from those of our patients: only 10% of our initial complete responders developed tumors staged T_2 or higher. The Somerville group reported that 3 of 6 patients with T_{is} developed muscle-invasive bladder cancer in contrast to only 3 of 21 in our series.

Issell et al. (1984) reported the data from a cooperative study on the use of mitomycin C as treatment for patients with superficial bladder cancer. All patients had failed intravesical thiotepa therapy and had evaluable disease. Fourteen of the patients had T_{is}, and their complete-response rate was 29%. This was lower than the complete-response rate of those with T_a (39%) or T_1 (70%) tumors.

Although these studies have used mitomycin C as *treatment*, it is preferable to use intravesical therapy as *prophylaxis* after resecting all tumor. Huland et al. (1984) performed a randomized prospective study comparing intravesical mitomycin C to no intravesical therapy following complete endoscopic resection. Mitomycin C was instilled at a dose of 20 mg in 20 ml solution beginning 4 weeks after tumor resection. All patients had a negative cytologic evaluation as prerequisite to acceptance onto the protocol. Notably, only 10% of those who received an intensive course of mitomycin C had a subsequent tumor, as compared with 51% of those who received no intravesical chemotherapy. In addition, those receiving mitomycin C prophylaxis had a much lower likelihood of progression or death from bladder cancer.

Recently, many clinicians have begun using intravesical BCG as treatment of superficial bladder tumors. To gauge its activity as contrasted to that of mitomycin C, we have analyzed our experience with intravesical BCG. Except for patients with T_{is}, a comparison between BCG and mitomycin C is invalid since my patients who received BCG therapy had had a more thorough resection and fulguration of evident tumor. Fifty-five patients received one vial of Tice-strain BCG weekly for 6 weeks and were evaluated 6 weeks after the last dose. The complete-response rate for patients with T_a, T_1, and T_{is} was 56% (31/55). Thirty-two percent (10/31) of the complete responders had received mitomycin C compared to 54% (13/24) of those who had persistent tumor despite BCG.

The complete-response rate was 58% (11/19) for those who received BCG for T_{is}. Only 33% of those receiving mitomycin C for T_{is} had a complete response, although an additional

48% had a partial response. The likelihood of having a subsequent cystectomy (14% after mitomycin C and 9% after BCG) or a tumor that invaded into the muscle (14% after mitomycin C and 27% after BCG) was approximately the same for the complete responders to either treatment (Table 2–5). The likelihood of having a cystectomy was much higher for the partial responders and failures following mitomycin C instillation than for those who failed BCG, 57% vs. 25%. This may simply reflect the longer mean follow-up period for those receiving mitomycin for T_{is} compared to those who received BCG, i.e., 33 vs. 18 months.

TABLE 2–5.
Bacille Calmette-Guérin vs. Mitomycin C for Carcinoma In Situ*

| Response Group | Agent | No. Treated | Responding Patients | | Cystectomy (%) | T_{2+} (%) |
			No.	%		
CR	MMC	21	7	33	14	14
CR	BCG	19	11	58	9	27
F	MMC	21	14	67	57	14
F	BCG	19	8	42	25	12

*T_{2+} = $\geq T_2$; CR = complete response; F = failure; MMC = mitomycin C; BCG = bacille Calmette-Guérin.

Haff et al.(1986) have also reported their results with intravesical BCG. They used the Pasteur strain, and among the 61 patients treated for superficial bladder cancer were 19 who had T_{is}. Three of these had associated papillary tumors. In eight (42%), tumor regressed completely and cytologic results converted to negative. In 3 of the 11 treatment failures, the T_{is} had resolved but superficial papillary tumors were present at the first evaluation. Nine patients received a second 6-week course of BCG, and five were rendered free of tumor after this second course. Thus, the overall complete-response rate for T_{is} was 68% (13 of 19).

One study in progress is comparing BCG and mitomycin C in a randomized trial. Debruyne and Van Meijden (1987) presented their preliminary data at the 1987 meeting of the American Urological Association. The BCG strain used in their study was produced in the Netherlands and is termed RIVM. All visible tumors were resected before patients with superficial bladder cancer were randomized to either BCG or mitomycin C, 40 mg weekly for 6 weeks. Of 329 patients studied, 13 (4%) had only T_{is}. Lesions of 58% were noninvasive papillary tumors (pT_a) and of 38%, lamina propria invasion (pT_1). Seventy percent of the patients had primary tumors. Of 103 evaluable patients, no significant difference was evident between treatments in the recurrence rate or toxicity.

In reviewing results with intravesical therapy at Memorial Sloan-Kettering Cancer Center, Herr (1987) emphasized the necessity for more randomized comparative trials among the currently used intravesical therapeutic agents: thiotepa, mitomycin C, Adriamycin, and BCG. A variety of end points can be used, namely, the number of recurrences, the recurrence rate per 100 patient months, and the incidence of tumor progression as indicated either by a change in the current local treatment or by muscle invasion.

Herr (1987), using muscle-invasive disease as an end point, analyzed his results with intravesical BCG and noted that 26 of 43 patients who had transurethral resection alone later required cystectomy, whereas only 5 of 43 of those randomized to BCG following transurethral resection of all evident tumor required a cystectomy. A more recent analysis of 221 patients treated with BCG indicated progression in 29%: change of the local treatment (19%), tumor penetration into the muscle (8%), and metastatic disease (2%).

Herr believes that candidates for intravesical therapy following transurethral resection of bladder tumors are those who are at greatest risk for recurrence and progression. This group includes those with invasion into the lamina propria, those with multifocal papillary tumors, and those with grade 2 or 3 lesions who either present with a minimum of four lesions or demonstrate three or more tumors at each of two prior cystoscopic examinations 3 months apart. Another group that should receive intravesical therapy comprises those patients with multifocal T_{is}, defined as tumor present in at least three areas of the bladder or over 25% of the estimated surface area of the bladder. It is Herr's view that, although intravesical therapy for other patients with superficial bladder cancer may be beneficial to some, a large percentage of these patients do not benefit because their disease is not likely to recur or progress, and thus repeated instillation of intravesical drugs adds toxicity and cost without additional result. I am more liberal in my use of intravesical therapy. I consider patients candidates for intravesical therapy if they have superficial tumors that are multiple or have recurred. Their risk of another tumor is quite high, and I therefore discuss with patients the potential benefit of intravesical therapy in terms of lessening their need for subsequent endoscopic resections.

CONCLUSION

To provide a more scientific basis to intravesical therapy, more information is needed in several areas. These include the optimal concentration of each drug, the optimal exposure time of the drug to the urothelial surface, and the optimal frequency of instillations. Another area to evaluate is whether combination or single-agent intravesical therapy is superior.

Our data indicate that therapeutic courses of intravesical mitomycin C and BCG are similar in terms of the likelihood of progression in tumor stage or requirement for a cystectomy. Persistence of tumor following a course of mitomycin C or BCG is an indication to consider a trial with the other agent—so long as the tumor has not progressed in stage or has not involved the prostatic ducts or stroma. The decision regarding which agent to use first as treatment or prophylaxis of superficial bladder cancer rests on such considerations as overall cost, cost to the patient, local and systemic toxicity, and the clinician's familiarity and comfort with the agent.

REFERENCES

1. Debruyne FJG, Van Meijden PM. 1987. BCG versus MMC intravesical therapy in patients with superficial bladder cancer: First results of a randomized prospective trial (abstract). *J Urol* 137:179A.
2. Friedell GH, Soloway MS, Hilgar AG, et al. 1986. Summary of workshop on carcinoma in situ of the bladder. *J Urol* 136:1047–1048.
3. Haff EO, Dresner SM, Ratliff TL, et al. 1986. Two courses of intravesical bacillus Calmette-Guerin for transitional cell carcinoma of the bladder. *J Urol* 136:820–824.
4. Herr HW. 1987. Intravesical therapy: A critical review. *Urol Clin North Am* 14:399–404.
5. Huland H, Otto U, Droese M, et al. 1984. Long-term mitomycin C instillation after transurethral resection of superficial bladder carcinoma: Influence on recurrence, progression, and survival. *J Urol* 132:27–29.
6. Issell BF, Prout GR Jr, Soloway MS. 1984. Mitomycin C intravesical therapy in noninvasive bladder cancer after failure on thiotepa. *Cancer* 53:1025–1028.
7. Soloway MS. 1984. Intravesical and systemic chemotherapy in the management of superficial bladder cancer. *Urol Clin North Am* 11:623–636.
8. Soloway MS. 1987. Selecting initial therapy for bladder cancer. *Cancer* 60:502–513.
9. Soloway MS. 1985. Treatment of superficial bladder cancer with intravesical mitomycin C: Analysis of immediate and long-term response in 70 patients. *J Urol* 134:1107–1109.

10. Soloway MS, Murphy WM, De Furia MD, et al. 1981. The effect of mitomycin C on superficial bladder cancer. *J Urol* 125: 646–648.

11. Somerville JJF, Newling DWW, Richard B, et al. 1985. Mitomycin C in superficial bladder cancer: 24-month follow-up. *Br J Urol* 57:686–689.

12. Torti FM, Lum BL. 1984. The biology and treatment of superficial bladder cancer. *J Clin Oncol* 2:505–531.

Chapter 3

Intravesical BCG Therapy: Memorial Sloan-Kettering Cancer Center Experience*

Harry W. Herr, M.D.

Among the estimated 45,000 new cases of bladder cancer to be diagnosed this year (Silverberg 1986), 75% to 85% will be superficial (category T_a, T_{is}, T_1). Superficial bladder tumors recur as a rule (in 70% to 95% of cases), and as a result they are probably the most commonly diagnosed tumor excluding skin cancer. Up to 30% of all patients who have superficial tumors may develop a muscle-infiltrating neoplasm within 5 years, and when the tumor is T_a or T_1 plus T_{is}, infiltration may occur in 50% to 80% of cases (Herr 1983).

The treatment of superficial bladder cancer has three objectives: to eradicate existing disease, to serve as prophylaxis against new occurrences, and to prevent progression to muscle invasion or metastasis. Endoscopic surgery (transurethral resection [TUR]) is the primary therapeutic modality. Intravesical therapy is employed as treatment when the location or multiplicity of tumors precludes complete resection (uncommon) or when coexisting residual flat carcinoma in situ (T_{is}) is identified. Surgery does little to prevent new tumor occurrences and may enhance their likelihood by facilitating dissemination and implantation of tumor cells (Soloway 1980). Intravesical therapy following TUR may be cytotoxic to occult carcinoma or premalignant mucosal lesions, and this potential benefit has led to its widespread therapeutic and prophylactic use against residual or recurring bladder tumors.

Historically, intravesical chemotherapy has resulted in modest, but largely unimpressive, results (Herr 1987). Recent interest has turned to investigating immunologic approaches using biologic response modifiers intravesically. One such agent is bacillus Calmette-Guérin (BCG). In 1976, Morales et al. reported the first successful use of BCG against superficial bladder cancer.

MSKCC EXPERIENCE WITH BCG

Three prospective randomized clinical trials have been conducted at the Memorial Sloan-Kettering Cancer Center (MSKCC) evaluating BCG in the management of superficial bladder cancer.

*This study was supported in part by Public Health Service grants CA-19267 and CA-08748 and contract N01-CB-74746 from the National Cancer Institute, National Institutes of Health, Bethesda, Md.

Study 1

Between 1978 and 1981, 86 patients with polychronotopic superficial bladder cancers (T_a or T_1, grades 2, 3, and T_{is}) were randomly allocated to receive TUR plus BCG (43 patients) vs. standard therapy with TUR alone (43 patients) (Pinsky et al. 1985). T_a grade 1 tumors are considered benign papillomas and are not generally included in our intravesical clinical trials. The average number of papillary tumors per patient month before treatment was 3.4 in the BCG group and 2.6 in the control arm over an average of 19 months. Two to 4 weeks after the TUR, BCG was given intravesically (Pasteur strain, 120 mg in 50 ml saline, retained for 2 hours) and intradermally (Tice strain, 5×10^6 viable units by multiple tine technique) once a week for 6 consecutive weeks. Patients in both arms were evaluated every 3 months with urine cytology, cystoendoscopy, and biopsy or resection, as necessary. Responses were considered complete or incomplete. A complete response was defined as negative results on cystoscopy, biopsy, and urine cytology. Complete responses only were considered significant.

After a minimum follow-up of 60 months (median, 75 months), 17 of 43 patients (40%) are free of disease (median time to recurrence, 21 months) vs. none of the TUR control patients (median time to recurrence, 6 months). Disease progressed in 14 of the 43 (33%) BCG-treated patients vs. 27 of 43 (63%) controls. Compared with TUR, BCG reduced the number of recurrent tumors and the rate of progression and prolonged the disease-free interval and time to progression ($P = .001$).

Bacillus Calmette-Guérin also proved effective therapy for diffuse, high-grade (grade 3) symptomatic flat T_{is} (Herr et al. 1986). Of the 86 patients, 49 (57%) had multifocal T_{is} (more than three discrete lesions or 50% or more mucosal involvement) associated with papillary tumors: 23 of 43 (54%) in the BCG group and 26 of 43 (61%) in the control group. Urinary cytologic studies were positive for all patients at the time of BCG treatment. Complete regression of T_{is} documented by negative bladder biopsy and cytology was seen in 15 of 23 (65%) of the BCG-treated patients for a median duration of 51 months (range, 37–75 months), as compared with 2 of 26 (8%) patients in the control group for a median duration of only 3 months. Many patients also reported improvement of T_{is}-induced symptoms of vesical irritability. Seventeen of the patients treated with TUR (65%) have required cystectomy for invasive carcinoma from 3 to 21 months after randomization, as compared with five (22%) of those treated with BCG (in three, the disease was confined to the prostatic epithelium and no tumor was found in the bladder specimen). Based on this encouraging experience, we treated with intravesical BCG alone a nonrandomized group of 24 patients who had primary T_{is} and were refractory to TUR and considered for cystectomy. Of these, 17 (71%) responded for a median duration of 45 months (range, 36–53 months).

Collectively, these data showed that therapeutic BCG was capable of producing long-term remissions of medium- to high-grade papillary and flat in situ cancers of the bladder in patients at high risk for persistent disease (Fig 3–1) and of preventing or delaying tumor progression necessitating cystectomy (Fig 3–2). Intravesical BCG was equally effective against primary T_{is}, T_{is} associated with papillary tumors, and T_{is} in patients who had failed prior intravesical chemotherapy. In addition, we were able to monitor successfully early response to BCG by flow cytometry of saline bladder irrigation specimens during therapy (Badalament et al. 1986), useful because loss of DNA aneuploidy often translated into a durable disease-free interval (Fig 3–3).

Study 2

In 1981, 88 patients received BCG either intravesically and percutaneously combined (42 patients) or intravesically alone (46 patients) (Herr et al. 1985). Many included were

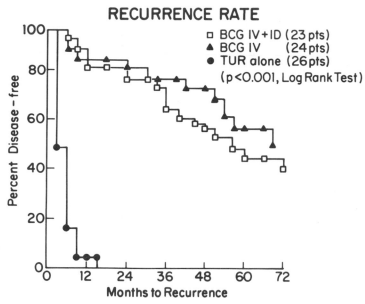

FIG 3–1.
Intervals free of carcinoma in situ of patients treated with transurethral resection (*TUR*) alone, TUR combined with intravesical (*IV*) plus intradermal (*ID*) BCG, or with intravesical BCG alone (*P*<.001, log rank test).

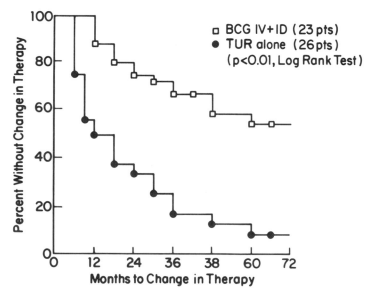

FIG 3–2.
Time to progression of carcinoma in situ after transurethral resection (*TUR*) alone or combined with BCG therapy (*P*<.01, log-rank test).

control patients crossed over from Study 1. The rationale was that (1) we and others had observed that intravesical BCG alone appeared to be effective (Herr et al. 1985, 1986); (2) a randomized trial using only intradermal administration had failed to demonstrate antitumor effect within the bladder (Stöber and Peter 1980); and (3) we had detected relapses of urothelial neoplasms involving the distal ureters and prostatic urethra despite absence of recurrent

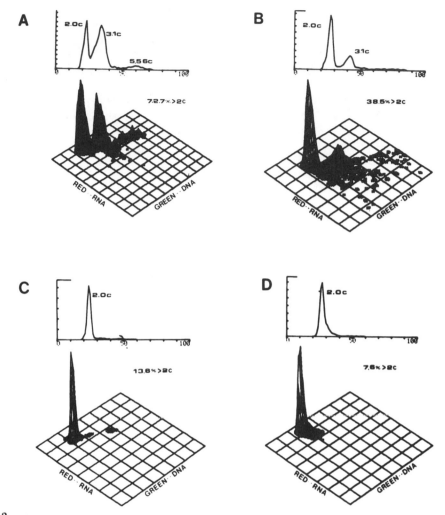

FIG 3–3.
Automated flow cytometry display of a patient monitored during treatment with intravesical BCG for diffuse in situ carcinoma. **A,** before treatment, two aneuploidal populations representing tumor cells are present. **B,** before the third dose of BCG, flow cytometry reveals a single aneuploidal cell line. **C,** flow cytometry after the fifth dose of BCG shows no evidence of aneuploidy. **D,** 6 weeks after BCG, flow cytometric results are entirely normal. Cystoscopy, biopsy, and urinary cytology revealed no evidence of in situ carcinoma, and the patient maintained his complete response for longer than 5 years.

disease within the bladder (Herr and Whitmore 1987). Of the first 66 patients with T_{is} who responded to BCG, 19 (29%) relapsed in the ureter and 9 (14%) in the prostatic urethra within 30 months. These observations suggest that systemic BCG does not add to the therapeutic effect, and contact between BCG and tumor-bearing urothelium is a critical factor.

Among the 46 patients who received only intravesical BCG, 23 (50%) remained tumor free, as compared to 17 of the 42 (41%) who received the combined BCG regimen; 37 of 46 (80%) and 27 of 42 (64%), respectively, remained progression free. We concluded that intravesical BCG administration produced responses similar to those of combined systemic and intravesical BCG. After 1981, intravesical BCG became the standard regimen.

Study 3

The first two studies did not define the optimal duration of BCG therapy. Between 1981 and 1984, 93 patients were entered into a third prospective randomized trial comparing nonmaintenance (46 patients) vs. maintenance (47 patients) BCG therapy once a month for 2 years (Badalament 1987b). Both groups received the standard induction 6-week intravesical BCG regimen and were randomized at the first follow-up cystoscopic evaluation 3 months later. After a minimum follow-up period of 24 months (range, 24–60 months), 32 of 46 (70%) nonmaintenance and 29 of 47 (62%) maintenance patients remained disease free (P = NS), and no difference in the degree or rate of progression between the two groups was seen (Fig 3–4). Maintenance BCG was associated with significantly increased local toxicity.

The beneficial effect of BCG on residual T_{is} is further demonstrated in this study, since 33 of the 93 patients (36%) had T_{is} when randomized to maintenance (17 patients) or nonmaintenance (16 patients). Of the 33, 22 (67%) were recurrence and progression free, as compared with 47 of 58 patients (81%) without T_{is} (Fig 3–5). There was also no difference in the response of T_{is} to maintenance or nonmaintenance BCG (76% vs. 56%, respectively), although the data suggested 6 weeks of intravesical BCG may not be sufficient for some patients with diffuse T_{is}.

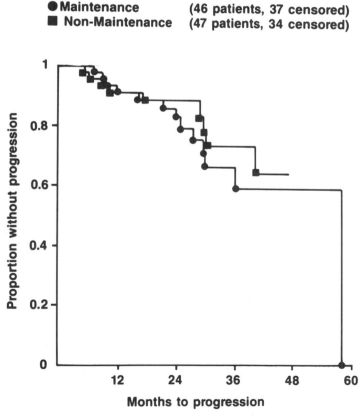

FIG 3–4.
Progression-free intervals for patients maintained on BCG vs. those not receiving maintenance therapy. Progression was not significantly different in the two groups.

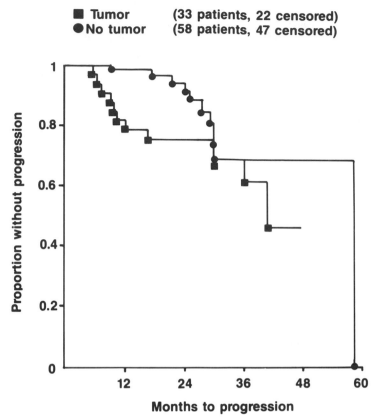

FIG 3–5.
Progression-free intervals for patients with and without carcinoma in situ following induction of BCG therapy. No significant difference in tumor recurrence rates emerged between patients treated therapeutically or prophylactically (*P* = .95).

MULTIVARIATE STATISTICAL ANALYSIS

Efficacy of intravesical therapy is usually measured by tumor recurrences. Tumor progression is, however, independent of the number of tumor recurrences (MacKenzie et al. 1981) and therefore represents a biologically more meaningful end point of intravesical therapy. Progression may be defined as muscle invasion, metastasis, or local extension requiring a change in therapy. To define significant variables for tumor progression, we performed a multivariate logistic regression analysis using data from the first 221 consecutive patients with superficial bladder tumors treated with intravesical BCG and monitored for more than 3 and up to 8 years (Badalament et al. 1987a). Variables were evaluated before and at 3 and 6 months after BCG administration. The aim was to define groups of patients at high or low risk for disease progression.

The only significant variables, in decreasing order, were a T_1 tumor category (grades 2 or 3), a positive result on urinary cytology, and a positive biopsy. Nonsignificant variables included grade 1 (papilloma) tumors, maintenance vs. nonmaintenance BCG, prior intravesical chemotherapy, presence or absence of granulomas histologically, purified protein derivative skin test reactivity before or after BCG treatment, evaluation at 3 or 6 months after receiving BCG, 6 or 12 weeks (a second course) of BCG in the case of apparent early nonresponders, and the number of tumors or duration of disease before BCG treatment.

Of the 221 patients, 76 (34%) had tumor progression (Fig 3–6)—local in 45 (59%), muscle-invasive (T_{2+}) in 25 (33%), and metastatic in 6 (8%) (Fig 3–7). Progression by tumor category showed significance only for T_1 tumors (Fig 3–8). Of the 111 patients who had T_{is}, 35 (32%) failed, but the median time to progression has not been reached (68% of patients have not required a change in therapy for more than 5 years). Half of the T_a and T_1 tumors had associated multifocal T_{is}, but the fact that subsequent recurrence and progression rates were independent of T_{is} provides additional strong evidence of the responsiveness of T_{is} to BCG.

The multivariate analysis permitted us to identify four separate risk groups for progression after BCG therapy. The probability of tumor progression between 6 months and 1, 3, and 5 years was as follows: for T_1 tumor, 73%, 100%, and 100%; for a positive result on biopsy and urine cytology, 50%, 87%, and 100%; for positive cytologic or biopsy result, 17%, 55%, and 74+%; and for a negative response on biopsy and cytology, 2%, 13%, and 27%, respectively. Evaluation at 6 months after BCG administration identifies patients at high and low risk for progression; those at high risk (nonresponders or incomplete responders) require alternative treatment strategies, whereas low-risk patients (complete responders) can be spared further therapy.

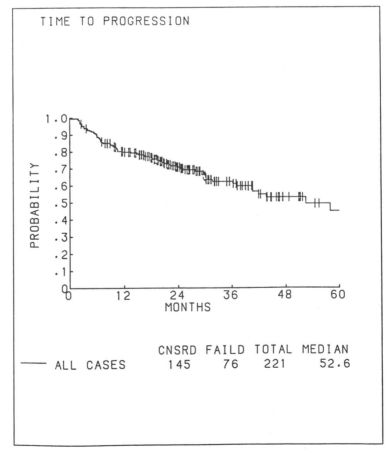

FIG 3–6.
Overall time to progression of 221 patients who had superficial bladder cancer treated with intravesical BCG. Seventy-six (35%) progressed, and 145 (66%) are disease free. CNSRD = censored: free of disease progression.

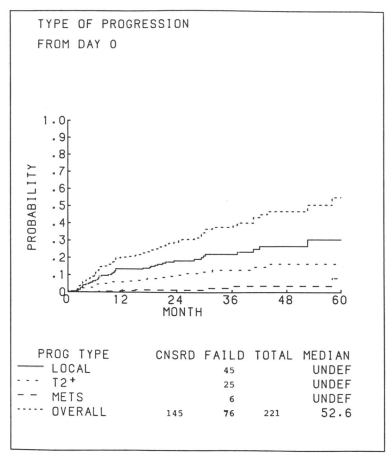

FIG 3–7.
Time to progression of superficial bladder cancer after BCG therapy. Progression was divided into local (progressive carcinoma in situ requiring a change in therapy), muscle invasion (T_{2+}), or distant metastasis (METS). Overall progression (in 76 patients) is indicated by the *upper dashed line*. Local progression occurred in 45 patients, muscle invasion in 25, and distant metastasis in 6. One hundred forty-five patients were censored (CNSRD): free of disease progression.

PATIENTS WHO REQUIRE INTRAVESICAL BCG

Patients at highest risk for tumor recurrence and progression may benefit most from intravesical BCG. This group includes those with T_1 papillary tumors (especially if multiple), multifocal papillary T_a tumors (grades 2 and 3), multifocal T_{is} (three or more discrete lesions or 25% or greater mucosal surface involvement), patients with symptomatic T_{is}, and any patient with a persistently positive result on voided urine cytology after a TUR. In the event that all papillary or flat in situ tumors cannot be resected or fulgurated, therapeutic BCG instillation is a reasonable approach, followed in 6 to 8 weeks by cystoscopic evaluation of response. Urine cytology and flow cytometry analyses (if available) are useful and should be performed every 3 months. Cytologic evaluation may be used to judge the completeness of TUR, to monitor effects of therapy, and as a useful guide to the frequency of endoscopic evaluation and changes in therapeutic strategy.

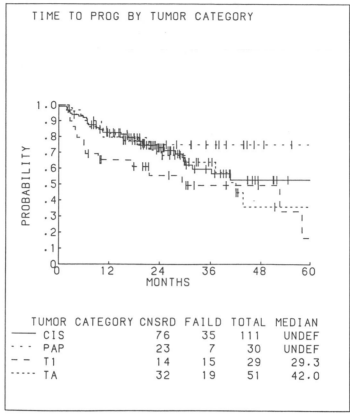

FIG 3–8.
Time to progression according to tumor category of superficial bladder cancer treated with intravesical BCG. Carcinoma in situ (*CIS*) progressed in 35 of 111 patients; papillary (*PAP*) tumors in 7 of 30; T_1 tumors in 15 of 29; and T_a tumors in 19 of 51. Significant progression rates were seen only for T_1 tumors ($P = .01$), as compared with carcinoma in situ, papilloma, or in situ papillary cancers. CNSRD = free of disease progression.

IMPACT OF BCG ON SURVIVAL

Results from the MSKCC clinical trials and multivariate analysis permit some speculation as to the potential impact of BCG on the quality of life and survival of patients with superficial bladder tumors. Of the 45,000 patients who develop new cases of bladder cancer each year, 75%, or 34,000, will present with superficial tumors. Some of these patients will develop muscle invasion (T_{2+}) or metastasis if treated by transurethral resection alone. Such progression probably varies between 30% (reported literature rate) and 60% (observed among the randomized controls in the first MSKCC BCG study). If we use the conservative figure of 30%, then 10,000 of the 34,000 patients with superficial tumors are at risk for developing life-threatening progressive disease. Of these, approximately 40%, or 4,000 patients, will be salvaged with cystectomy, and the other 6,000 will eventually die of bladder cancer.

Data from the multivariate study shows that 25% (56/221) of patients will progress to tumors of grade T_2 or higher or to metastasis despite the BCG therapy, but 75% (165/221) will not. Thus, if the 10,000 patients at risk receive BCG, 75%, or 7,500, may survive with their bladders intact and 60% (34/56), or 1,500, of the 2,500 failures will be salvaged with cystectomy (the higher survival rate after cystectomy in this situation is because more patients are operated for T_{is} refractory to BCG than for progression over time to grade T_2 or higher disease). Overall, this translates into 9,000 patients alive over 5 years after receiving BCG, most of whom retain the bladder, as compared with 4,000 patients alive after TUR and subsequent cystectomy. For high-risk patients with superficial bladder cancer, BCG may significantly improve the quality of life in terms of bladder function and save more than 5,000 lives each year.

RISK ASSOCIATED WITH INTRAVESICAL BCG

Is there a significant risk associated with conservative intravesical therapy for T_{is}? Probably not, if patients are closely observed, as evidenced by the 145 of 221 (66%) patients who sustained durable disease-free intervals. More than 60% of such patients (as defined by the control group in Study 1) progress to muscle invasion if treated by TUR alone. Moreover, because response to BCG cannot be predicted, we use it for most patients. Since we have not witnessed progression from in situ to muscle invasion or metastasis during therapy or during the 3 months thereafter, the response attests to the feasibility and practicality of an initial conservative approach.

Is there a significant risk associated with continued intravesical therapy for T_{is} that fails to respond initially or later to BCG? Of 45 patients with T_{is} who failed locally after BCG, 20 (44%) received additional BCG or another intravesical agent and have remained free of tumor for a median of 37 months; 20 (44%) had a cystectomy (mostly for symptomatic T_{is}), only 3 of whom had microfoci of submucosal invasion; and 5 (11%) received either radiotherapy or systemic chemotherapy in an effort to preserve the bladder. Only 1 of these patients has died of bladder cancer, and out of the total of 221 patients treated with BCG and followed for more than 3 years, only 9 (4%) have died of tumor-related causes. These data suggest that appropriately selected patients with persistent or relapsing T_{is} may benefit from continued intravesical BCG therapy. Others can be salvaged with cystectomy.

Overall, for patients with superficial bladder cancer, intravesical BCG achieves durable responses and prevents or delays progression of disease requiring cystectomy in the majority of patients. Bacillus Calmette-Guerin appears to be the agent of choice for carcinoma in situ of the bladder.

REFERENCES

1. Badalament RA, Gay H, Herr HW, et al. 1986. Monitoring intravesical BCG treatment of superficial bladder cancer by flow cytometry. *Cancer* 58:2751–2757.
2. Badalament RA, Herr HW, Amato D, et al. 1987a. Superficial bladder cancer treated with BCG: A multivariate analysis of factors affecting tumor progression (abstract). *Proc Am Soc Clin Oncol* 6:98.
3. Badalament RA, Herr HW, Wong GY, et al. 1987b. A prospective randomized trial of maintenance versus nonmaintenance intravesical bacillus Calmette-Guerin therapy of superficial bladder cancer. *J Clin Oncol* 5:441–449.
4. Herr HW. 1983. Carcinoma in situ of the bladder. *Semin Urol* 1:15–22.
5. Herr HW. 1987. Intravesical therapy: A critical review. *Urol Clin North Am* 14:399–404.
6. Herr HW, Whitmore WF. 1987. Ureteral carcinoma in situ after successful intravesical therapy for superficial bladder tumors: Incidence, possible pathogenesis and management. *J Urol* 138:292–294.
7. Herr HW, Pinsky CM, Whitmore WF Jr, et al. 1985. Experience with intravesical bacillus Calmette-Guerin therapy of superficial bladder tumors. *Urology* 25:119–123.
8. Herr HW, Pinsky CM, Whitmore WF Jr, et al. 1986. Long-term effect of intravesical bacillus Calmette-Guérin on flat carcinoma in situ of the bladder. *J Urol* 135:265–267.

9. MacKenzie N, Torti FM, Faysal M. 1981. The natural history of superficial bladder tumors (abstract). *Proc Am Assoc Cancer Res* 22:198.

10. Morales A, Eidinger D, Bruce AW. 1976. Intracavitary bacillus Calmette-Guerin in the treatment of superficial bladder tumors. *J Urol* 116:180–183.

11. Pinsky CM, Camacho FJ, Kerr D, et al. 1985. Intravesical administration of bacillus Calmette-Guerin in patients with recurrent superficial carcinoma of the urinary bladder: Report of prospective, randomized trial. *Cancer Treat Rep* 69:47–53.

12. Silverberg E. 1986. Cancer statistics—1986. *CA* 36:19–35.

13. Soloway MS. 1980. Rationale for intensive intravesical chemotherapy for superficial bladder cancer. *J Urol* 123:461–466.

14. Stöber V, Peter H. 1980. BCG immunotherapy for prevention of relapse in patients with bladder cancer. *Therapiewoche* 30:60–67.

Intravesical Thiotepa and Mitomycin C Treatment as Prophylaxis: Long-Term Follow-up to Recurrence, Progression, and Survival

Horst Zincke, M.D.

Sabri E. Sen, M.D.

Ralph C. Benson, Jr., M.D.

Previous studies at the Mayo Clinic have shown the propensity of superficial bladder tumors (T_a, T_{is}) to recur and progress with a wide spectrum of biologic aggressiveness, extending from single grade 1 stage T_a papillary transitional cell cancer (Greene et al. 1973) to high-grade carcinoma in situ (T_{is}) (Zincke et al. 1985b) of the urinary bladder. The concept of tumor cell implantation at the time of instrumentation and the associated traumatization of the urothelial surface during the transurethral removal of bladder tumors has attracted attention recently (Soloway 1984; Zincke et al. 1983). The prophylactic intravesical use of chemotherapeutic agents has been successful in preventing recurrences in a prospective, controlled setting (Huland et al. 1984; Soloway 1984; Zincke et al. 1983, 1985a).

This treatment was particularly effective for patients with recurrent multiple-stage T_a papillary tumors and was less effective for patients with T_{is} or high-grade disease (Zincke et al. 1983). A single instillation of thiotepa or doxorubicin (Adriamycin) at the end of a complete transurethral resection of a bladder tumor (T_a and T_{is}) decreased the recurrence rate from 71% in the control group to 30% in the treatment group ($P<.01$). In a prospective, randomized study with crossover design, we instilled thiotepa or mitomycin C immediately after transurethral resection and at intervals afterward; this decreased the rate of bladder tumor recurrence at 3 months to 7% using thiotepa and to 2.4% using mitomycin C. At 1 year, 78% and 67% of patients were free of cancer after receiving intravesical thiotepa and mitomycin C, respectively. The crossover results were inconclusive because of the small number of patients observed over only a short time (3 to 36 months; mean, 16.1 months; median, 15.5 months). The study seemed to indicate that the drugs were equally effective in decreasing bladder tumor recurrence when used prophylactically. However, that study did not determine the effect of the treatment on long-term recurrence, progression, and survival.

In this chapter, we present the long-term follow-up data on recurrence, progression, and survival for 82 of the patients who, at the time of transurethral resection and later, underwent prophylactic instillation of thiotepa and mitomycin C for superficial (stages T_a and T_{is}) bladder cancer (Zincke et al. 1985a).

MATERIAL AND METHODS

At the beginning, 105 patients were eligible for this study. Criteria for eligibility and follow-up were strict. All patients had histologically proved transitional cell cancer of grade 1, 2, 3, or 4 that was truly superficial—namely, stage T_a or T_{is}, without any evidence of invasion. Only patients in whom all visible tumor had been completely resected were included. Patients were excluded if their leukocyte count was less than $3,500/\mu l$ or their platelet count was less than $130,000/\mu l$ or if they had been previously treated systemically or intravesically with chemotherapeutic or immunotherapeutic agents. Also excluded were patients who had had previous pelvic radiotherapy and had limited bladder capacity (<75 ml) or urinary incontinence, who had another malignancy other than nonmelanomatous skin cancer, or who failed to sign the informed consent form.

Cystoscopy and endoscopic tumor resection included biopsy of at least five sites (adjacent to any visible lesion, trigone, posterior and both lateral walls, dome, and prostatic urethra). Either when T_{is} was present or to ensure that all tumor had been resected, we obtained an additional urine specimen for cytologic study 2 weeks after resection and before the first follow-up treatment.

On the basis of frozen-section studies, patients were stratified by tumor grade, histologic appearance (papillary vs. T_{is}), and interval between diagnosis and treatment (<1, 1–12, or >12 months).

Immediately after transurethral resection, the 105 patients were randomized to receive either 60 mg thiotepa in 60 ml distilled water or 40 mg of mitomycin C in 40 ml distilled water. The drug was left indwelling for 30 minutes. Additional intravesical instillations were performed biweekly for a total of five treatments, during which the patient was asked to retain the agent for 2 hours and to void spontaneously afterward.

Repeat cystoscopy and urine cytologic study were performed every 3 months for 1 year after initiation of therapy, twice a year for another 2 years when no tumor was present, and annually thereafter when no recurrence was found. Patients were considered to have recurrence when visible tumor was identified by biopsy or a urine cytologic result was positive. If no tumor was present at the first 3-month assessment, the treatment interval was lengthened from biweekly to every 4 weeks for 6 months. If recurrent bladder tumor was still not evident, the patient was observed regularly without further treatment. If tumor recurred during treatment with the assigned primary drug, the patient was crossed over to the other drug. If tumor recurred on the crossover medication, the patient was taken off the study and was treated as deemed necessary. Treatments included transurethral resection, agents other than mitomycin C and thiotepa (e.g., intravesical bacillus Calmette-Guérin or, in rare cases, hematoporphyrin derivative [HPD] phototherapy), and, in some cases, partial cystectomy or radical cystoprostatectomy.

Of the original 105 patients randomized to receive thiotepa or mitomycin C, only 83 were included in the present long-term analysis. The reasons for exclusion are presented in Table 4–1. Among the 83 were 71 men and 12 women whose ages ranged from 25 to 89 years (mean, 64 years). The follow-up period ranged from 20.7 to 67.1 months (mean $\pm$ SD, 45.5 ± 12 months; median, 43.3 months). One patient who underwent mitomycin C treatment

TABLE 4–1.
Reasons for Exclusion of Randomized Patients

Reason for Exclusion	Thiotepa (n = 54)	Mitomycin C (n = 51)
	No. of Patients/Treatment	
Invasive carcinoma	3	1
No pathologic evidence of carcinoma	1	1
At least 1 other primary carcinoma in last 5 yr	2	1
Incomplete tumor resection	0	1
Previous treatment with a study agent	5	1
Previous radiation therapy	1	1
Failure to sign consent form	1	3
Total	13	9
Included in analysis	41	42*

*One patient was lost to follow-up.

was lost to follow-up. Seventeen patients received a crossover regimen (12 crossed to mitomycin C and 5 to thiotepa). Follow-up for these patients ranged from 11.3 to 60 months (mean, 35.4 ± 14 months; median, 35.7 months). This follow-up time compares favorably with that in the progression studies performed by the National Bladder Cancer Cooperative Group (Heney et al. 1983) and that of Green and associates (1984).

Because of the randomization and stratification design, the patients were equally distributed among the variables of interest (Table 4–2). The variables were studied separately

TABLE 4–2.
Characteristics of Patient Groups With Superficial (T$_a$, T$_{is}$) Bladder Tumors

Characteristic	Mitomycin C (n = 41) No.	%	Thiotepa (n = 41) No.	%	Total Patients (n = 82) No.	%
Sex						
Male	34	83	36	88	70	85
Female	7	17	5	12	12	15
Recurrent tumor	21	51	19	46	40	48
Progression to higher stage (≥T$_1$)	7	14	1	2	8	10
Grade						
1	15	37	13	32	28	34
2	23	56	24	59	47	57
3, 4	3	7	4	10	7	9
Histologic type						
Papillary	37	90	36	88	73	89
T$_{is}$	4	10	5	12	9	11
Crossover to						
Thiotepa	5		—		5	
Mitomycin C	—		12		12	

and by multiple regression to assess their prognostic significance. Kaplan-Meier analysis was performed to quantitate rates of recurrence and progression.

RESULTS

Recurrence

Tumor recurred in 19 of 41 patients in the thiotepa group and in 21 of 41 patients in the mitomycin C group. At 1 year, 82% of the patients receiving thiotepa and 73% of those receiving mitomycin C were free of disease (Fig 4–1). At 3 years, 54% in both groups were free of recurrence, and at 5 years 54% and 33% of each group, respectively, were free of cancer; this difference was not statistically significant ($P = .46$). As in our preliminary report (Zincke et al. 1985a), most of the variables studied (see Table 4–2) did not show significant differences, except that interval from diagnosis to treatment appeared to be strongly prognostic for recurrence (Fig 4–2). At 1 year, 92% of the patients with a first tumor and 65% of those who had had a previous bladder tumor had no recurrence. Intravesical treatment conferred a favorable effect on those patients younger than 65 years or of the female gender. In a multiple regression analysis, only a history of bladder tumor was found to be prognostically significant; recurrence rate did not differ by type of treatment.

Tumor grade did not affect recurrence significantly (Fig 4–3), nor did histologic appearance (in situ vs. papillary) (Fig 4–4), although the 9 patients with T_{is} tended to have a high recurrence rate. The lack of significance of tumor grade in these 9 patients might be explained on the basis of small sample size: tumors in 7 of the 9 patients were grades 3 and 4.

Crossover Treatment

Only 5 patients who crossed to the thiotepa group and 12 who crossed to the mitomycin C group were evaluable (Fig 4–5). There was no significant difference in decreasing recurrence rate ($P = .91$). At 1 year, 60% of the patients who were now in the thiotepa group and 55% of the patients currently in the mitomycin C group were free of recurrent tumor; at 2 years these values were 40% for the thiotepa group and 43% for the mitomycin C group.

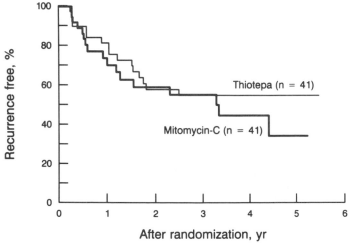

FIG 4–1.
Recurrence according to treatment.

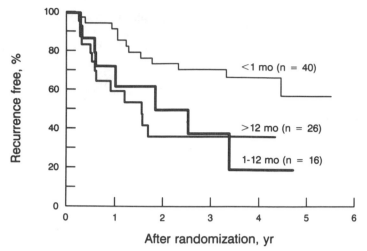

FIG 4–2.
Recurrence according to time from first diagnosis to randomization. $P = .01$ for difference between <1 month and the other two groups.

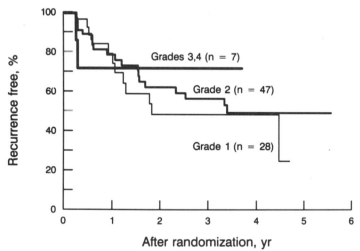

FIG 4–3.
Recurrence according to tumor grade.

Progression

Progression was defined for this analysis as tumor progressing to a higher stage—i.e., T_1 or higher. Nonprogression rates for the thiotepa and mitomycin C groups at 1 year were 100% and 88%, respectively (no significant difference) (Fig 4–6). Nonprogression rates were extremely favorable for patients with no previous bladder tumor history; at 1, 3, and 5 years, disease in 98% of these patients had not progressed to a higher stage. This rate was significantly ($P = .02$) superior to that of patients whose tumors had recurred previously (Fig 4–7). The grade of lesion made no significant difference in progression rate (Fig 4–8). In this study, disease did not progress in any of the nine patients with T_{is}. However, progression did occur in patients with papillary cancer, although 90% were still progression free at 5 years (Fig 4–9).

Overall, progression occurred in a total of 8 patients. Of these, 5 initially received mitomycin C (1 had thiotepa initially), and all progressed to a higher stage during that course. In the 2 patients who received thiotepa initially and had recurrences, progression occurred during their secondary regimen with mitomycin C. Among the 8 with progression, disease still was grade 2 in 2 and had developed to grades 3 and 4 in the others. Three progressed to T_1 disease, 2 to T_2 disease, and 3 to T_3 disease or greater. Five patients underwent cystoprostatectomy, and 1 patient underwent partial cystectomy.

Crossover Regimen

In none of the 5 patients who received thiotepa after mitomycin C treatment failed did

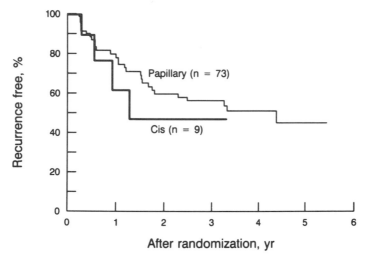

FIG 4–4.
Recurrence according to histologic appearance (*Cis* = carcinoma in situ).

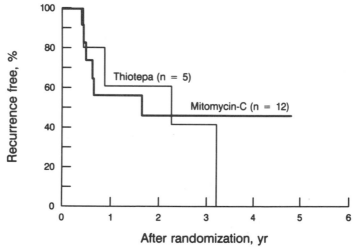

FIG 4–5.
Recurrence during crossover (secondary) treatment.

disease progress during follow-up, but progression occurred in 2 of the 12 patients who received mitomycin C as the secondary regimen. The 2-year nonprogression rate on a cross-over regimen was 67% (Fig 4–10).

Cancer Deaths

Two patients died of metastatic transitional cell cancer after having undergone cystectomy for deeply infiltrating tumor. Disease progressed in one during his primary mitomycin C treatment and in the other during his secondary mitomycin C treatment.

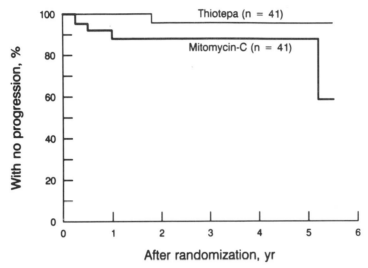

FIG 4–6.
Nonprogression according to treatment.

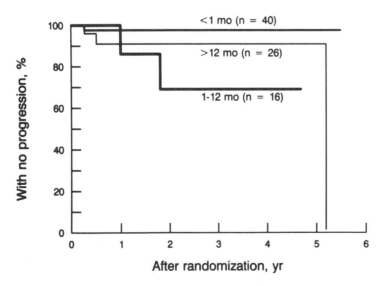

FIG 4–7.
Nonprogression according to time from first diagnosis to randomization. $P = .02$ for difference between <1 month and the other two groups.

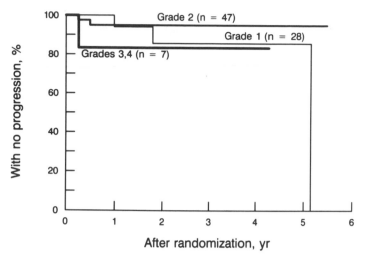

FIG 4–8.
Nonprogression according to tumor grade.

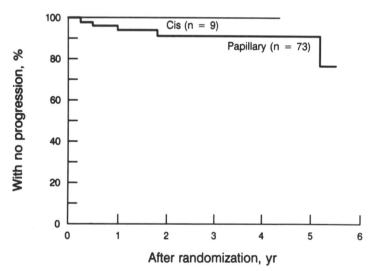

FIG 4–9.
Nonprogression according to histologic appearance (*Cis* = carcinoma in situ).

DISCUSSION

To be considered effective, an intravesical chemotherapy regimen not only should decrease morbidity, bladder trauma, and cost of treatment but also should significantly decrease recurrence rate. Even more important, it should, depending on the characteristics of the primary tumor, delay or prevent the progression that occurs with conventional therapy (that is, transurethral resection only). Finally, by definition, preventing progression should prevent death due to transitional cell cancer. We qualified "progression" to mean a first-invasion event ($\geq T_1$) because, in our opinion, stage T_1 disease has an entirely different biologic potential from that of truly superficial cancer (e.g., noninfiltrating cancer, stages T_a and T_{is}).

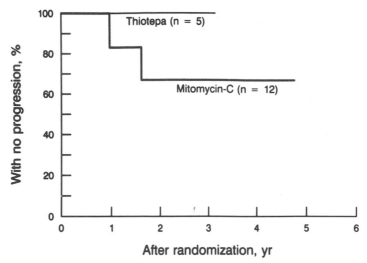

FIG 4–10.
Nonprogression during crossover (secondary) treatment.

A previous study at the Mayo Clinic (Zincke et al. 1985a) included, in addition to randomization, carefully designed stratification criteria. Furthermore, patients were entered in our prophylactic-regimen study only after undergoing a complete transurethral resection of the tumor and a urine cytologic study with a negative result. The design of the present study—initiating intravesical therapy immediately after transurethral resection—should prevent, at least to some degree, tumor cell implantation. That this preventive concept can be successful has been shown in two previous studies at our institution (Zincke et al. 1983, 1985a,b). We were also able to demonstrate that a prophylactic regimen using either mitomycin C or thiotepa can significantly decrease the recurrence rate of disease below that achieved with only a one-time instillation of the drug (5% vs. 30%). From these two studies, one can conclude that combination treatment (i.e., at the time of surgery and afterward) appears to be more effective than a single treatment.

Previous studies by the Bladder Cancer Cooperative Group (Heney et al. 1983) have shown that, for patients treated by conservative means only for stage T_a disease and monitored for a prolonged period, the progression rate was 2% if their disease was grade 1 but 25% if it was grade 3. We could not verify this finding, probably because of the small number of patients with high-grade disease in our study. Another possibility is that the biologic pattern of disease—its grade—is altered over time by therapy. Previous controlled studies (Green et al. 1984; Huland et al. 1984; Soloway 1984; Zincke et al. 1983, 1985a) have clearly demonstrated the highly beneficial effect of prophylactic intravesical chemotherapy in preventing tumor recurrence. Recurrence rates decreased significantly, particularly for patients with low-grade disease. In the present study, neither drug proved superior to the other, and progression rates were low (10%) (see Table 4–2). Particularly gratifying were the results when thiotepa was the primary or the crossover drug—only one patient progressed (primarily).

Although several investigators have clearly shown, in prospective randomized controlled studies, that intravesical chemotherapy used prophylactically can decrease bladder tumor recurrences, its effect on progression has been less clear (Prout et al. 1983). In an extension of a European Organization on Research and Treatment of Cancer (EORTC) protocol reported by Green and associates (1984), patients who received intravesical chemotherapy for at least 1 year had a significantly lower incidence of tumor progression than those who were treated conservatively; death from transitional cell cancer occurred in 3% and 19%, respectively, of these patients. Soloway (1984) analyzed data from his patients who had received mitomycin C treatment intravesically according to progression, number of patients who required cystectomy, and number of patients who died of bladder cancer. After a mean follow-up of 2 years, disease had progressed in 8% of the complete responders and 11% of the partial responders; 19% of the patients whose mitomycin C treatment had failed had progressing disease; and 7% of the patients had died of metastatic transitional cell cancer.

Indirect proof that intensive intravesical therapy with mitomycin C might prevent death was provided by Huland and associates (1984). A prospective randomized study with a mean follow-up of 30 months identified significant differences in rates of recurrence, progression, and death between the treatment and control groups. However, this study did not follow both groups prospectively to progression and death; when the control group's follow-up was terminated, one fourth of the patients had been monitored for less than 12 months. Some of these patients subsequently received other forms of treatment, and some were lost to follow-up. Nevertheless, a regimen of mitomycin C given intravesically every 2 weeks for the first year and every 4 weeks for the second and third years resulted in a recurrence rate of only 10.4%, progression in only 1 of 48 patients, and no cancer death, whereas in the control group disease progressed in 8 of 31 patients and 5 patients died.

The excellent response rate in recurrence and progression reported in Huland and associates' study (1984) could not be confirmed in our analysis. For instance, after a mean follow-up of almost 4 years, tumor had recurred in 21 of our 41 patients who received mitomycin C treatment. After a minimum of 9 months of intravesical administration of drugs, the percentage of patients recurrence-free was only 73% for those receiving mitomycin C and 82% for those receiving thiotepa. Our recurrence-free rate of about 50% at later dates suggests, however, that a prolonged regimen of intense intravesical therapy like that in the Huland et al. study (1984) might be beneficial. We could not establish this conclusively in our study because the patients received the intensive course of intravesical chemotherapy for only 9 months, were observed beyond this time only as long as they were free of cancer, and were crossed over to the alternative drug in case of failure as early as 3 months after the study began.

That neither drug is superior to the other in preventing recurrence after primary drug failure has been demonstrated in this study. Our numbers are similar to those found by Issell and associates (1984)—a complete-response rate of 42% among patients in whom thiotepa had failed and secondary treatment was with mitomycin C.

Of the variables examined in our long-term study, only previous tumor history had a significant association with tumor recurrence and progression. In particular, T_{is} and tumor grade were not associated with a significantly higher incidence of recurrence or progression. However, we draw this conclusion guardedly because the numbers in the categories of T_{is} and high-grade tumor were small.

Progression occurred mainly (7 of 8) in patients who were receiving mitomycin C treatment (initial or crossover); it occurred in only 2 patients who began on thiotepa and were given mitomycin C as a crossover. The fact that none of the 5 patients who received thiotepa secondarily had progressing disease, as compared with 2 of the 12 who were given mitomycin C secondarily, is only suggestive and should be confirmed in larger studies.

CONCLUSION

Conclusions from this long-term study must be derived with caution. On one hand, the patients were taken off the study when muscle invasion became evident and required more aggressive treatment or when their secondary regimen had failed. On the other hand, half the patients had no recurrence and thus can be used for a long-term study because no additional treatment was administered. The conclusions to be drawn from this study are limited to the following:

1. Intravesical therapy with thiotepa and mitomycin C can decrease the rate of bladder tumor recurrence equally effectively when given as first- and second-line treatments, as in this study, for about 12 months.

2. The overall progression rate can be limited to less than 10% and is particularly low after thiotepa treatment (2%).

3. Intravesical mitomycin C used as a second treatment after failure of thiotepa is associated with a higher progression rate, but not vice versa. More effective alternative treatment modalities, perhaps bacillus Calmette-Guerin, may have to be used earlier.

REFERENCES

1. Green DF, Robinson MR, Glashan R, et al. 1984. Does intravesical chemotherapy prevent invasive bladder cancer? *J Urol* 131:33–35.
2. Greene LF, Hanash KA, Farrow GM. 1973. Benign papilloma or papillary carcinoma of the bladder? *J Urol* 110:205–207.
3. Heney NM, Ahmed S, Flanagan MJ, et al. 1983. Superficial bladder cancer: Progression and recurrence. *J Urol* 130:1083–1086.
4. Huland H, Otto U, Droese M, et al. 1984. Long-term mitomycin C instillation after transurethral resection of superficial bladder carcinoma: Influence on recurrence, progression and survival. *J Urol* 132:27–29.
5. Issell BF, Prout GR Jr, Soloway MS, et al. 1984. Mitomycin C intravesical therapy in noninvasive bladder cancer after failure on thiotepa. *Cancer* 53:1025–1028.
6. Prout GR Jr, Koontz WW Jr, Coombs LJ, et al. 1983. Long-term fate of 90 patients with superficial bladder cancer randomly assigned to receive or not to receive thiotepa. *J Urol* 130:677–680.
7. Soloway MS. 1984. Intravesical and systemic chemotherapy in the management of superficial bladder cancer. *Urol Clin North Am* 11:623–635.
8. Zincke H, Benson RC Jr, Hilton JF, et al. 1985a. Intravesical thiotepa and mitomycin-C treatment immediately after transurethral resection and later for superficial (stages Ta and Tis) bladder cancer: A prospective, randomized, stratified study with crossover design. *J Urol* 134:1110–1114.
9. Zincke H, Utz DC, Farrow GM. 1985b. Review of Mayo Clinic experience with carcinoma in situ. *Urology* 26(suppl 4):39–46.
10. Zincke H, Utz DC, Taylor WF, et al. 1983. Influence of thiotepa and doxorubicin instillation at time of transurethral surgical treatment of bladder cancer on tumor recurrence: A prospective, randomized, double-blind, controlled trial. *J Urol* 129:505–509.

Chapter 5

CISCA Chemotherapy for Disseminated Bladder Carcinoma

Christopher J. Logothetis, M.D.

CISCA chemotherapy has been employed at The University of Texas M. D. Anderson Cancer Center since 1977 to treat advanced urothelial tumors. During that period, we have gained extensive experience in its use.

CISCA consists of cyclophosphamide at 650 mg/m², doxorubicin (Adriamycin) at 50 mg/m², and cisplatin at 70 to 100 mg/m². The dose of cisplatin is always given with adequate pre-hydration and simultaneous forced mannitol diuresis.

Since we introduced CISCA at UT M. D. Anderson Cancer Center, many researchers have used this combination with varying success rates. In general, response rates to the combination of cyclophosphamide, Adriamycin, and cisplatin have been higher than to combinations using cisplatin and one other agent, as documented in numerous series. Despite this, most investigators have been unwilling to accept that the CISCA combination is superior.

The differences between UT M. D. Anderson Cancer Center experience with CISCA chemotherapy and experiences reported by other cooperative groups can be attributed to numerous variables. The first, and perhaps the most important, is the probable difference in study populations. Patients treated at UT M. D. Anderson Cancer Center may differ significantly from those treated at other institutions. Differences in chemotherapy dosages are also very significant. In studies by both the Southeastern Oncology Group and the Eastern Cooperative Oncology Group, the dosages of CISCA were significantly lower than those we employ (Troner and Hemstreet 1981; Khandekar et al. 1985). The single report by Kedia et al. (1981) of a study that employs a dose of CISCA similar to that used at our institution achieves a very comparable result.

RETROSPECTIVE REVIEW

To evaluate better the ultimate effect of CISCA chemotherapy on urothelial tumors, we believed it was very important to assess variables that may predict for response and to identify those tumor features that could be employed to evaluate the effectiveness of treatment in future prospective trials. Accordingly, we undertook a retrospective review of 97 cases where adequate clinical data and pathologic tissue were available for reevaluation. Each of the 97 patients had unresectable urothelial tumors treated at UT M. D. Anderson Cancer Center between 1977 and 1985. The clinical characteristics and primary therapy of these 97 patients are summarized in Table 5–1.

The prognostic variables identified were type of prior therapy (irradiation or cystectomy), tumor cell type (transitional cell carcinoma, mixed tumors, squamous cell carcinoma), and extent of tumor spread (local-regional disease with either nodal involvement or direct pelvic invasion only vs. distant visceral involvement). Each of the variables had previously been identified as significant in predicting responses to subsequent therapy.

Tables 5–2 and 5–3 indicate that histologic type and extent of tumor spread predicted for the likelihood of achieving a complete response (CR), but treatment-related variables

TABLE 5–1.
CISCA Chemotherapy for Disseminated Bladder Cancer, 1977–1987

Variable	Patients (n = 97) No.	%
Sex		
Female	24	25
Male	74	75
Age (yr)		
Mean	63.8	
Median	66	
Range	33–82	
Race		
Black	6	7
White	91	92
Histologic tumor type*		
TCC	74	75
Mixed	20	21
SCC	3	4
Tumor spread at treatment		
Nodal metastasis	62	63
Visceral	35	36
Prior treatment		
Cystectomy	28	29
Partial cystectomy	5	6
Chemotherapy	0	0
Radiation	45	56

*TCC = transitional cell carcinoma; SCC = squamous cell carcinoma.

TABLE 5–2.
Influence of Histologic Type on Response to CISCA*

Cell Type	No. of Patients	PR No.	PR %	CR No.	CR %	Overall %
TCC	74	22	31	23	39	70
TCC + spindle cell	3	1	33	1	33	60
TCC + adenocarcinoma	6	0		1	17	
TCC + squamous cell	11	5	45	3	27	72

*PR = partial response; CR = complete response; TCC = transitional cell carcinoma.

TABLE 5–3.
Influence of Previous Treatment on Response to CISCA

Prior Therapy	No. of Patients	Response[†]			
		PR		CR	
		No.	%	No.	%
Cystectomy	33	8	24	10	30
No cystectomy	64	19	30	15	23
Radiation*	45	11	24	17	37
No radiation	51	16	31	17	33

*History incomplete for radiation in one patient.
[†]PR = partial response; CR = complete response.

(prior cystectomy or prior radiation) did not. Patients whose metastasis was nodal only had the highest CR rate (45.2%).

The influence of tumor cell type on the response rates of these 97 patients was analyzed retrospectively. Patients with pure transitional cell carcinoma had higher CR and partial response (PR) rates than those with the pathologically easily identified mixed tumors. A closer analysis of the patients with mixed tumors, however, shows that those patients whose primary tumors contain adenomatous elements are the ones responsible for the significantly lower response rate. Patients with squamoid elements in addition to transitional cell carcinoma have a response rate equivalent to that of patients with pure transitional cell carcinoma.

The significance of a CR can be most reliably assessed by its durability (Table 5–4). Patients who achieved a CR can be divided into two broad groups, those whose CR was durable (alive and disease-free >100 weeks) and those whose CR was early and short term (disease-free survival <100 weeks). No significant factor could be found in these two groups that predicted durability. We interpret this as demonstrating that, although histologic type and extent of tumor dissemination predicted for the likelihood of achieving a response, they did not predict the likelihood of CRs being durable. Similarly, the relative frequency of a cystectomy and radiation therapy was equal in these two groups of patients.

TABLE 5–4.
Survival Analysis of Patients in Complete Remission*

Patient Status	No.	%
Alive + disease-free	13	38
Died of recurrent tumor	18	51
Lost to follow-up	1	3
Died of secondary primary cancer	3	9
Total	35	

*Mean survival 300.8 weeks, median 296 weeks, range 135–496 weeks.

Death of patients in CR for less than 100 weeks was overwhelmingly caused by recurrent urothelial tumors (16 of 17, 94%), whereas only 2 of the 18 patients in CR for more than 100 weeks (11%) have relapsed after a follow-up of over 300 weeks. These patients with a "durable" CR have potentially achieved cures, despite the fact that they have had unresectable disease.

DISCUSSION

We conclude from our retrospective analysis of these select patients that the response to CISCA chemotherapy does include a relatively high frequency of CR. The pessimistic interpretation of the results of Adriamycin/cisplatin based combination chemotherapy does not appear to be warranted. The assertion that some patients should be treated only if they have symptomatic metastasis is also not justified by these data and appropriate interpretation of the published data.

Although we believe that our review confirms that CISCA chemotherapy can achieve a CR that occasionally can be durable, these data must be interpreted cautiously. The results achieved in these select patients can only be extrapolated to patients with comparable clinical presentations treated with a similar intensity. For this retrospective analysis, we have selected only patients who were treated at UT M. D. Anderson Cancer Center, which may create a selection bias that is influencing response rates. Nevertheless, we believe that predictors of response that include histologic type and degree of tumor dissemination have been reliably identified and should be factors in subsequent trials conducted to evaluate the effectiveness of treatment.

The lack of effect of prior treatment on response should probably be considered as interesting only. These patients were treated in the era of preoperative radiation therapy plus cystectomy, and therefore the results may not predict for the likelihood of response of patients with persistent tumor within radiated fields. The absence of an impact on survival of a prior cystectomy, however, is an important finding. Although this result may suggest that a cystectomy is not required in all patients who achieve a CR following CISCA chemotherapy, it does not yet offer firm evidence that these patients can avoid a cystectomy. Patients presenting with disseminated bladder cancer at the outset differ inherently from patients whose cancer has metastasized after a cystectomy. Too few patients remain in a durable CR who have not had a cystectomy to allow a firm statement about its benefit or lack of benefit.

The most important predictor of long-term disease-free survival in this total population was response to therapy. However, this retrospective analysis of selected patients cannot determine the relative response rates to CISCA chemotherapy and to the more recent methotrexate/cisplatin combinations. Similarly, the results of CISCA chemotherapy in this select patient group cannot be compared to those reported with similar combinations given at different dosages in other trials.

CONCLUSION

This retrospective review of our experience with CISCA chemotherapy confirms the ability of this combination to induce CRs. The CRs occur most frequently in patients with local-regional disease. The recent optimism that has followed the development of the methotrexate/cisplatin combination could be the result of an increased response rate that, in part, can be attributed to the treatment of more patients with only local-regional disease (Logothetis et al. 1985). The benefit of the methotrexate/cisplatin combinations (Sternberg et al. 1986) and their possible superiority over the Adriamycin/cisplatin combinations can only be evaluated in a prospective random fashion.

To evaluate prospectively the significance of the prognostic variables that we have identified in this study and the effectiveness of the methotrexate/cisplatin combination relative to CISCA, we are now engaged in a prospective randomized trial at UT M. D. Anderson

Cancer Center. In this study, we will incorporate all patients who have urothelial tumors and will stratify them according to the histologic and clinical variables that we have identified. The regimens compared are CISCA chemotherapy as employed at UT M. D. Anderson Cancer Center and M-VAC (methotrexate, vinblastine, Adriamycin, cisplatin) chemotherapy as has been reported by the Memorial Sloan-Kettering Cancer Center (Sternberg et al. 1986).

REFERENCES

1. Kedia KR, Gibbons C, Persky L. 1981. The management of advanced bladder carcinoma. *J Urol* 125:655–658.
2. Khandekar JD, Elson RJ, DeWys WD, et al. 1985. Comparative activity and toxicity of cis-diammine-dichloroplatinum (DDP) and a combination of doxorubicin, cyclophosphamide, and DDP in disseminated transitional cell carcinoma of the urinary tract. *J Clin Oncol* 3:539–545.
3. Logothetis CJ, Samuels ML, Ogden S, et al. 1985. Cyclophosphamide, doxorubicin and cisplatin chemotherapy for patients with locally advanced urothelial tumors with or without nodal metastasis. *J Urol* 134:460–464.
4. Sternberg CN, Yagoda A, Scher HI, et al. 1986. Surgical staging and long term survival in patients with advanced transitional cell carcinoma (TCC) of the urothelium treated with M-VAC (abstract). *Proc Am Soc Clin Oncol* 5:101.
5. Troner MB, Hemstreet G III. 1981. Cyclophosphamide, doxorubicin, and cisplatin (CAP) in the treatment of urothelial malignancy: A pilot study of the Southeastern Cancer Study Group. *Cancer Treat Rep* 65:1–2.

M-VAC for Advanced Urothelial Tumors*

Alan Yagoda, M.D.

Cora N. Sternberg, M.D.

Howard I. Scher, M.D.

Robin C. Watson, M.D.

Harry W. Herr, M.D.

Victor Reuter, M.D.

Michael J. Morse, M.D.

Pramod C. Sogani, M.D.

Nancy L. Geller, Ph.D.

Neil Bander, M.D.

William R. Fair, M.D.

Willet F. Whitmore, Jr., M.D.

In a series of phase II disease-site–specific trials for advanced urothelial cancer at Memorial Sloan-Kettering Cancer Center (MSKCC) in patients selected for bidimensionally measurable indicator lesions, cisplatin, methotrexate, doxorubicin (Adriamycin), and vinblastine sulfate administered singly induced complete (CR) and partial (PR) response in 30%, 29%, 17%, and 18%, respectively (Yagoda 1988). Combinations of methotrexate and vinblastine and of cisplatin and Adriamycin, with or without cyclophosphamide, produced responses in 39%, 48%, and 46%, respectively, but less than 5% to 10% of patients achieved CR status: the median

*This work has been supported in part by NCI grant 5P01-CA05826-25 and contract NO1-CM57732 from the National Cancer Institute, Bethesda, Md., and the Isidore Komanoff/Solid Tumor Service Funds.

survival duration for responders varied from 48 to 92 weeks, as compared with 13 to 22 weeks for nonresponders. The most active combinations, methotrexate plus vinblastine and cisplatin plus Adriamycin, were combined into the M-VAC regimen. This chapter summarizes the results of 92 "consecutive-sampled" patients who received M-VAC between February 1983 and August 1985 (Sternberg et al. 1988).

MATERIALS AND METHODS

Patient Data

All protocol data, x-rays, and pathologic material of 88 patients treated at MSKCC and 4 at North Shore University Hospital were reviewed at MSKCC. Protocol eligibility required the presence of at least one indicator lesion such as involved lymph nodes, cutaneous or subcutaneous masses identified by physical examination, parenchymal pulmonary lesions visible on chest x-ray, or mediastinal, intra-abdominal, pelvic, or hepatic masses identified by computerized transaxial tomography (CT). All other evaluable and unidimensional disease parameters were also monitored; these included masses with indistinct borders, bone metastases, and abnormal tumor-related biochemical and biologic markers. A total of 149 disease sites, including both bidimensional and unidimensional lesions, were available for evaluation. Entry criteria required no recent irradiation to the indicator lesion, Karnofsky performance score above 30%, more than 3,500 white blood cells (WBC) per microliter, a platelet count higher than 150,000/μl, a serum creatinine level (Cr) less than 1.7 mg/100 ml, blood urea nitrogen (BUN) less than 30 mg/100 ml or a creatinine clearance rate (Ccr) higher than 50 ml/minute, a New York Heart Association Functional Class below III, and a serum bilirubin level less than 1.5 mg/100 ml.

All patients were evaluated by a complete history and physical examination, and the longest perpendicular diameters of all measurable lesions were generally recorded by two observers. Computed transaxial tomographic scans, x-rays, and sonograms were reviewed independently (R.C.W.). Laboratory tests included automated blood and platelet counts, serum multiple analysis (SMA-12), and determinations of Cr and 12-hour Ccr; chest x-rays and appropriate scans were performed to define measurable disease. Transurethral resection of the bladder (TURB), bimanual examination of the patient under anesthesia, and urinary cytology were performed initially and repeated at 3- to 6-month intervals for patients with an intact bladder. Weekly blood counts were requested. Methotrexate levels were determined 24 hours after the day-1 dosage, but measurement was discontinued when 122 evaluated levels in 46 patients all remained in the nontoxic range.

During a 3- to 5-day hospitalization, patients underwent diagnostic studies and received M-VAC (Table 6–1). Methotrexate, 30 mg/m^2 intravenously, was administered on day 1, followed by intravenous hydration with 5% dextrose with .5N saline to assure a urinary output greater than 100 ml/hour. Approximately 24 hours later, vinblastine, 3 mg/m^2, Adriamycin, 30 mg/m^2, and cisplatin, 70 mg/m^2, were administered; most patients received 12.5 g mannitol before the cisplatin. The only planned dose modification was for Adriamycin, which was decreased to 15 mg/m^2 for patients who had received irradiation of more than 2,500 cGy in 5 days to the whole pelvis or in whom two or more bone-marrow–containing sites had been irradiated. Standard MSKCC antiemetics were employed. When the WBC count was above 2,500 cells/μl, the platelet count above 100,000/μl, and there was no evidence of mucositis, methotrexate and vinblastine were administered on days 15 and 22. Every attempt was made to repeat the cycle beginning on day 28, but scheduling of hospital admission and surgical

TABLE 6–1.
M-VAC Regimen*

Drug (mg/m²)	1	2	15†	22†	29
Methotrexate	30		30	30	R
					E
Vinblastine		3	3	3	C
					Y
Adriamycin		30			C
		(15 after			L
		prior			
		irradiation)			
Cisplatin		70			E

*M-VAC = methotrexate, vinblastine, Adriamycin, cisplatin.
†No drugs were administered when mucositis was present, white blood cell count was less than 2,500/µl, or platelet count was less than 100,000/µl.

evaluation, as well as myelosuppression, resulted in the median cycle length being increased to 5 or more weeks.

An analysis of patient characteristics (Table 6–2) showed the median age to be 62 years and the median Karnofsky performance score 80%. Most patients (77%) originally had a primary urinary bladder tumor of the transitional cell variety (98%). Prior therapies included irradiation in 58%, systemic cytotoxic drugs in 14%, laparotomy in 58%, and surgical resection in 45%; within 6 weeks before beginning M-VAC, 83% of the patients underwent 87 diagnostic procedures for pathologic confirmation of disease. Ninety patients (98%) had an indicator lesion that could properly be monitored for response. The other two patients are considered to have had only evaluable disease. Both had documented disease at surgery, prior to the first M-VAC cycle; after three and five M-VAC cycles, respectively, they are surviving 15 + and 27 + months without evidence of disease.

Initial laboratory values indicated that some patients entered the study with abnormalities greater than the MSKCC norm: an abnormal level of BUN in 21%, of Cr in 19%, and an abnormal Ccr in 60% (median 66 ml/minute, below MSKCC norm of >85 ml/minute). However, the percentage of patients entering with values above protocol criteria was only 4% for BUN, 3% for Cr, and 9% for Ccr. Of note, the recorded BUN, Cr, and Ccr values varied considerably depending on the extent of intravenous hydration and the accuracy of urine collections. A first-cycle carcinoembryonic antigen (CEA) measurement, which was obtained for 55 patients (60%), was abnormal in 13% (median, 23 ng/µl); CEA was measured in 25% of patients in subsequent cycles.

Response Criteria

An adequate trial was defined as (1) a 1-month survival with appropriate follow-up and (2) administration of a minimum of one standard dosage on days 1 and 2, plus either initial doses repeated once or therapy administered on day 15 or 22 or both. Standard phase II response criteria (Table 6–3) included those suggested by the First International Consensus Development Conference on Bladder Cancer (Yagoda 1985; Van Oostrom et al. 1986). Of note, in the TNM (tumor, nodes, metastasis) classification of the International Union Against Cancer (UICC), the subscript "c" denotes a clinical (not a surgical) staging that includes TURB. In addition, since the prefix "s" is employed in the UICC TNM system for patients who undergo surgical staging before definitive therapy, "s" is used here as a *postscript* to

TABLE 6–2.
Patient Characteristics

Characteristic	Patients (n = 92)	
	No.	%
Age (yr)		
Median, 62		
Range, 23–77		
Karnofsky performance score		
Median		80
Range		30–90
Males		76
Primary tumor		
Urinary bladder		77
Renal pelvis		10
Ureter		5
Urethra		8
Pathology		
Transitional cell	90	98
Adenocarcinoma	1	1
Squamous cell	1	1
Prior therapy		
Chemotherapy		28
Systemic		14
Intravesical		14
Irradiation		58
2,500 cGy		36
2,500 cGy		22
None		42
Laparotomy	53	
Surgical resection	41	
Radical cystectomy	25	
Partial cystectomy	5	
Nephrectomy	7	
Ureterectomy	3	
Urethrectomy	1	
Neck dissection	1	
Restaging within 6 wk	76	
Laparotomy	19	
Cystectomy	3	
Nephrectomy	2	
TURB*	30	
Biopsy		
Lung, thoracotomy	5	
Bone	3	
Liver	4	
Lymph nodes	16	
Pelvic/abdominal masses	5	
Primary indicator lesion	90	
Lung	24	
Nodes, abdominal or pelvic masses by CT*	50	
Nodes on physical examination	6	
Liver	5	
Bladder masses	4	
Urethral mass	1	

(Continued)

TABLE 6–2 (cont.).
Patient Characteristics

	Patients (n = 92)	
Characteristic	No.	%
Stage (83 patients)		
N_+M_0	19	
$N_{0/+}M_+$	64	

*TURB = transurethral resection of the bladder; CT = computed transaxial tomography.

indicate that no disease remained after surgical resection of residual masses. This proposed system is, in essence, already used for other solid tumors such as ovarian and testicular cancers. However, it is important to realize that, in our study, the $_cCR$ (clinical CR) $+ _pCR$ (pathologically confirmed CR) is equivalent to the "true" CR rate after chemotherapy alone; the CR_s category really denotes a combination regimen of chemotherapy plus surgery.

TABLE 6–3.
Response Criteria

Complete remission (CR)
    Complete disappearance of all evidence of tumor by physical examination, x-rays, radionuclide scans, CT scans, sonography, tumor-related biochemical and biologic marker parameters, urine cytology, cystoscopy and biopsy, including no T_{is}, for >1 month.
        $_cCR$ = Clinically proved, defined by criteria listed above.
        $_pCR$ = Pathologically proved at laparotomy, thoracotomy, or by biopsy of previous sites of known disease.
        CR_s = Surgical removal of all residual disease required to attain CR status.
Partial remission (PR)
    >50% decrease of the summed products of the longest perpendicular diameters of all measured lesions by diagnostic tests defined in CR without simultaneous increase in size of any lesion or appearance of new lesions for >1 month. (PR should also be used for CR patients with positive cytology or T_{is}.)
Minor response (MR)
    25%–49% decrease in tumor size as defined in PR for >1 month.
Stabilization (STAB)
    <25% change in tumor size as defined in PR for >3 months.
Progression (PROG)
    >25% increase in tumor size as defined in PR; STAB <3 months; appearance of new lesions; or a mixed response.

The effect on time to relapse and on survival of this combined modality, chemotherapy or surgery and/or irradiation, is of major interest. Theoretically, one would expect the patients classified $_pCR$ to fare better than those in the $_cCR$ category, and that the least successful group would be the CR_s. Data from an MSKCC study of 134 patients with P_{1-4} disease found that, after radical cystectomy with or without irradiation, only 54% survived 1 year and 19% 2 years (Smith and Whitmore 1981).

RESULTS

Patient Response

Of 92 patients, 5% are considered inadequately treated, 2% had a non-transitional cell tumor, both of whom progressed with M-VAC therapy, and 2% had only evaluable disease, as previously discussed. Among the remaining 83 patients who had bidimensionally measurable transitional cell carcinoma evaluable for response, 11 achieved a $_c$CR, 10 a $_p$CR, and 10 a CR$_s$; the overall CR rate was 37% (95% confidence interval [CI], 27%–48%). Median response duration was 37 months (range, 8–47+), and since 17 patients (55%) are still alive, median survival cannot yet be reported after a median follow-up of 40 months. The estimated probabilities of surviving 2 and 3 years, respectively, are 71% (95% CI, 55%–87%) and 54% (95% CI, 35%–73%) (Table 6–4).

Among the 11 patients (13%; 95% CI, 6%–21%) who achieved $_c$CR status, 7 had a primary bladder tumor, 2 a renal pelvis tumor, and 2 a ureteral tumor. Metastatic disease initially was documented in the lung in three patients and subcutaneous lymph nodes in four; CT scan identified abdominal or pelvic masses in eight and bone metastasis in two. After a median of five M-VAC cycles, all refused surgical staging. Six patients relapsed, one with a new T$_{is}$ lesion at 8 months, another with a new renal pelvis tumor at 23 months, one at 19 months in the retroperitoneal lymph nodes, and three in the brain, two of whom also relapsed in bone.

Among the 10 patients (12%; 95% CI, 5%–19%) who achieved a $_p$CR, 7 had a bladder primary tumor and 1 each had a renal pelvis, a ureteral, and a urethral primary tumor. Median follow-up is currently 43 months, median duration of response exceeds 24 months, and median survival exceeds 33 months. Of note, two who achieved a $_c$PR subsequently were categorized as $_p$CR after biopsy proved the residual masses noted on a CT scan to be only fibrosis. In one patient categorized with progressing disease ($_c$PROG), all retroperitoneal and nodal masses completely disappeared, but a pelvic cystic mass was enlarging; laparotomy showed it to be a necrotic lymphocele.

Among the 10 patients (12%; 95% CI, 5%–19%) who achieved a CR$_s$ status, 9 had a

TABLE 6–4.
Response Rate to M-VAC*

	Patients (n = 92)			Survival Rate in Yr (%)		
	No.	%	95% CI (%)	1	2	3
Inadequate	5	5		0	0	0
Non-TCC	2	2		0	0	0
Adequate TCC for evaluation of						
Survival	85	92				
Response	83	90		52†	27†	20†
Response						
CR + PR	57	69	59–79	72	40	31
CR	31	37	27–48	94	71	55
$_c$CR	11	13	6–21	91	73	58
$_p$CR	10	12	5–19	90	70	58
$_c$CR + $_p$CR	21	25	16–34	—	—	—
CR$_s$	10	12	5–19	90	70	50
PR	26	31	21–41	46	4	0
MR	7	8	2–14	29	0	0
PROG	19	23	14–32	11	0	0
N_+M_0	10/19	53	31–75	—	—	—
$N_{0/+}M_+$	21/64	33	22–45	—	—	—

*M-VAC = methotrexate, vinblastine, Adriamycin, cisplatin; CI = confidence interval; TCC = transitional cell carcinoma; CR = complete remission; PR = partial remission; MR = minor response; PROG = progressive disease; $_c$CR = clinical CR; $_p$CR = pathologic CR; CR$_s$ = CR achieved surgically.
†CR + PR + MR for 83 patients.

primary bladder tumor and 1 a renal pelvis cancer. The median CR_s survival duration has been reached at 27 months, and the median follow-up is currently 39 months (range, 12–48+). Before receiving M-VAC, six patients in this CR_s group had had a laparotomy and exhibited unresectable disease ($_sT_{3-4b}$). The median number of M-VAC courses before follow-up laparotomy (nine patients) and thoracotomy (one patient) was five (range, 3–6). All patients who achieved a CR_s were initially categorized as $_cPR$; however, one was found to have only residual P_{is}. Seven of nine with N_{3-4} disease were downstaged to N_0 and one to N_1. The original intention was to administer four cycles of M-VAC to be followed by surgery and, if disease was found, to administer a minimum of two additional cycles; however, 4 of 10 patients refused further treatment.

Thirty-one percent of patients achieved a PR (95% CI, 21%–41%); the median time for response duration was 8 months (range, 4–15) and for survival, 11 months (range, 4–24). The PR group received a median of six M-VAC cycles (range, 3–7). In 16 of this group, disease relapsed in sites other than those involved at presentation: brain in four, bladder with T_{is} in one, lung in one, liver in three, bowel in two, subcutaneous lymph nodes in three, and bone in two. All of these patients initially had extensive disease—9 in the lung, 13 in retroperitoneal lymph nodes documented by CT scan, 5 in the liver, 8 in subcutaneous lymph nodes or masses, 4 in pelvic or abdominal masses, and 5 in bone.

Eight percent of the patients (95% CI, 2%–14%) had a minimal response that lasted a median of 4 months (range, 2–9). All these patients have died after a median of 11 months (range, 4–22), a period similar to the survival duration of patients with a PR. They had received a median of four M-VAC cycles (range, 2–4). Twenty-three percent (95% CI, 14%–32%) of patients had progressing disease; their median survival was 7 months (range, 2–18). In almost all of them, tumor progression was evident within the first cycle, which explains the median of two M-VAC cycles (range, 1.5–5). These patients had presented with metastases in the lung (4), lymph nodes and abdominal and pelvic masses documented by CT scan (14), subcutaneous tissues (2), bone (9), and liver (3). New disease progression was observed in bone in two patients, liver in two, and subcutaneous lymph nodes in one.

Response Correlation

M-VAC caused tumor to regress at all metastatic sites, including 66% of metastatic nodes and pelvic masses, 77% of pulmonary lesions, 64% of hepatic lesions, 90% of subcutaneous masses or nodes, 73% of primary bladder lesions, and 100% of urethral lesions. Evaluable response occurred in 55% of osseous metastases. However, CR was much rarer, occurring in only 30% of subcutaneous masses and lymph nodes, 28% of abdominal and pelvic masses and lymph nodes, 29% of bladder lesions, 23% of osseous metastases, and 9% of hepatic lesions. Among the 16 patients who had abnormal CEA levels, 6% had a CR and 44% a PR; CEA levels decreased appropriately during remission and increased at relapse.

Nineteen patients began therapy with N_+M_0 and 64 with $N_{0/+}M_+$ disease. In the N_+ group, 53% achieved CR (2 $_cCR$, 4 $_pCR$, 4 CR_s) vs. 33% in the M_+ group (9 $_cCR$, 6$_pCR$, 6 CR_s); however, the true CR ($_cCR$ + $_pCR$) rate was 32% vs. 23%, respectively, for the two groups. The true PR incidences for the two groups (CR_s + $_cPR$) were similar, 42% for those with N_+ as compared with 44% for those with M_+.

Among eight patients with renal pelvis transitional cell carcinoma, four (50%) had a CR, one (13%) a PR, two a minimal response, and one progressing disease. Three of the four (75%) with adequately treated ureteral cancer had a CR and one had progressing disease. Among six patients with urethral tumors, one (17%) had a CR, three (50%) a PR, and two progressing disease.

Three of six patients who achieved $_c$CR in the urinary bladder underwent laparotomy; one of them achieved $_p$CR and another, who had presented with $_sT_{4b}N_4M_0$, was reclassified $P_{is}N_0M_0$. The last patient in the $_c$CR group died from brain metastases at 47 months. One patient categorized $_c$PR because of a persistent urethral mass was found to be $_p$CR, since the mass contained only fibrotic tissue. Seven patients were classified CR_s after surgery or cystoprostatectomy, and one after radical nephrectomy. Surgical restaging was performed in 24 selected patients who had responded to chemotherapy and in one who had $_c$PROG by CT scan. When the clinical vs. the pathologic (T vs. P) response rates were correlated, it was surprising that there was no understaging or overstaging in the $_c$CR group, but 28% of the $_c$PR group was clinically understaged (T < P).

Fifty-three patients had had prior irradiation, among whom we considered 49 adequately treated; 33% achieved a CR and 27% a PR. In the CR group, 12 had received less than 2,400 cGy and four had received more than 3,900 cGy, whereas in the PR group, nine had received less than 2,000 cGy and four more than 4,000 cGy. Four patients (8%) who showed a minimal response had received more than 3,000 cGy. In comparison, among the 14 patients (29%) whose disease progressed, nine had received less than 2,000 cGy, four had more than 4,000 cGy, and one had had chest wall irradiation. Thirteen patients (14%) had received prior systemic chemotherapy. Two of these had nontransitional cell tumors, and two were inadequately treated. Among the remaining nine patients, three each (27%) achieved CR or PR. Among the 74 evaluable patients who had no prior chemotherapy, 36% achieved a CR and 31% a PR. Remission was unaffected by prior intravesical chemotherapy.

Major dose modifications occurred. The initial cisplatin dose was divided between days 2 and 3 in eight adequately treated patients; 13% achieved a CR and 26% a PR. Cisplatin was discontinued in a subsequent cycle because of renal dysfunction in five instances. Thirteen patients never received the Adriamycin dose prescribed for the extent of their prior irradiation; in this group, four (31%) each achieved a CR or PR. Among the 92 patients studied, the Adriamycin dose was incorrectly increased in 1% to 8% of cycles and decreased in each of the first 6 cycles in 25%, 26%, 36%, 27%, 34%, and 29% of patients, respectively, and in cycles 7 through 11 in 7%. The Adriamycin dose was decreased in half or more of the subsequent cycles in 18 patients (10 because of a significant cardiovascular history); seven (39%) achieved a CR and four (22%) a PR. Ten (56%) of these 18 patients had either hypertension, cardiac valvular disorder, or a history of myocardial infarction, cardiac arrhythmia, or coronary artery bypass.

Relapse Pattern

At present, 10 (12%) of the adequately treated patients with transitional cell carcinoma have developed brain metastases, 6 while in CR and 4 in PR; when these are compared with the 57 classified CR + PR, the incidence of brain metastasis increases to 18%. Brain metastases were observed at a median of 11 months (range, 6–42), and the median survival time after diagnosis was 2 months (range, 1–21), despite attempts to salvage some patients with whole-brain irradiation, surgery, and intrathecal methotrexate via an Ommaya shunt. In approximately half, the brain was the only site of relapse. Five of the patients who developed brain metastasis (50%) had presented initially with pulmonary lesions, and they had either achieved a $_c$CR (three patients) or were still responding in the lung (two $_c$PR) at the time of brain relapse. In one patient, the brain mass was only discovered at autopsy. Two patients who presented with liver disease and achieved a $_c$PR also developed central nervous system disease.

Fourteen patients progressed in bone, and eight eventually developed liver metastases. The overall survival duration from the start of M-VAC therapy for patients whose disease was progressing in the liver was 10 months (range, 6–15).

Toxicity

A total of 420 M-VAC cycles (median, 4 per patient; range, 1–11) were administered. Nausea and vomiting were universal despite antiemetics, and mucositis occurred in 41% of the patients but was categorized +3 in only 4% (Table 6–5). Neurotoxicity was noted in 4% of patients, 31% experienced +1 renal dysfunction, 11% had hepatic toxicity, 3% a local reaction, 6% diarrhea, and 4% a drug-related death.

For each of six cycles, the WBC median nadirs were 2,600 to 3,000 cells/μl (range, 100–10,000); overall, 8% to 32% of cycles caused more than a +3 (<2,000 cells/μl) toxicity. Only 2% to 5% of patients demonstrated more than +3 platelet toxicity. Hemoglobin decreased by more than 20 g/L and more than 40 g/L, respectively, in 42% and 34% of the 92 patients treated by M-VAC. Median cycle lengths were 35 to 37 days for cycles one through four and 36 to 41 days for cycles five through seven; cycles varied from 24 to 86 days because of delays in hospitalization and clinic scheduling. Only 70% to 81% and 61% to 100% of patients, respectively, had one interim dose in cycles 1 through 4 and 5 through 11. For these cycles, in fact, only 30% to 56% and 38% to 80%, respectively, could receive both interim doses. Such toxicity has now been significantly ameliorated with granulocyte colony-stimulating factor (G-CSF). Gabrilove et al. (1988a,b) studied 22 patients who received G-CSF in doses of 1 to 60 μg/kg before and during the first cycle followed by no G-CSF in the second cycle. Myelosuppression was almost negated with doses greater than 3 μg/kg, and of note, the

TABLE 6–5.
M-VAC Toxicity*

Variable	Overall Level (%)				Cycles		
	+1	+2	+3	+4	1–3	4–6	7–11
No. of patients per cycle					91–65	49–22	17
White blood cell count (%)							
+4 (<1,000 cells/μl)					0–7	2–5	6
+3 (<2,000 cells/μl)					18–25	18–21	12
+2					19–40	26–37	29
+1					19–22	24–36	41
Platelets (%)							
+4 (<25,000 cells/μl)					2–4	0–5	0
+3 (<50,000 cells/μl)					0–1	0–6	24
+2					2–8	9–18	18
+1					13–34	20–23	12
Hemoglobin	42[†]	34[‡]					
Nausea/vomiting	34	21	4	0			
Mucositis	19	18	4	0			
Renal	31	3	3	0			
Hepatic	9	0	2	0			
Neurologic	3	0	0	0			
Local reaction	3	0	0	0			
Ototoxicity	2	0	0	0			
Nadir sepsis				19			

*M-VAC = methotrexate, vinblastine, Adriamycin, cisplatin.
[†]Decrease <2 g/100 ml.
[‡]Decrease <4 g/100 ml. Drug-related death, 4%.

incidence of mucositis was also markedly decreased from 44% in the nontreated group to 11% in those receiving G-CSF.

DISCUSSION

M-VAC seems to be effective against transitional cell carcinoma of the urothelium, inducing a significant response rate—37% CR and 31% PR. Based on data from the present study (Sternberg et al. 1988) and that from our neoadjuvant trial (Scher et al. 1988a; 1988b), M-VAC does not appear to be effective against nontransitional cell types or T_{is} or in preventing de novo T_{is} tumors elsewhere in the urothelium. The 18% brain relapse incidence in patients who had achieved CR or PR is disturbing, particularly since half did not relapse systemically; the median survival following brain relapse was 2 months. In addition, although hepatic metastases responded, tumor regression was transient and disease progressed.

The suggested new response criteria are useful and will help in comparing the efficacy of regimens in published studies, particularly in delineating more clearly the specific effect of chemotherapy in achieving a CR status. In the present trial, 53% of the 19 patients with N_+M_0 disease achieved a CR, as compared with 33% of 64 who had $N_{0/+}$ M_+ disease. The effect of surgical debulking of remaining disease on the relapse pattern and survival duration will be of interest as further cases are evaluated. Without the availability of an effective salvage regimen, the CR_s status may not be useful; however, in the present series, such patients ($_cPR$ to CR_s) did survive 27 months vs. 11 months for those with PR or MR.

Toxicity was significant, and not all patients could receive the regimen as planned. The introduction of G-CSF, which ameliorates myelosuppression and mucositis, may permit greater adherence to the dosage schedule.

At present, M-VAC does seem to be more efficacious than single agents and other combination regimens that have been evaluated at MSKCC. However, the prospective randomized studies that have been undertaken comparing M-VAC to cisplatin, to methotrexate, and to CISCA (cisplatin, cyclophosphamide, and Adriamycin) will determine the true efficacy of this regimen.

ACKNOWLEDGMENT

The author gratefully acknowledges the editorial assistance of Ms Martha Gold.

REFERENCES

1. Gabrilove JL, Jakubowski A, Fain K, et al. 1988a. A study of human recombinant granulocyte colony stimulating factor in cancer patients at risk for chemotherapy-induced neutropenia: A preliminary report. *N Engl J Med* 318:1414–1420.
2. Gabrilove JL, Jakubowski A, Scher H, et al. 1988b. A study of human recombinant granulocyte colony stimulating factor in cancer patients at risk for chemotherapy-induced neutropenia. *J Clin Invest* (in press).
3. Scher HI, Yagoda A, Herr HW, et al. 1988a. Neoadjuvant M-VAC (methotrexate, vinblastine, doxorubicin and cisplatin) effect on the primary bladder lesion. *J Urol* 139:470–474.
4. Scher HI, Yagoda A, Herr HW, et al. 1988b. Neoadjuvant M-VAC (methotrexate, vinblastine, doxorubicin and cisplatin) for extravesical urinary tract tumors. *J Urol* 139:475–477.
5. Smith JA, Whitmore WF. 1981. Regional lymph node metastasis from bladder cancer. *J Urol* 126:591–593.

6. Sternberg CN, Yagoda A, Scher HI, et al. 1988. M-VAC (methotrexate, vinblastine, doxorubicin and cisplatin) for advanced transitional cell carcinoma of the urothelium. *J Urol* 139:461–469.

7. Van Oosterom AT, Akaza H, Hall R, et al. 1986. Response criteria phase II/phase III invasive bladder, in Denis L, Niijima T, Prout G, et al (eds): *Proceedings of the First International Development Conference on Guidelines for Clinical Research in Bladder Cancer.* New York, Alan R. Liss, pp 301–310.

8. Yagoda A. 1988. Chemotherapy of urothelial tract cancer: Memorial Sloan-Kettering Cancer Center experience, in DeVita VT, Hellman S, Rosenberg SA (eds): *Important Advances in Oncology—1988.* Philadelphia, JB Lippincott, pp 143–160.

9. Yagoda A. 1985. Progress in the treatment of advanced urothelial tract tumors. *J Clin Oncol* 3:1448–1450.

Chapter 7

CMV for Metastatic Urothelial Tumors

Richard K. Lo, M.D.

Fuad S. Freiha, M.D.

Frank M. Torti, M.D.

The 5-year survival rate for persons with locally advanced bladder tumors has remained disappointingly low at around 50%. Occult and unrecognized metastases account for the majority of the fatalities. Heretofore, chemotherapy has been ineffective against these tumors. Recently, however, several cancer centers have reported moderate success in treating metastatic transitional cell carcinomas, using programs with cisplatin-based combination chemotherapy (Samuels et al. 1979; Harker et al. 1985; Sternberg et al. 1985). Herein, we report the results of the Stanford University-Northern California Oncology Group (NCOG), which used the cisplatin-methotrexate-vinblastine (CMV) combination.

Cisplatin is the mainstay of combination chemotherapy for metastatic transitional cell carcinoma of the bladder. It is the most active single agent, inducing partial response rates of 20% to 43% (Soloway et al. 1981). Methotrexate, too, has induced partial response rates of up to 38% (Natale et al. 1981). Other agents that have shown activity against metastatic transitional cell carcinoma include vinblastine and doxorubicin (Adriamycin); vinblastine, administered as a single agent to heavily pretreated patients, has been active in 18% (Blumenreich et al. 1982).

In 1981, encouraged by reports of synergistic activities in some combination regimens and by the Stanford experience of nonadditive nephrotoxicity when cisplatin and methotrexate were used together for patients with head and neck cancers (Jacobs et al. 1983), we combined the three drugs with the most proved activity—cisplatin, methotrexate, and vinblastine (CMV)—to treat advanced metastatic transitional cell carcinoma of the urothelium (Harker et al. 1985; Meyers et al. 1985, 1987).

MATERIALS AND METHODS

Between 1981 and 1984, 71 eligible patients with metastatic transitional cell carcinoma of the bladder, renal pelvis, and ureter were entered into a cooperative phase II trial of a three-drug CMV regimen conducted by the NCOG. Eligibility criteria included (1) measurable metastatic tumor identified by physical examination, chest roentgenogram, or computerized tomographic (CT) examination of the chest, abdomen, or pelvis; (2) no prior systemic chemotherapy; (3) a creatinine clearance rate of more than 50 ml/minute, a leukocyte count higher than 4,000/ml, a platelet count higher than 100,000/ml, and a serum bilirubin value less than 2 mg/dl; and (4) a Karnofsky performance status of 40% or more. All patients were assessed initially by physical examination, hematologic and liver function tests, serum creatinine and 24-hour urinary creatinine clearance tests, chest roentgenogram, radionuclide bone scan, and CT examination of the abdomen and pelvis.

The CMV combination, as piloted at Stanford, was administered in 21-day cycles as follows: methotrexate, 40 mg/m², and vinblastine, 5 mg/m², intravenously on days 1 and 8. These doses were modified later to methotrexate, 30 mg/m², and vinblastine, 4 mg/m² (Table 7–1), owing to occasional hematologic toxicity in the first 22 patients. Cisplatin, 100 mg/m², was administered on day 2 as a continuous 4-hour infusion, with prehydration a prerequisite. The 24-hour creatinine clearance rate was assessed before each cycle to determine the need for any dose modification of cisplatin or methotrexate.

The hematologic parameters for methotrexate and vinblastine dose modification are shown in Table 7–2. In addition, methotrexate dose adjustments were made for renal function: no methotrexate was administered when the creatinine clearance rate decreased below 45 mg/minute or when the serum creatinine level increased to more than 2.0 mg/dl. Cisplatin was administered at full dose when the measured creatinine clearance rate was more than 60 ml/minute. The cisplatin dose was reduced 50% for a creatinine clearance rate between 45 and 60 mg/minute, and no cisplatin was administered when the creatinine clearance rate decreased to less than 45 ml/minute. The cisplatin dosage was not modified for hematologic toxicity. To facilitate maximum drug doses, delays for bone marrow recovery of up to 2 weeks were allowed before beginning each new chemotherapy cycle.

TABLE 7–1.
Cisplatin, Methotrexate, and Vinblastine (CMV) for Metastatic Transitional Cell Carcinoma

Drug	Schedule*		
	Day 1	Day 2	Day 8
Cisplatin (100 mg/m²)		X	
Methotrexate (30 mg/m²)	X		X
Vinblastine (4 mg/m²)	X		X

*The cycle repeats in 21 days.

TABLE 7–2.
Parameters and Modified Doses of Methotrexate and Vinblastine (CMV Protocol)*

WBC	Platelets per ml (%)			
	>150,000	100,000–149,999	75,000–99,999	<75,000
>3,500	100	100	50†	0
3,000–3,499	75‡	75‡	50	0
2,500–2,999	50	50	0§	0
<2,500	0	0	0	0

*CMV = cisplatin, methotrexate, vinblastine; WBC = white blood cells.
†If the dose indicated at day 1 of a subsequent cycle (day 22) falls below 50%, delay the cycle up to 2 weeks.
‡Administer 100% of the calculated dose on day 8 when platelet and WBC counts are at this level.
§Administer 50% of calculated dose on day 8 when platelet and WBC counts are at this level.

Response criteria were defined as follows: (1) Complete response (CR)—complete disappearance of all disease determined by physical examination, blood chemistry, or roentgenogram for a minimum of 4 weeks. Bone abnormalities were required to show evidence of healing or partial resolution on bone scan. (2) Partial response (PR)—at least 50% reduction of the product of the two longest perpendicular diameters of all measurable lesions for at least 8 weeks. A bone response consisting of recalcification of a lytic bone metastasis was included as a PR providing no disease progression occurred elsewhere. (3) Nonresponse (NR)—all others, including stable disease, disease progression, and mixed responses. Patients found to have bladder involvement during the initial evaluation underwent cystoscopic examination of the bladder, biopsies, and urine cytologic evaluation after two to four cycles of chemotherapy. For the bladder to be designated as a site of CR required that both the biopsies and cytologic studies be negative.

RESULTS

Of 71 patients initially enrolled in the CMV study, 62 were considered evaluable. Sixteen of these (26%) achieved a CR with chemotherapy alone. Using the Memorial Sloan-Kettering Cancer Center criteria for responses after surgical consolidation, we achieved an overall response rate (CR + CR_s) of 34%.

There were no significant characteristic differences between the responders and nonresponders. Prior pelvic irradiation (preoperative or curative) had no effect on the response rate. Patients who achieved CR with CMV received a median of six cycles of chemotherapy (range, 4–10); the majority showed an objective response by the end of the fourth cycle. In addition to the CRs achieved by CMV therapy alone, four patients achieved CR status after surgical consolidation. Three patients with bladder or pelvic masses were rendered operable after CMV therapy, and indeed no disease or only microscopic disease remained in the resected specimen. Among the 16 patients who achieved CR, 12 relapsed; relapses occurred as late as 16 months after therapy. The median survival duration of this group was 14 months, although two patients continued in unmaintained remission at 18+ and 35+ months.

Toxicity of the CMV regimen was moderate. All patients had nausea, vomiting, and alopecia. In 15 patients, the serum creatinine level rose to more than 2 mg/dl. Thirty-one patients required a dose modification owing to their decreased creatinine clearance rate; none of these, however, had progressive renal insufficiency or required dialysis. Fourteen patients developed severe leukopenia (white blood cell count <1,000/ml) and were hospitalized. Six of them also had gram-negative bacteremia, and two died. These two had received the higher doses of methotrexate and vinblastine before we made the dose adjustments mentioned earlier. Since introduction of the slightly lower doses of methotrexate (30 mg/m²) and vinblastine (4 mg/m²), efficacy has not decreased, although toxicity has diminished markedly. Other minor gastrointestinal symptoms were also reported.

DISCUSSION

We have demonstrated that CRs can be achieved with CMV combination chemotherapy in a substantial minority of patients with metastatic urothelial tumors of the bladder, renal pelvis, and ureter. Similar success has been shown by the Memorial Sloan-Kettering group using a similar regimen plus Adriamycin (M-VAC: methotrexate, vinblastine, Adriamycin, and cisplatin). In a recent update of their experience with M-VAC, they reported a 37% CR rate (Sternberg et al. 1983), which is similar to ours.

When metastases were in the bone and liver, sites traditionally refractory to chemotherapy, CMV still demonstrated respectable response rates of 20% and 38%, respectively. Furthermore, responses also occurred in patients with metastases in multiple sites, again a population usually unresponsive to chemotherapy.

Two other features in our series of patients should be emphasized. Seventeen had not undergone a cystectomy before beginning CMV therapy. Eleven, including 6 of 12 whose treatment was CMV alone, achieved a CR. Response in all instances was pathologically confirmed by cystoscopy and bladder biopsies. Resection of a residual pelvic mass in one patient showed fibrosis only. Five of five patients who had pretreatment radiotherapy also achieved CR. The median survival duration of this group was 24 months.

The demonstrated activity of CMV against the primary tumor is encouraging, since primary tumors, because of their bulk and their heterogenous nature, are often more refractory to chemotherapy than are metastatic tumors. This activity against the primary tumor has prompted us to initiate a program of neoadjuvant CMV chemotherapy for locally advanced (stages C and D_1) tumors, to be consolidated by radical cystectomy. Similarly, when responses between the distant and primary sites are discordant and residual tumor remains in the bladder, cystectomy should be recommended because of the success at the distant sites.

We also saw discordant responses in a group of patients who achieved a CR at the systemic sites, only to relapse in the central nervous system. As it is with most other tumors, the central nervous system appeared to be a privileged site, resistant to chemotherapy; therefore aggressive resection of an isolated intracranial metastasis might be indicated for patients who have demonstrated a CR in other sites.

CMV may constitute the chemotherapeutic approach to advanced metastatic urothelial carcinoma that has the best therapeutic index, that is, when current doses are employed, responses equal or exceed others reported in the literature. In addition, toxicity has been moderate in this easily administered 3-week regimen. Given the success of this and other programs in managing metastatic disease, we need to define further and extend the potential roles of adjuvant and neoadjuvant chemotherapy, using the same agents, for locally advanced bladder transitional cell carcinoma.

REFERENCES

1. Blumenreich MS, Yagoda A, Natale RB, et al. 1982. Phase II trial of vinblastine sulfate for metastatic urothelial tract tumors. *Cancer* 50:435–438.
2. Harker WG, Meyers FJ, Freiha FS, et al. 1985. Cisplatin, methotrexate, and vinblastine (CMV): An effective chemotherapy regimen for metastatic transitional cell carcinoma of the urinary tract. A Northern California Oncology Group study. *J Clin Oncol* 3:1463–1470.
3. Jacobs C, Meyers F, Hendrickson C, et al. 1983. A randomized phase III study of cisplatin with or without methotrexate for recurrent squamous cell carcinoma of the head and neck: A Northern California Oncology Group study. *Cancer* 52:1563–1569.
4. Meyers FJ, Palmer JM, Freiha FS, et al. 1985. The fate of the bladder treated with cisplatin, methotrexate, and vinblastine: A Northern California Oncology Group study. *J Urol* 134:1118–1121.
5. Meyers FJ, Palmer JM, Hannigan JF. 1987. Chemotherapy of disseminated transitional cell carcinoma, in Williams RD (ed): *Advances in Urologic Oncology,* vol 1. New York, Macmillan Publishing Co, pp 183–192.
6. Natale RB, Yagoda A, Watson RC, et al. 1981. Methotrexate: An active drug in bladder cancer. *Cancer* 47:1246–1250.

7. Samuels ML, Moran ME, Johnson DE, et al. 1979. CISCA combination chemotherapy for metastatic carcinoma of the bladder, in Johnson DE, Samuels ML (eds): *Cancer of the Genitourinary Tract.* New York, Raven Press, pp 101–106.
8. Soloway MD, Ikard M, Ford K. 1981. Cis-diaminedichloroplatinum (II) in locally advanced and metastatic urothelial cancer. *Cancer* 47:476–480.
9. Sternberg CN, Yagoda A, Scher HI, et al. 1988. M-VAC (methotrexate, vinblastine, doxorubicin and cisplatin) for advanced transitional cell carcinoma of the urothelium. *J Urol* 139:461–469.
10. Sternberg CN, Yagoda A, Scher HI, et al. 1985. Preliminary results of M-VAC (methotrexate, vinblastine, doxorubicin and cisplatin) for transitional cell carcinoma of the urothelium. *J Urol* 133:403–407.

Chapter 8

Intra-arterial Chemotherapy for Localized Carcinoma of the Bladder*

James E. Montie, M.D.

Ronald M. Bukowski, M.D.

J. Edson Pontes, M.D.

Ram Ganapathi, Ph.D.

Charles E. Pippenger, Ph.D.

Roxanne E. Steinle, M.D.

Marian Lee, M.D.

Barbara Risius, M.D.

Michael Geisinger, M.D.

Margaret Zelch, M.D.

Improvement in the results of chemotherapy for bladder cancer is chiefly dependent on identifying new agents that have antitumor activity, but alterations in the dose, timing, or route of delivery of agents already known to be effective may also prove valuable. Intra-arterial infusion is one such option. However, although clinical research using regional intra-arterial infusion chemotherapy has been conducted for more than two decades, no evidence conclusively confirms its superiority over an intravenous route of administration. Most clinical studies of intra-arterial chemotherapy do not include a clear end point allowing comparison of results with those of intravenous therapy.

Regional chemotherapy is logical; giving the most drug to the area of highest tumor burden makes sense (Chen and Gross 1980). Specifically, intra-arterial infusion of the bladder is logical based on the relatively low blood flow to a muscular organ, the probability that a

*This study was supported in part by a grant from Bristol-Myers Corp.

significant amount of the drug is extracted during the first pass through the infused organ, and the rapid elimination of the best agent, cisplatin, through renal excretion (Campbell et al. 1983; Logothetis and Samuels 1984; Stewart et al. 1987). This reasoning must be confirmed, however, by properly designed studies; unfortunately there are many variables that interact but are often uncontrolled.

In this chapter, we review our experience at the Cleveland Clinic using intra-arterial chemotherapy in three different trials. We concentrate on the preliminary results of a study to determine the maximum tolerated dose of intra-arterial cisplatin within the methotrexate, vinblastine, doxorubicin (Adriamycin), and cisplatin (M-VAC) combination.

MATERIALS, METHODS, AND RESULTS

Study I

Based on preliminary data from The University of Texas M. D. Anderson Cancer Center on intravenous CISCA (cisplatin, Adriamycin, and cyclophosphamide) and on intra-arterial chemotherapy protocols in the pelvis (Logothetis et al. 1982; Wallace et al. 1982), we initiated a phase II trial of CISCA in 1982. Cisplatin and Adriamycin were administered intra-arterially and cyclophosphamide intravenously. We treated 17 patients, selecting those with large tumors in an effort to facilitate the clinical assessment of response to therapy. Noteworthy for future studies was the fact that the dose of cisplatin was 40 to 75 mg/m^2 in normal saline infused in 30 minutes. Complete results have been published, but in summary, 14 of 16 evaluable patients (87.5%) were considered to have responded at least partially (Maatman et al. 1986). Three of 13 patients who underwent a cystectomy had a pathologically confirmed complete response (CR). A conclusion drawn from that study was that the local toxicity of this regimen was significant; it included buttock pain, skin erythema, ulceration, and plexopathy. Adriamycin was believed to be the agent most responsible for the local toxicity.

Study II

To confirm the clinical judgment that the majority of toxicity from the above protocol was due to the intra-arterial Adriamycin, we conducted a limited study of intra-arterial cisplatin alone. The dose was 70 to 100 mg/m^2 in normal saline over 30 minutes. Toxicity was substantially less; only one patient developed a temporary plexopathy. However, in only 3 of 8 patients did the treatment appear clinically to have a salutary effect, and no patient had a CR.

Study III

As the above studies were completed, data from Yagoda and colleagues on the M-VAC regimen were released suggesting that this combination was the best available (Sternberg et al. 1985). Our earlier studies had emphasized two points: first, the evaluation of a response less than a pathologic CR in the bladder was difficult and subjective, making comparison of "response rates" between studies at different institutions very suspect, and second, the amount of cisplatin that could be safely administered intra-arterially was not entirely established. We elected to pursue a trial asking the following questions: (1) what is the maximum tolerated dose of intra-arterial cisplatin when incorporated into M-VAC (MVA intravenously), and (2) what are the relative concentrations between peripheral venous and common iliac venous levels of cisplatin after intra-arterial infusion?

Twenty-one patients have been entered into this study. Criteria for patient eligibility are shown in Table 8–1, and the treatment schedule and dose escalation are listed in Table 8–2. Varying doses of cisplatin in 150 ml 3% saline were infused by either a right or left internal iliac artery catheter on day 2 over 30 minutes after previous hydration with normal saline; mannitol 12.5 gm was given intravenously before therapy. The study schema is shown in Figure 8–1.

All patients who achieved a clinically apparent CR were advised to have either a partial or a total cystectomy to confirm the staging pathologically, but several refused and have only been observed by periodic radiologic studies, cystoscopy, examination of the patient under anesthesia, and biopsy.

Toxicity was graded according to standard Eastern Cooperative Oncology Group (ECOG)

TABLE 8–1.
Phase I Intra-arterial M-VAC: Patient
Eligibility Criteria*

Locally advanced bladder carcinoma, clinical
   stages T_{2-4} N_{X-2} M_0
Measurable or evaluable lesion at cystoscopy
Previous therapy
Systemic chemotherapy—none
Intravesical chemotherapy allowed
Pelvic radiotherapy allowed
No prior malignancy within past 5 yr
Performance status 0–1 (ECOG)
Laboratory requirements

WBC	$\geq$4,000/μl
Platelets	$\geq$100,000/μl
Serum total creatinine	$\leq$1.5 mg/ml
Serum total bilirubin	$\leq$1.5 mg/ml
Creatinine clearance	$\geq$60 ml/min

*M-VAC = methotrexate, vinblastine,
Adriamycin, cisplatin; ECOG = Eastern
Cooperative Oncology Group; WBC = white
blood cells.

TABLE 8–2.
Intra-arterial M-VAC Treatment Schedule

Chemotherapy (repeated every 28 days)*	
M — Methotrexate	30 mg/m² IV days 1, 15, 22
V — Vinblastine	3 mg/m² IV days 2, 15, 22
A — Adriamycin	30 mg/m² IV day 2
C — Cisplatin	60–140 mg/m² IV day 2

Dose Escalation Scheme	
Level	Dose Cisplatin (mg/m²)
I	60
II	80
III	100
IV	120
V	140

*Courses are repeated at 28-day intervals, with clinical and
pathologic restaging following two and four courses of
treatment.

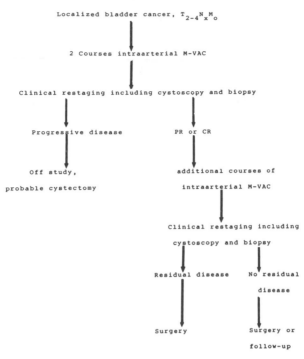

FIG 8–1.
Study schema for intra-arterial *M-VAC* (methotrexate, vinblastine, Adriamycin, cisplatin) phase I–II trial. *PR* = partial response; *CR* = complete response.

criteria. The determination of the maximum tolerated dose was based on the following: (1) gastrointestinal toxicity: intractable (grade 3) vomiting in 2 of 4 patients treated at any dose level; (2) renal toxicity: grade 2 or greater toxicity in 2 of 4 patients, not returning to normal before the next course of treatment; (3) neurologic toxicity: grade 2 or greater toxicity, including paresthesias, decreased muscle strength, or pain on the infused side, in 2 of 4 patients, not returning to normal before the next course of treatment; or (4) grade 3 or grade 4 toxicity not otherwise specified occurring in 3 of 6 patients at any dose level.

Course number two and subsequent courses were administered on day 28 if the leukocyte count was above $4,000/\mu l$, platelet count above $100,000/\mu l$, and creatinine level less than or equal to 1.5 mg/100 ml. Doses of myelosuppressive agents (methotrexate, vinblastine, or Adriamycin) were modified as required by, and subsequent courses were based on, hematologic toxicity, as established by the following nadir counts:

Leukocytes	Platelets	Dose Change
$>2,000/\mu l$	$>50,000/\mu l$	None
$1,000-1,999/\mu l$	$25,000-54,000/\mu l$	Decreased 25%
$<1,000/\mu l$	$<25,000/\mu l$	Decreased 50%

Chemotherapy on days 15 and 22 of any cycle was administered if the leukocyte count was above $3,000/\mu l$, platelet count above $100,000/\mu l$, and creatinine level less than or equal to 1.5 mg/100 ml. Seventeen patients have completed treatment at this time. Their median age is 58 years (range, 44–75 years). A mean of 2.7 courses of chemotherapy has been administered per patient. Two patients were considered to be a poor risk based on age (>70 years) and

15 were considered good risks. The frequency of treatment modifications on days 15 and 22 is presented in Table 8–3.

Toxicity data are presented in Table 8–4. Preliminary observations indicate that the maximum tolerated dose would be 100 mg/m.[2]

Although the number of patients receiving any individual dose is too small to draw meaningful conclusions, response data based on post-treatment clinical restaging is shown in Table 8–5. At the time of the 2- or 4-month evaluation, 69% of those treated had evidence of downstaging, although the relationship of this observation to long-term benefit is debatable. The number of patients who underwent surgery at this point is small (7/17). However, it is noteworthy that of 3 patients who achieved a clinical CR, 2 were found to have residual microscopic cancer at surgery.

Pharmacokinetic data are preliminary. Heparinized blood was obtained from a peripheral vein and from the common or internal iliac vein on the infused side following the initiation of cisplatin infusion via the hypogastric artery. The peripheral venous samples were obtained at 0, 15, 30, 60, 90, 120, 150, 180, and 240 minutes, and samples from the iliac vein were obtained at 0, 15, 30, 60, 90, and 120 minutes. An aliquot of the plasma sample was saved to analyze total platinum levels, and the remainder of the platinum sample was centrifuged at 850 g for 30 minutes at 4°C through an Amicron Centriflo CF-25 cone (25,000 molecular weight cut-off) to obtain the ultrafiltrate for analyzing free platinum levels. Plasma and ultrafiltrate samples were frozen at −20°C prior to analysis by atomic absorption spectrophotometry. Analysis of the platinum samples was carried out using a Perkin-Elmer model 5000 atomic absorption spectrophotometer equipped with an HGA-500 graphite furnace. The platinum in the samples was quantified by comparing the value of the platinum absorbance peak area to a standard curve of platinum peak area vs. platinum concentration that was developed using dilutions of a 1-mg/ml platinum (1,000 ppm) standard of platinic chloride in a plasma or ultrafiltrate matrix. Pharmacokinetic data are presented in Figure 8–2. We believed that the pharmacokinetic data suggested a 1.5- to 2.0-fold increase in cisplatin in the iliac vein as compared to the peripheral venous concentration.

TABLE 8–3.
Treatment Modification for Myelosuppression on Days 15 and 22

Dose level of Cisplatin (mg/m²)	No. Patients Treated	MTX and VBL Omitted, D15 and/or D22* (% Courses)
60	4	11.5
80	3	37.5
100	3	30.0
120	7	22.5

*MTX = methotrexate; VBL = vinblastine; D15, D22 = day 15, day 22.

DISCUSSION

Evidence confirming the value of intra-arterial infusion chemotherapy over similar intravenous chemotherapy is lacking. Certainly for bladder cancer the data favoring the intra-arterial approach are anecdotal.

To evaluate the effectiveness of intra-arterial chemotherapy, one must first define the

TABLE 8–4.
Intra-arterial M-VAC: Toxicity Results*

Dose Level of Cisplatin (mg/m²)	Patient No.	Risk Status	No. of Courses	Cystectomy	Toxicity Grade (Highest)						Response	
					N/V	Leukopenia	Thrombocytopenia	Neurologic	Ototoxicity	Renal	Clinical	Pathologic
60	1	Good	4	No	2	1	1	—	—	—	CR	—
	2	Good	2	Yes	2	2	—	1	—	2	NR	NC
	3	Good	3	Yes	3	3	1	1	—	1	CR	DS
	6	Good	4	Yes	3	2	—	2	—	—	CR	DS
80	4	Good	2	Yes	2	3	—	—	—	—	PR	DS
	5	Good	4	No	2	2	—	—	—	1	NR	—
	7	Good	4	No	2	3	2	—	—	1	CR	—
100	8	Good	2	No	1	2	—	1	—	—	NR	US
	9	Good	2	Yes	2	4	4	—	—	1	NR	DS
	10	Good	1	No	2	—	—	—	—	—	PD	PD
	22	Good	1+	TE	—	—	—	—	—	—	TE	TE
120	11	Good	4	Yes	3	1	—	3	—	1	CR	CR
	12†	Good	4	Yes	2	1	—	—	—	1	PR	DS
	13	Good	2	Refused	2	1	3	1	—	—	NR	—
	14	Good	4	Yes	2	2	2	2	—	2	CR	DS
	15	Good	4	Refused	2	2	—	1	—	1	CR	—
	16	Good	4	Yes	3	1	—	1	1	1	CR	NC
	17	Good	4	Pending	2	2	3	—	1	1	PR	TE
	18	Good	4	Pending	2	3	2	2	—	1	CR	TE
	20	Good	2+	TE	1	3	1	2	—	1	TE	TE
140	21	Good	2+	TE	2	2	—	—	1	1	TE	TE
	19	Good	2+	TE	2	3	1	1	—	1	TE	TE

*M-VAC = methotrexate, vinblastine, Adriamycin, cisplatin; N/V = nausea and vomiting; CR = complete remission; PR = partial response; NR = no response; PD = progressive disease; TE = too early; NC = no change; DS = downstaged; US = upstaged.
†Cisplatin intravenously.

TABLE 8–5.
Restaging After M-VAC for Transitional Cell Bladder Carcinoma

No. Eligible Patients (n = 17)	Clinical Stage*						
	Pretreatment	Post-treatment					
		T_4	T_3	T_2	T_{is}	T_0	Too early
1	T_2			1			
7	T_3		2		1	3	1
9	T_4	3			1	4	1

*Clinical downstaging occurred in 9 of 15 patients (60%).

goals of treatment. Improved survival rate can be one goal when investigators integrate intra-arterial therapy with cystectomy or definitive radiation therapy; this is a form of preemptive or "neoadjuvant" therapy. Evaluating this regimen requires comparing it with surgery or radiation therapy alone, with neoadjuvant intravenous treatment, and with classical adjuvant therapy after surgery or irradiation. Indeed, if the target of the treatment is systemic, undetected micrometastases present at the time of treatment, intra-arterial therapy could possibly be inferior to intravenous treatment because it could produce lower systemic drug levels.

Another goal of intra-arterial treatment might be to lower systemic toxicity, possible because a proportion of the medication is absorbed during the initial pass through the infused area. This decrease in toxicity may allow an adequate dose of the chemotherapy to be administered more safely or comfortably. This goal has not been a prominent one in bladder cancer intra-arterial treatment.

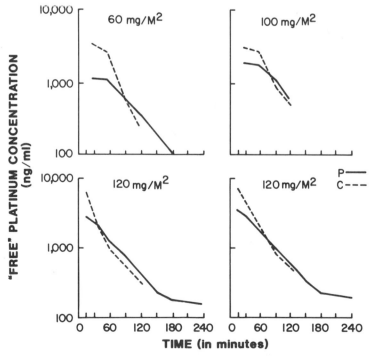

FIG 8–2.
Pharmacokinetic data for four patients, comparing peripheral (*P*) and common (*C*) internal iliac venous levels.

A third possible goal of intra-arterial treatment is to use it as primary therapy. Pathologically confirmed CRs in the bladder have been documented with CISCA, M-VAC, and CMV (cisplatin, methotrexate, and vinblastine) protocols, thus introducing the possibility of using chemotherapy to avoid a cystectomy. These data cannot be interpreted to mean that chemotherapy has an advantage over definitive radiation therapy or a very aggressive transurethral resection, both of which also render the bladder disease free in selected patients. However, the concept that increasing the effective dose of chemotherapy by using an intra-arterial route can improve the potential of primary chemotherapy is intriguing. The major limitation to using it as primary chemotherapy is the uncertain accuracy of restaging endoscopic and radiographic procedures in differentiating a true CR from a partial response where only residual microscopic disease remains. This difficulty has not been overcome.

The present study indicates that the maximum tolerated dose of intra-arterial cisplatin in M-VAC is 100 mg/m^2. This trial employed hypertonic saline with the cisplatin, and one could argue that this contributes to the possibility of using this large dose of cisplatin. The standard dose of cisplatin in M-VAC as described by Yagoda (Sternberg et al. 1985) is 70 mg/m^2 and was arrived at empirically. A study evaluating 100 mg/m^2 cisplatin intravenously with M-VAC in either 0.9% or 3% saline is unavailable.

We have compared the cisplatin concentration in the common or internal iliac vein (immediately distal to the primary venous drainage of the region infused intra-arterially) with the peripheral venous concentration. The results suggest a higher dose of cisplatin is being delivered to the pelvis and, presumably, the tumor. Flow in the infused artery, catheter position and dynamics, and vascularity of the tumor are all variables not controlled.

The pharmacokinetic variables that may be critical to the success of a chemotherapy program are generally discounted in clinical therapy. The complexity of this situation, even for intravenous therapy, has been recently highlighted by a study by Rodman et al. (1987). The steady-state plasma concentration of the drug used in their study (teniposide [VM-26]) varied as much as four- to sixfold among patients receiving the same dose schedule. If an antitumor response is significantly dose-dependent, as is currently accepted, variations in concentration may be very important. Delivering an effective target plasma concentration could be a possible goal for treatment, much the same as the dose of antibiotics, theophylline, or phenytoin (Dilantin) are titrated for therapeutic levels. The additional variable of route of administration, specifically the intra-arterial approach, further complicates this situation. Multiple modifications on the intra-arterial theme, such as stop-flow or pulsatile infusion; the addition of vasoconstrictors such as angiotensin; chemoembolization; hyperthermia; or concomitant radiation therapy have also been proposed.

Animal studies suggest that intra-arterial administration has an advantage over intravenous chemotherapy in some selected systems, but the evaluation becomes exceedingly difficult in human studies. Only large, difficult, randomized trials offer a hope of defining the role of intra-arterial treatment.

REFERENCES

1. Campbell TN, Howell SB, Pfeifle CE, et al. 1983. Clinical pharmacokinetics of intraarterial cisplatin in humans. *J Clin Oncol* 1:755–762.
2. Chen HSG, Gross JF. 1980. Intra-arterial infusion of anticancer drugs: Theoretic aspects of drug delivery and review of responses. *Cancer Treat Rep* 64:31–40.
3. Logothetis CJ, Samuels ML. 1984. Intra-arterial chemotherapy for malignant urothelial tumors. *Cancer Bull* 36:47–52.
4. Logothetis CJ, Samuels ML, Wallace S, et al. 1982. Management of pelvic complications of malignant

urothelial tumors with combined intra-arterial and iv chemotherapy. *Cancer Treat Rep* 66:1501–1507.

5. Maatman TJ, Montie JE, Bukowski RM, et al. 1986. Intra-arterial chemotherapy as an adjuvant to surgery in transitional cell carcinoma of the bladder. *J Urol* 135:256–260.

6. Rodman JH, Abromowitch M, Sinkule JA, et al. 1987. Clinical pharmacodynamics of continuous infusion teniposide: Systemic exposure as a determinant of response in a phase I trial. *J Clin Oncol* 5:1007–1014.

7. Sternberg CN, Yagoda A, Scher HI, et al. 1985. Preliminary results of M-VAC (methotrexate, vinblastine, doxorubicin and cisplatin) for transitional cell carcinoma of the urothelium. *J Urol* 133:403–407.

8. Stewart DJ, Eapen L, Hirte WE, et al. 1987. Intra-arterial cisplatin for bladder cancer. *J Urol* 138:302–305.

9. Wallace S, Chuang VP, Samuels M, et al. 1982. Transcatheter intraarterial infusion of chemotherapy in advanced bladder cancer. *Cancer* 49:640–645.

Chapter 9

Postoperative Adjuvant CISCA Chemotherapy for High-Risk Invasive Bladder Cancer

Christopher J. Logothetis, M.D.

CISCA chemotherapy (cisplatin, cyclophosphamide, doxorubicin [Adriamycin]) as employed at The University of Texas M. D. Anderson Cancer Center has been effective as treatment for patients with metastatic urothelial tumors. Although we achieve a high response rate, however, the relative frequency of complete responses is low. Complete remissions occur most frequently among those patients with local-regional nodal metastases (Logothetis 1985), and these patients also have the highest likelihood of achieving durable responses. Because, in the majority of patients, bladder carcinoma spreads systematically from the primary tumor to lymph nodes followed by distant visceral metastases, we interpret this finding as evidence of increased effectiveness when CISCA chemotherapy is introduced earlier in the evolution of the disease.

These conclusions led us to a trial of combination cystectomy followed by adjuvant CISCA chemotherapy for those patients at high risk for relapse. The patients selected for adjuvant CISCA chemotherapy were those who had transitional cell carcinomas, squamous cell carcinomas, and mixed tumors (transitional cell carcinomas with elements of squamous carcinoma, adenocarcinoma, or spindle cells). Excluded were patients with mixed mesodermal tumors and those with adenocarcinoma of the bladder. Mixed mesodermal tumors were considered a rare subtype, and we have previously reported that adenocarcinomas were refractory to cisplatin-based chemotherapy (Logothetis et al. 1985).

Between March 1981 and March 1986, cystectomy was performed in 339 patients at UT M. D. Anderson Cancer Center. Of these 339 patients, 206 had favorable pathologic findings—either high-grade diffuse superficial disease or minimally invasive disease without lymphatic or vascular invasion—and were considered at low risk for recurrence (Table 9–1). The remaining patients were considered to be at high risk for relapse. This category included those with evidence of perivesicular tumor involvement (pathologic stage C), direct invasion of the vagina or prostate (pathologic stage D_1), nodal metastases (pathologic stage D_1), or those with lymphatic or vascular invasion in their primary tumor.

Of the total population at high risk for relapse, 62 either refused adjuvant CISCA chemotherapy, were not offered the treatment by the surgeons, or had medical contraindications that precluded the use of adjuvant CISCA chemotherapy. These patients constitute a high-

TABLE 9–1.
Outcome of Study Patients by Category

Outcome	Low-Risk (Control)	High-Risk (Control)	High-Risk Adjuvant
Alive + disease-free	138	19	44
Died of unrelated disorder	11	3	6
Lost to follow-up	8	1	0
Died of disease	39	34	14
Fatal complication of treatment	5	2	3
Alive with disease	5	3	4
Totals	206	62	71

risk control group. Seventy-one high-risk patients received adjuvant CISCA chemotherapy and constitute a high-risk adjuvant group. A comparison of these two groups of patients (Table 9–2) indicates that the frequency of the histologic subtypes and the degree of invasion into pelvic viscera were essentially the same. Only the frequency of nodal metastases was higher in the high-risk adjuvant group than in the high-risk control group.

Adjuvant therapy was begun approximately 6 weeks following the cystectomy and was delivered for a planned total of five monthly courses. Survival comparisons were made between the three broad groups of patients: those who received adjuvant CISCA chemotherapy (n = 71), those at high risk for relapse who did not receive adjuvant chemotherapy (n = 62), and those at low risk for relapse (n = 206) (Table 9–3). A very significant difference

TABLE 9–2.
Comparison of Clinical Characteristics Between High-Risk Groups

Characteristic	High-Risk Control (n = 62)		Adjuvant (n = 71)	
	No.	%	No.	%
Cell type*				
TCC	39	63	46	65
Mixed	19	31	24	34
SCC	4	7	1	1
Pathologic stage				
Lymphatic invasion	20	32	17	24
Perivesicular	27	44	23	32
Pelvic visceral	11	18	11	16
Nodal metastasis	4	7	20	28

*TCC = transitional cell carcinoma; SCC = squamous cell carcinoma.

TABLE 9–3.
Comparison of Disease-Free Survival Rates

Patient Group	No. of Patients	Survivors		P Value
		No.	%	
Low-risk control	206	157	76 }	.0001
High-risk control	62	23	37	
Low-risk control	206	157	76 }	.33
Adjuvant	71	50	70	
High-risk control	62	23	37 }	.0012
Adjuvant	71	50	70	

in survival exists between the low-risk controls and patients at high risk for relapse who did not receive adjuvant chemotherapy ($P = .0001$). This first comparison confirms the significance of the pathologic findings and their ability to predict the likelihood for relapse. The second comparison, between those patients who received adjuvant chemotherapy and those in the low-risk group, reveals no significant difference in survival rate. Finally, a comparison between those patients who had equivalent and poor prognostic findings but did not receive adjuvant CISCA chemotherapy and the adjuvant patients indicated a highly significant difference in survival rate (Table 9–3).

Patients were further subclassified by histologic subtype and degree of invasion in the primary tumor, and survival rates were compared (Table 9–4). Survival rates were significantly higher for patients with pelvic visceral invasion or perivesicular tumor involvement who received adjuvant CISCA chemotherapy. Survival rates were also higher for patients with pure transitional cell carcinomas and mixed transitional cell carcinomas. The most improved survival rates occurred among those with chemotherapy-sensitive pure transitional cell carcinomas.

The only subgroup not benefitting from adjuvant CISCA chemotherapy comprised those with lymphatic/vascular invasion from the primary tumor. The cure rate among the patients who did not receive adjuvant chemotherapy but who had lymphatic/vascular invasion only from the primary tumor was better than anticipated (50%). Therefore, although 65% of patients receiving adjuvant chemotherapy for lymphatic/vascular invasion remained alive and disease free, the improvement in survival rate was not statistically significant.

We tabulated the causes of death in the study patients. Very few patients were lost to follow-up, and the majority of patients who died did so of recurrent disease. The frequency of fatal complications was low in all three groups of patients (see Table 9–1). Treatment-related deaths, therefore, did not influence the outcome of our study.

The intensity of the therapy was maintained throughout; dosages were not reduced. Sixty-seven percent of the patients received a full five courses of chemotherapy, 22% received four courses of chemotherapy, and 5.5% received only three courses of chemotherapy. Only two patients refused further treatment after two courses of chemotherapy.

These data establish the feasibility of adjuvant CISCA chemotherapy following a cystectomy. In addition, our study now includes an adequate number of adjuvant patients (71) with a long enough follow-up to make firm statements about long-term disease-free survival. Follow-up of the disease-free patients is 28 to 310 weeks (mean, 118 weeks), which carries them beyond the published major risk for recurrence. Time to recurrence in most studies indicates that bladder cancer most often relapses within the first year following a cystectomy. Since the majority of patients alive and disease free have been monitored for longer than a

TABLE 9–4.
Comparison of Disease-Free Survival Rates by Pathologic Findings and Treatment

	High-Risk Control			Adjuvant			
	Total	Survivors		Total	Survivors		
Findings	No.	No.	%	No.	No.	%	P Value
Lymphatic vascular invasion	20	10	50	17	11	65	.15
Perivesicular invasion	27	1	4	23	16	70	.10
Pelvic visceral invasion	11	1	9	11	10	91	.0001
Nodal metastasis	4	1	25	20	13	65	—

year, it is very likely that a larger cure fraction has been achieved in this study population.

No other trial exists that has an adequate follow-up and an adequate number of patients for comparison. A trial by Daniels et al. (1983), using cyclophosphamide/cisplatin and CISCA, failed to confirm an increased cure fraction with cisplatin-based chemotherapy. A small single-armed trial using cisplatin-based chemotherapy (Roemeling et al. 1987) has suggested an increased cure fraction, but that study involves too few patients to confirm or refute our data. Whether the addition of more recent methotrexate/cisplatin combinations will increase the cure rate among our patients remains to be seen. Such a study is currently going on at our institution.

We believe that these data confirm the benefit of adjuvant combination chemotherapy as treatment for bladder carcinoma. Patients with pure transitional cell carcinoma benefit the most, but patients with mixed tumors derive some benefit from the treatment. Patients with pathologic stage C disease and those whose pelvic viscera are involved demonstrated a clear survival benefit compared to their counterparts treated during the same period of time who did not receive adjuvant therapy. Although potential selection biases exist between these groups, a careful analysis of the various prognostic variables reveals that these two populations were very comparable. Each of these populations was treated during the same study period by the same physicians. We also believe that patients with nodal metastases benefit with increased survivals. Their survival rates with adjuvant CISCA chemotherapy are superior to those reported in the literature for patients who receive only a cystectomy and pelvic lymph node dissection. In our series, too few patients with nodal metastases did not receive adjuvant CISCA chemotherapy for us to draw a comparison.

We recommend adjuvant cisplatin-based combination chemotherapy for patients at high risk for recurrence following a cystectomy. Patients benefitting from adjuvant chemotherapy include those with pathologic stage C and pathologic stage D_1 (visceral invasion, nodal metastasis) bladder carcinoma.

REFERENCES

1. Daniels JR, Skinner DG, Lieskovsky G, et al. 1983. Carcinoma of the bladder: Chemotherapy of advanced disease and rational design of adjuvant programs, in Skinner DG (ed): *Urological Cancer.* New York, Grune & Stratton, pp 217–235.
2. Logothetis CJ. 1985. Perioperative chemotherapy for the management of primary local regional urothelial tumors, in Wagener DJ, Blijham GH, Smeets JBE, et al (eds): *Primary Chemotherapy in Cancer Medicine.* New York, Alan R. Liss, pp 359–366.
3. Logothetis CJ, Samuels ML, Ogden SL. 1985. Chemotherapy for adenocarcinomas of bladder and urachal origin: 5-Fluouracil, doxorubicin, and mitomycin-C. *Urology* 26:252–255.
4. Roemeling RV, Hrushesky WJM, Fraley EE. 1987. Long-term control of locally advanced transitional cell bladder cancer (TCCB) by high-dose intensity, circadian-based adjuvant chemotherapy, in Salmon SE (ed): *Adjuvant Therapy of Cancer V.* New York, Grune & Stratton, pp 571–580.

Chapter 10

Preemptive (Neoadjuvant) Cisplatin Chemotherapy for High-Risk Invasive Bladder Cancer*

Derek Raghavan, M.B.B.S., Ph.D., F.R.A.C.P.

Bruce Pearson, M.B.B.S., F.R.C.S., F.R.A.C.S.

Peter Duval, M.B.B.S., F.R.C.R., F.R.A.C.R.

John Rogers, M.B.B.S., F.R.A.C.S., F.R.C.S.

W. Hunter Watt, M.B.B.S., F.R.A.C.S.

Nory Teriana, B.Sc.

Hedy Mameghan, B.M., B.Ch., F.R.C.R.,
      F.R.A.C.R.

John Boulas, M.B.B.S., F.R.A.C.S.

Invasive bladder cancer still constitutes a major problem in management. The published long-term survival figures of less than 50% for stage T_2–T_4 (B_2–D_1) transitional cell carcinoma (TCC), whatever treatment is used, give little cause for satisfaction (Bloom et al. 1982; Skinner and Lieskovsky 1984; Richie 1988; Rose and Shipley 1988). From clinical and autopsy data, it appears that micrometastases are often present at the time of first diagnosis (Skinner 1980; Whitmore 1980; Raghavan 1985). Recurrence, metastases, or both appear within 12 to 18 months in more than half the patients, whether treated initially by radical radiotherapy, cystectomy, or a combination of the two. Although the pelvis is the commonest site of recurrence in patients treated by radical radiotherapy, metastases are often found in distant lymph nodes, bones, lungs, or liver, and less commonly in other sites (Skinner 1980; Raghavan 1985).

*This work has been supported in part by grants from New South Wales Women's Bowl for Others Club, the Penrith Lions Club, and the Merrion Rawlinson Cancer Fund.

In an effort to improve the cure rate of invasive, clinically nonmetastatic bladder cancer, several investigational programs have been initiated, combining preemptive (neoadjuvant) intravenous cytotoxic chemotherapy with definitive treatment (radical radiotherapy, surgery, or a combination of these). The rationale for these programs has been reviewed in detail elsewhere (Raghavan 1985, 1988; Soloway 1985).

We report here the results from a series of 100 patients with invasive TCC who were treated with preemptive intravenous cisplatin followed by radiotherapy, cystectomy, or both.

PATIENTS AND METHODS

Patient Population

An initial series of 50 patients (Raghavan et al. 1985) was treated between August 1981 and November 1983, which allowed for a follow-up time of 4 to 6 years. Subsequently, another 50 patients were entered into this study until March 1987. The characteristics of the patients and their tumors are summarized in Tables 10–1 and 10–2. An apparent stage migration (Raghavan 1988; Tonkin and Tannock 1988) occurred during the study, with a higher proportion of patients with stage T_2 (B_2) tumors being referred between November 1983 and March 1987.

TABLE 10–1.
Patient Characteristics (n = 100)

Characteristic	% of Total
Sex	
M:F, 81:19	
Age (yr)	
Mean, 63.26	
SD, 7.9	
Median, 64	
Range, 29–79	
≥70	23
Social	
Smokers	85
Analgesic abuse	20
Other	
Renal dysfunction	45
Prior radiotherapy	0
Prior systemic chemotherapy	0

TABLE 10–2.
Tumor Characteristics (n = 100)

Characteristic	% of Total
Grade	
1	0
2	16
3	84
Stage	
T_2/T_{2+}	42
T_3	38
T_4	20

The referred patients were typical of Western populations with bladder cancer (Skinner 1980; Russell et al. 1988): elderly (median age, 64 years), a high proportion of smokers with intercurrent diseases, concomitant renal tract dysfunction, and belonging predominantly to lower socioeconomic groups. An unusual feature of Australian patients with TCC is a history of excessive intake of phenacetin-containing analgesic compounds and an associated chronic renal dysfunction (McCredie et al. 1983).

Staging Protocol

Patients underwent an intensive program of noninvasive staging, including full physical examination; cystoscopy, biopsy, and bimanual examination performed under anesthesia; assessment of tumor markers (serum levels of carcinoembryonic antigen and human chorionic gonadotropin); CT (computerized tomographic) scan of the abdomen and pelvis; chest x-ray; and radionuclide scans of bone, if indicated. The details of the program have been reported elsewhere (Raghavan et al. 1984, 1985; Pearson and Raghavan 1985). An attempt was made to allocate tumor stage according to the TNM (tumor, node, metastasis) classification (UICC 1980). As the staging program did not involve routine cystectomy, it often was difficult to distinguish between T_2 and T_3 tumors; where this distinction was not well defined, tumors were classified arbitrarily as "T_2/T_{2+}" and included within the T_2 grouping. A higher T stage was not allocated on the basis of a CT scan alone—i.e., these scans were used merely to confirm the results of clinical staging and biopsy and to demonstrate distant metastases. Enlarged pelvic nodes on CT scan did not preclude entry into the study.

Treatment Protocol

This approach has been described previously (Pearson and Raghavan 1985; Raghavan et al. 1985). In brief, patients were treated with two doses of intravenous cisplatin (100 mg/m² 3 weeks apart) and an aggressive hydration regimen including forced diuresis. This required meticulous medical and nursing supervision to avoid fluid overload in these elderly patients. Appropriate dosage reductions were applied for patients with severely impaired renal function (e.g., serum creatinine level >1.5 times the upper limit of normal) and for some patients over the age of 70 years (Raghavan et al. 1988a). After cisplatin treatment, tumors were restaged with repeat cystoscopy and biopsy. An apparent reduction of tumor mass on CT scan alone was not classified as a response. There are no perfect criteria for objective assessment of response with noninvasive staging. However, we attempted to assess objectively a greater than 50% reduction of tumor mass (Raghavan et al. 1985). We made no attempt to distinguish artificially between complete and partial remission after cisplatin treatment because of the inadequacies of the noninvasive staging protocol.

Patients were then referred for definitive treatment, which reflected the patterns of clinical practice among referring clinicians. Radical radiotherapy alone was administered to 75 patients; the rest underwent radical cystectomy with or without preoperative radiotherapy.

The standard radiotherapy regimen consisted of 4,500 to 5,000 cGy to the pelvis, with a boost yielding a total of 6,000 cGy to the bladder. Planning for irradiation was carried out with the aid of localizing CT scans. Multiple fields were used, and radiotherapy was delivered by 4 to 10 MeV linear accelerators.

The tumors were reassessed 6 to 8 weeks after completion of radiotherapy. Patients were then monitored routinely by the referring urologic surgeons, and they made intermittent visits to the treatment centers. Two patients (2%) have been lost to long-term follow-up.

RESULTS

All patients were assessed for the acute toxicity of preemptive cisplatin and of the definitive treatment. An attempt was made to document objective response after cisplatin for 96 patients (in 4 cases, different urologic surgeons performed the pretreatment and post-treatment cystoscopies). Response was evaluated in all patients after the completion of definitive treatment. Long-term survival data were available for the first 50 patients (treated before November 1983).

Toxicity

More than 90% of patients suffered severe nausea, vomiting, or both, despite the use of haloperidol, lorazepam, and dexamethasone. Other common side effects included transient auditory dysfunction (tinnitus, audiogram changes, or high-tone hearing loss); acute diarrhea or cystitis during radiotherapy; and acute renal dysfunction (although dialysis was not required). Other occasional toxic effects have been reported previously, including cardiac arrhythmias, Mallory-Weiss syndrome (one case), and dehydration (in an insulin-dependent diabetic patient) (Pearson and Raghavan 1985; Raghavan et al. 1985). There were no treatment-related deaths. Despite these problems, the use of preemptive chemotherapy did not compromise the planned dosage of irradiation, and there were no unexpected complications in patients who underwent cystectomy.

The extent of chronic toxicity is more difficult to define because the schedule of follow-up of long-term survivors was more varied. The commonest late side effects after radiotherapy included mild chronic diarrhea or chronic cystitis. In a quality-of-life survey of 38 patients treated before November 1984, 15% noted frequent post-treatment diarrhea, and one third suffered occasional symptoms of cystitis (although in some instances these may have been caused by recurrence of disease). Another feature of importance was a deterioration in sexual function after treatment in one third of respondents. These data have been reported in detail previously (Raghavan et al. 1988b).

Response

After preemptive cisplatin treatment, 61% of the tumors showed an objective response, and 30% were unchanged. In five patients, progressive tumor was present after cisplatin administration, and in four patients, objective reassessment was not carried out after cisplatin treatment. After completing definitive treatment, 86% showed a reduction in tumor mass, 11% had residual stable disease, and 3% continued to progress (one each in the bladder, liver, and supraclavicular nodes). It should be noted, however, that in some instances, definitive treatment consisted of radiotherapy followed by early elective cystectomy, with complete remission being achieved by the final treatment step.

More than 70% of patients with malignant cystitis experienced a dramatic amelioration of their symptoms within 3 weeks of the first dose of cisplatin. Whether this correlated with tumor response or was simply a function of "flushing" of the bladder by the forced diuresis during drug administration is not clear.

Survival

The pattern of survival of the first 50 patients, after a minimum follow-up of 4 years, is shown in Figure 10–1. Twenty-nine of these patients have died of cancer, with the majority

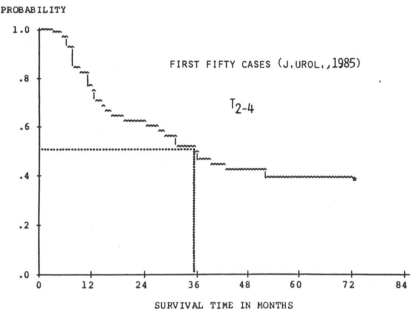

FIG 10–1.
Updated 6-year actuarial survival rates of first 50 patients (treated between August 1981 and November 1983); this series first reported in *J Urol* 133:399–402, 1985.

of deaths occurring within the first 18 months.

Actuarial survival curves for the complete series of 100 patients, divided according to T stage, are plotted in Figure 10–2. Log-rank analysis showed T stage to be a statistically significant prognostic variable. It should be emphasized that the survival curves for the total series of 100 patients are not yet mature.

DISCUSSION

Our data, and those of others (Fagg et al. 1984; Soloway 1985; Rose and Shipley 1988), show substantial activity of preemptive intravenous cisplatin against invasive TCC of the bladder. Our study was designed simply to assess the safety and efficacy of this approach rather than to investigate survival benefit in a randomized fashion, and thus its true utility has not yet been defined. The large accrual of patients occurred either while a randomized study to test our hypothesis was being designed or as a result of the refusal of some clinicians to enter patients into this randomized trial once accrual had been opened. Despite the entry of 100 patients, this study is essentially a phase I–II trial, and our data should not be misinterpreted as representing a phase III study.

We have previously reported preliminary survival figures merely to illustrate that this approach does not obviously compromise survival (Raghavan et al. 1985). This cautious, preliminary report of an actuarial 2-year survival rate of 80% has been taken out of context; in fact, our more recent data show, not surprisingly, a reduction of the actuarial survival rate to 42% at 6 years. Whether this represents an advance is unclear, since this has not been a randomized study. Our data do show that preemptive high-dose intravenous cisplatin can be administered safely to elderly patients with impaired renal function, provided meticulous and experienced medical and nursing supervision is available. The acute symptoms of malignant cystitis usually resolve rapidly after this treatment. A response rate of 60% after preemptive cisplatin has been demonstrated in several studies (Fagg et al. 1984; Raghavan et al. 1985), as has a total response rate of greater than 80% after the completion of the program. It also appears that long-term toxicity is not increased by this approach.

As noted above, a randomized multicenter trial has been initiated, under the auspices of the Australian Bladder Cancer Study Group, to assess the possible survival benefit from preemptive chemotherapy. This trial involves randomization to one of the following (Raghavan 1988):

1. Radical radiotherapy (6,000 cGy to the tumor in 6 weeks, using 200-cGy fractions and multiple fields, delivered via a linear accelerator after defining tumor volumes by CT scan);

2. Preemptive intravenous cisplatin (100 mg/m^2, two doses 3 weeks apart), followed by the schedule of radical radiotherapy described above.

Although 100 patients have been randomized to date, accrual has suffered from the biases of referring clinicians who believe either that preemptive chemotherapy represents the state of the art and hence that randomization is not appropriate, or that this approach has already been proved to be a failure because of the proportion of patients relapsing in the pilot studies. In view of the problems that beset the use of historically controlled trials (Raghavan 1988; Tonkin and Tannock 1988), these biases are clearly inappropriate.

At present, preemptive chemotherapy of invasive, clinically nonmetastatic bladder cancer is investigational only and requires validation by well-designed, controlled trials. Whether it is appropriate to use more toxic combination chemotherapy regimens (with higher initial response rates) in this context is not yet clear, partly because these regimens themselves require further evaluation. To date, no treatment-related deaths have been reported from

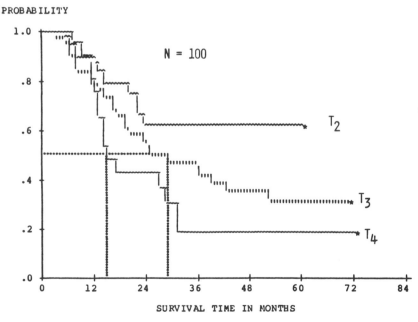

FIG 10–2.
Actuarial survival rates of total series of 100 patients. Note stage groupings of T_2/T_{2+}, T_3, and T_4, with a statistically significant difference ($P<.05$) between survival rates of patients with T_2 and T_3 disease.

single-agent preemptive chemotherapy programs, but a potential hazard exists if aggressive combination chemotherapy regimens are used for preemptive treatment in an unstructured and unevaluated fashion.

From the available data, it is clear that progress is being made in the management of invasive bladder cancer. However, the results are not yet good enough to allow us to be complacent. If this disease is to be cured in the majority of patients, we must continue to question our methods and to test the apparent advances in well-structured trials.

Acknowledgments

We are grateful to Ms Lesley Duncan, Ludwig Institute for Cancer Research, Sydney Branch, for assistance with statistical analysis and to our colleagues for referring patients for this program.

REFERENCES

1. Bloom HJG, Hendry WF, Wallace DM, et al. 1982. Treatment of T3 bladder cancer: Controlled trial of pre-operative radiotherapy and radical cystectomy versus radical radiotherapy. Second report and review. *Br J Urol* 54:136–150.
2. Fagg SL, Dawson-Edwards P, Hughes MA, et al. 1984. Cis-diamminedichloroplatinum (DDP) as initial treatment of invasive bladder cancer. *Br J Urol* 56:296–300.
3. McCredie M, Stewart JH, Ford JM, et al. 1983. Phenacetin-containing analgesics and cancer of the bladder or renal pelvis in women. *Br J Urol* 55:220–224.
4. Pearson BS, Raghavan D. 1985. First-line intravenous cisplatin for deeply invasive bladder cancer: Update on 70 cases. *Br J Urol* 57:690–693.
5. Raghavan D. 1985. First-line intravenous cisplatinum for invasive clinically non-metastatic bladder cancer, in Garnick M (ed): *Genitourinary Cancer.* New York, Churchill Livingstone, Inc, pp 193–207.
6. Raghavan D. 1988. Review: Pre-emptive intravenous chemotherapy for invasive bladder cancer. *Br J Urol* 61:1–8.
7. Raghavan D, Greenaway TJ, Grundy R, et al. 1988a. Pre-emptive intravenous cisplatin plus radical radiotherapy for fit septuagenarians with bladder cancer: Age itself is not a contraindication. *Br J Urol.*
8. Raghavan D, Grundy R, Lancaster L. 1988b. Assessment of quality of life in long-term survivors treated by first-line intravenous cisplatin for invasive bladder cancer, in Smith PH, Pavone-Macaluso M (eds): *E.O.R.T.C. Genitourinary Group Monograph 4: Management of Advanced Cancer of Prostate and Bladder.* New York, Alan R. Liss, pp 625–631.
9. Raghavan D, Pearson B, Coorey G, et al. 1984. Intravenous cisplatinum for invasive bladder cancer: Safety and feasibility of a new approach. *Med J Aust* 140:276–278.
10. Raghavan D, Pearson B, Duval P, et al. 1985. Initial intravenous cisplatinum therapy: Improved management for invasive high risk bladder cancer? *J Urol* 133:399–402.
11. Richie JP. 1988. Radical cystectomy: Innovations and results, in Raghavan D (ed): *The Management of Bladder Cancer.* London, Edward Arnold, pp 140–153.
12. Rose MA, Shipley WU. 1988. Radiation therapy in invasive bladder cancer: Principles, results, patient selection and innovations, in Raghavan D (ed): *The Management of Bladder Cancer.* London, Edward Arnold, pp 154–173.
13. Russell PJ, Raghavan D, Gregory P, et al. 1986. Bladder cancer xenografts: A model of tumor cell heterogeneity. *Cancer Res* 46:2035–2040.
14. Russell PJ, Raghavan D, Phillips J, et al. 1988. Biology of urothelial cancer, in Raghavan D (ed): *The Management of Bladder Cancer.* London, Edward Arnold, pp 1–41.

15. Skinner DG. 1980. Current perspectives in the management of high grade invasive bladder cancer. *Cancer* 45:1866–1874.

16. Skinner DG, Lieskovsky G. 1984. Contemporary cystectomy with pelvic node dissection compared to preoperative radiation therapy plus cystectomy in management of invasive bladder cancer. *J Urol* 131:1069–1072.

17. Soloway M. 1985. Learning to integrate systemic chemotherapy into a treatment plan for patients with advanced bladder cancer. *J Urol* 133:440–441.

18. Tonkin K, Tannock I. 1988. Evaluation of response and morbidity following treatment of bladder cancer, in Raghavan D (ed): *The Management of Bladder Cancer.* London, Edward Arnold, pp 228–244.

19. U.I.C.C. 1980. *Union Internationale contre le Cancer TNM Classification of Malignant Tumours,* ed 4. Geneva, International Union Against Cancer.

20. Whitmore WF Jr. 1980. Integrated irradiation and cystectomy for bladder cancer. *Br J Urol* 52:1–12.

Chapter 11

Phase I-II Trial of Neoadjuvant M-VAC for Primary Urothelial Tumors*

Alan Yagoda, M.D.

Howard I. Scher, M.D.

Harry W. Herr, M.D.

Cora N. Sternberg, M.D.

Victor Reuter, M.D.

D. David Dershaw, M.D.

George J. Bosl, M.D.

Michael J. Morse, M.D.

Pramod C. Sogani, M.D.

Robin C. Watson, M.D.

Nancy L. Geller, Ph.D.

E. Darracott Vaughan, M.D.

Willet F. Whitmore, Jr., M.D.

William R. Fair, M.D.

The 5-year survival rate for patients presenting with high-grade, high-stage bladder cancer after radical cystectomy, radiation therapy, or a combination of both is approximately 30%

*This study was supported in part by NCI Grant 5P01-CA05826-25 and contract NO1-CM57732 from the National Cancer Institute, Bethesda, Md., and the Isidore Komanoff/Solid Tumor Service Funds.

to 50% (Richie et al. 1985). In a study by Skinner and Lieskovsky (1988), 5-year survival rates were 29% and 22% for patients with P_{3b} and P_4 disease, respectively. Despite 70% to 93% of patients achieving local tumor control by radical cystectomy, the majority die from disseminated disease. The overall prognosis is dismal for patients who have $_pN_+$. Smith and Whitmore (1981) reported a Memorial Hospital study of 134 patients with pathologically proved nodal disease and found only 54% surviving 1 year and 17% 2 years; less than 7%, primarily those with a single microscopically involved lymph node, survived 5 years. Since 82% of patients with N_+M_0 disease died from a cancer-related cause, many because of disseminated disease, the theoretical role for adjuvant or neoadjuvant chemotherapy is obvious.

Results of a phase II trial of M-VAC (methotrexate, vinblastine, doxorubicin [Adriamycin], and cisplatin) for advanced urothelial tumors of the renal pelvis, ureter, urethra, prostatic ducts, and urinary bladder conducted at Memorial Sloan-Kettering Cancer Center (MSKCC) were encouraging (Sternberg et al. 1985; 1988). M-VAC induced a 69% response (95% confidence interval, 59%–79%) in 83 adequately treated patients with advanced disease, and 37% (95% confidence interval, 27%–47%) achieved a complete remission (CR) for a median duration that has not been reached at 36 months (Sternberg et al. 1988). Therefore, this regimen was chosen for a phase I-II study in a neoadjuvant setting (Scher et al. 1988a; 1988b).

MATERIALS AND METHODS

The neoadjuvant M-VAC regimen (Table 11–1), in contrast to that employed for advanced disease, has no Adriamycin dose reduction. The intent of this pilot study was to evaluate the extent of tumor regression after one to five M-VAC cycles, and the first transurethral resection of the bladder (TURB) was performed in 48 of 61 patients (79%) after cycle one or two of the M-VAC regimen. When CR was documented pathologically ($_pCR$), no further therapy was administered, whereas for those found to have residual disease pathologically ($_pPR$), two additional M-VAC cycles were suggested.

All patients required documentation of muscle-infiltrating tumor (T_{3-4}) by the Department of Pathology, Memorial Hospital. Additional workup was required to prove the absence of nodal (N_0) and metastatic (M_0) disease. Initial and follow-up TURBs, as well as restaging procedures, were performed at MSKCC or New York Hospital, except for three patients who, after repeated TURBs, only had pathologic review of submitted cystectomy specimens.

TABLE 11–1.
M-VAC Regimen*

Drug (mg/m²)	Day				
	1	2	15[†]	22[†]	29
Methotrexate	30		30	30	R
					E
Vinblastine		3	3	3	C
					Y
Adriamycin		30			C
					L
Cisplatin		70			E

*M-VAC = methotrexate, vinblastine, Adriamycin, cisplatin.
[†]No drugs were given when mucositis was present, white blood cell count was less than 2,500 cells/μL, or platelet count was less than 100,000 cells/μl.

All initial and follow-up roentgenographic (R.C.W. and D.D.D.) and pathologic (V.R.) materials were reviewed independently. Clinical evaluation of T stage was assessed visually, by biopsy, and by physical examination (bimanual palpation) with the patient under anesthesia at the time of TURB. Noninvasive diagnostic "T" staging included computerized tomography (CT), ultrasonography, urine cytology with flow cytometry in many instances, and physical examination. Surgical "P" staging involved either cystectomy or laparotomy with biopsy of the external aspect of the bladder at the site of the original tumor and a selected or a retroperitoneal lymph node dissection.

Sixty-one patients were entered in the study, of whom 50 had a primary urinary tumor and 11 an extravesical tumor (Table 11–2). Six patients with a urinary bladder tumor had received prior intravesical chemotherapy and immunotherapy. Two patients had an adenocarcinoma, and one each had a small cell and a transitional cell carcinoma with squamous cell components. In the 11 extravesical cases, four tumors originated from the prostate, two from the prostatic urethra, four from the urethra, and one from the ureter. Of four urethral tumors, one was transitional cell and adenocarcinoma and three were squamous cell carcinoma. Overall, 8 (13%) of 61 patients presented with an atypical histology.

Staging for extravesical disease employed the American Joint Committee on Cancer Staging system, and the TNM (tumor, nodes, metastasis) system of the International Union Against Cancer was used for primary bladder lesions. Response criteria (Table 11–3) incorporated the suggestions of the First International Consensus Development Conference on Guidelines for Clinical Research in Bladder Cancer (Van Oosterom et al. 1986; Yagoda 1985). Initially, downstaging by two or more T categories was the criterion for a partial response (PR); however, as the trial continued, only downstaging to T_{is} or T_0 was considered significant. Responses less than CR and PR were classified as incomplete (IR), since most lesions were really only evaluable rather than bidimensionally measurable. A clinically proved PR ($_cPR$) required a greater than 50% decrease in the size of lesions on TURB and on noninvasive

TABLE 11–2.
Patient Characteristics

Characteristic		Bladder (n = 50)	Extravesical (n = 11)
		Tumor Location	
Age (yr)	Median	61	61
	Range	31–78	48–63
Males (%)		90	91
Karnofsky performance score (%)	Median	80	80
	Range	60–90	80–90
Initial stage (%)			
T_4		28	8
T_3		56	46
T_2		14	46
T_{is}		2	0
Prior intravesical therapy (%)		12	18
Pathology (%)			
Transitional cell		90	64
Plus adenocarcinoma		4	9
Plus squamous cell		2	0
Small cell		2	0
Squamous cell		0	27

TABLE 11–3.
Neoadjuvant Response Criteria

Complete remission
  Clinical ($_cCR$)
    Clinically proved disappearance of all tumor including T_{is} by physical
      examination, radiographically, cytologically, and cystoscopically both
      visually and by biopsy, as defined by the UICC* TNM staging system.
  Pathologic ($_pCR$)
    Pathologically proved complete remission at laparotomy, as defined by the
      UICC TNM staging system. (Surgical staging may include either a
      radical or partial cystectomy and/or pelvic lymph node sampling with
      deep biopsy via the serosal surface of the bladder.)
  Surgical (CR_s)
    All remaining disease is believed to be surgically removed, and there is
      no evidence of disease after laparotomy. (Such patients were initially
      $_pPR$.)
Partial remission
  Clinical ($_cPR$)
    Greater than 50% decrease in the size of measurable lesions by
      cystoscopy, noninvasive staging, or both plus downstaging by two or
      more T categories, or T_0 cystoscopically, as defined in $_cCR$, with a
      persistent abnormality such as any bladder thickening seen by
      noninvasive staging or persistently positive urinary cytology.
  Pathologic ($_pPR$)
    Less than three microscopic foci of tumor or in situ disease observed on
      cystoscopy or in the surgical specimen obtained at laparotomy.

*UICC = International Union Against Cancer.

---

staging in addition to downstaging by a minimum of two or more T categories, or attainment of T_0 on TURB with a persistent T abnormality, such as bladder-wall thickening by CT or sonography or positive urinary cytology. A pathologically proved PR ($_pPR$) indicated that less than three microscopic tumor foci or in situ disease were noted in the surgical specimen. Although every attempt was made to restage patients surgically, many (12 of the initial 24) refused cystectomy because of complete disappearance of signs and symptoms and concern about future deterioration in quality of life from an ileal conduit. Patients were therefore urged to undergo laparotomy for lymph node dissection with a deep biopsy via the serosal surface of the bladder.

Two patients with a primary bladder tumor and two with primary extravesical tumor were excluded from the response evaluation because of probable total resection via TURB prior to receiving M-VAC or for refusal of any clinical restaging procedure. In addition, one patient had only diffuse T_{is} disease and another was found to have both a T_4N_0 transitional cell carcinoma and a local prostatic adenocarcinoma.

RESULTS

Response to M-VAC

Twelve percent of patients received one cycle, 27% two cycles, 15% three cycles, 39% four cycles, 5% five cycles, and 2% six cycles of M-VAC. For 17 selected bladder cancer patients exhibiting significant downstaging ($_cPR$) on TURB after two M-VAC cycles, therapy was continued to evaluate the incidence of $_cCR$ status. Of note, T_0 disease was observed in

24% and T_{is} in 35% of patients given two or less cycles, whereas 82% achieved T_0 and 18% T_{is} after three or more cycles ($P = .001$).

Fifty-four of 61 patients (89%), including those with atypical histologies, could be evaluated for a final clinical (T) response documented by TURB, cytology, sonography, and CT scans. Of these patients, 24% achieved $_cCR$ status, 15% with T_4, 19% with T_3, and 56% with T_2 lesions (Table 11–4). In addition, 39% of patients attained a $_cPR$, 46% with T_4, 39% with T_3, and 33% with T_2 disease. Overall, 63% of patients exhibited significant tumor regression.

Among 10 bladder cancer patients, 4 with $_cCR$ refused surgery and remained in CR in the final analysis; two relapsed with T_{is} and T_3 at 8 and 12 months, respectively, while two continue to be disease free at $8+$ and $19+$ months. Among five extravesical cases, 3 patients (60%) with a prostatic or prostatic urethral tumor achieved a $_cCR$, and 1 additional T_0 patient with prostatic enlargement seen on CT remains $_cPR$. In the final analysis, 5 of 10 patients (50%) with extravesical disease responded, in addition to 1 whose disease was downstaged from T_4 to T_2. However, for both the primary and extravesical tumors, all patients with a pure or mixed nontransitional cell histology failed to achieve CR; in fact, not infrequently, when the histology was mixed, the transitional cell component completely disappeared leaving only the adenocarcinoma or the squamous cell component. Additionally, data from the neoadjuvant and advanced-disease M-VAC studies (Sternberg et al. 1988) suggest that M-VAC is ineffective against established T_{is} and in the prevention of new T_{is} lesions.

Adequate cytologic examination was obtained in 56 of 61 patients (92%); among 42 (75%) who had a positive cytology, 26 (62%) converted to normal. Of 14 (25%) patients who initially had a negative cytology, 3 (21%) became positive.

Pretreatment clinical vs. postchemotherapy clinical (T-vs.-T) staging by TURB found 54% of patients achieving T_0 and an additional 9% having only T_{is} (Table 11–5). Thirty-eight percent of those with T_4 achieved T_0 status, as did 50% with T_3 and 90% with T_2.

In the T-vs.-P evaluation, which was possible in 36 (59%) of the 61 patients, 28% achieved P_0 status and 8% P_{is} (Table 11–6). Thus, significant downstaging was observed in 36%, a CR rate similar to that achieved with M-VAC for advanced disease. A comparison with the post–M-VAC TURB stage immediately prior to P staging (T vs. P) indicated that 72% were correctly staged (T = P), 28% were understaged (T < P), and none was clinically overstaged (T > P). In many instances, CT scans remained abnormal, possibly a result of a recent TURB procedure. For example, 3 of 6 patients who had bladder-wall thickening on CT scan were found pathologically to have fibrosis. Such results indicate that CT scans within 4 to 6 weeks after TURB can be extremely inaccurate for evaluating CR status. Considering the TURB evaluation just prior to radical cystectomy, 8 of 12 patients (66%) with stage T_0 were in fact P_0. The remaining 4 patients had residual muscle-infiltrating disease, and 3 of them also had an

TABLE 11–4.
Overall Clinical Response

Initial T Stage	No. of Patients	Clinical Response* (%)		
		$_cCR$	$_cPR$	$_cIR$
T_4	13	15	46	39
T_3	31	19	39	42
T_2	9	56	33	11
T_{is}	1	0	0	100
Total	54	24	39	37

*$_cCR$ = clinically proved complete response; $_cPR$ = clinically proved partial response; $_cIR$ = clinically proved incomplete response.

TABLE 11–5.
Initial T vs. Post-treatment T Response Rates on TURB (T-T)*

| | Stage Before M-VAC Treatment | | Stage After M-VAC Treatment (%) | | | | | |
T	No.	%	T_0	T_{is}	T_1	T_2	T_3	T_4
T_4	13	24	38	8	8	8	0	38
T_3	30	55	50	10	3	7	27	3
T_2	10	19	90	0	0	10	0	0
T_{is}	1	2	0	100	0	0	0	0
Total	54	100	54	9	4	7	15	11

*TURB = transurethral resection of the bladder; M-VAC = methotrexate, vinblastine, Adriamycin, cisplatin.

abnormality identified by a noninvasive staging procedure. Although the latter 3 patients were $_c$CR on TURB, they were considered to be $_c$PR in the final clinical (T) analysis (see Table 11–4).

Ten of 19 patients (53%) staged $_c$PR underwent laparotomy: 2 of 5 with T_4 tumors, 7 of 11 with T_3, and 1 of 3 with T_2 at presentation. One $_c$PR T_4 patient remained P_4 ($_p$IR) but was able to be completely resected (CR_s). The second $_c$PR T_4 patient was downstaged to T_{is} and was P_{is} ($_p$PR). Of 7 $_c$PR patients with T_3 lesions, 5 were T_0 on TURB but still had bladder-wall thickening on noninvasive tests (3 had fibrosis and were reclassified as $_p$CR, 1 had P_{is} and remained $_p$PR, and 1 remained $_p$PR because of residual pure adenocarcinoma; of note, review of the original biopsy found only transitional cell carcinoma). The remaining 2 $_c$PR T_3 patients had residual T_{is} prior to surgery and remained $_p$PR because of residual muscle-invading (1) or superficial (1) disease. Thus, 4 $_c$PR T_3 patients were completely resected and categorized in the final analysis as CR_s. One $_c$PR T_2 patient remained T_2 because of unresectable pure adenocarcinoma.

Of the 16 patients classified IR (see Table 11–4), 3 T_4 and 6 T_3 could be completely resected (CR_s), 2 of whom had an atypical histology. Among the remaining 7 patients with IR, 2 were unresectable, 1 had a positive urethral margin, and 1 had only diffuse T_{is}. Among 12 CR_s patients, only 3 are disease-free at 11+, 12+, and 25+ months, respectively (Table 11–7). Five patients are alive with disease at 5+, 14+, 17+, 20+, and 23 months, respectively, while 4 died within 7 to 14 months. Median time to relapse was approximately 10 months. Of note, 4 patients refused additional M-VAC administration after surgery.

TABLE 11–6.
Initial vs. Pathologic Response Rates (T vs. P)

| | Stage Before M-VAC Treatment | | Stage After M-VAC Treatment (No.) | | | | | |
T	No.	%	P_0	P_{is}	P_1	P_2	P_3	P_4
T_4	8	22	1	1	0	0	1	5
T_3	25	69	9	1	1	1	12	1
T_2	2	5	0	0	0	1	1	0
T_1	0	0	0	0	0	0	0	0
T_{is}	1	3	0	1	0	0	0	0
Total	36	100 (%)	28 (%)	8 (%)	3 (%)	5 (%)	39 (%)	17 (%)

*M-VAC = methotrexate, vinblastine, Adriamycin, cisplatin.

TABLE 11–7.
Status of CR_s Patients*

T Stage	Post-treatment Response			Status (mo.)
	TURB	Clinical	Pathologic	
T_4	T_4	$_cIR$	P_4N_0	Alive (20 +)
T_4	—	$_cIR$	P_4N_1	Alive (14 +)
T_3	T_3	$_cIR$	P_4N_2	Dead (12)
T_3	T_{is}	$_cPR$	P_3N_0	Dead (14)
T_3	T_{is}	$_cPR$	P_3N_0	Alive (17 +)
T_3	T_1	$_cPR$	P_1N_0	NED (25 +)
T_3	T_3	$_cIR$	P_3N_0	Dead (9)
T_2	T_0	—	P_3N_0	Dead (7)
$T_2{}^\dagger$	T_2	$_cIR$	P_2N_0	NED (12 +)
$T_3{}^\dagger$	T_3	$_cIR$	P_3N_0	Alive (23 +)
$T_4{}^\dagger$	T_3	$_cIR$	P_3N_0	Alive (5 +)
$T_2{}^\dagger$	T_3	$_cPR$	P_2N_0	NED (11 +)

*TURB = transurethral bladder resection; NED = no evidence of disease.
†Extravesical.

Forty-one primary bladder cancer patients had pure transitional cell carcinoma, of whom 10 were $_cCR$, 16 were $_cPR$, and 15 were $_cIR$ (see Table 11–7). Of 27 patients who underwent surgery, 6 were $_cCR$, 5 of whom became $_pCR$ and 1 $_pPR$. Of 9 $_cPR$ patients, 3 were $_pCR$, 4 $_pPR$, and 2 $_pIR$. Incomplete response was documented pathologically in 5 $_cIR$ patients. In the final analysis, there were 12 CR (4 $_cCR$ and 8 $_pCR$), 11 PR (7 $_cPR$ and 4 $_pPR$), and 15 IR (12 $_pIR$ and 3 $_cIR$). In the group with extravesical disease, 4 with urethral primary tumors refused operative intervention and 2 exhibited local progression of disease at 8 months. The three $_cCR$ patients with prostatic and prostatic urethral cancer developed a new T_{is} lesion at 10, 15, and 16 months, respectively; all remain disease free at 14 +, 16 +, and 29 + months. The $_cCR$ patient surviving 29 + months eventually underwent radical surgery 23 months after M-VAC for recurrent $P_{is}N_0M_0$ disease.

Toxicity

Although no patient died of drug-related causes, nadir-level sepsis occurred in 10% of 61 patients or 3% of 183 cycles. Median platelet counts were consistently above 200,000 cells/μl throughout all cycles, with the range varying from 70,000 to 801,000 cells/μl (Table 11–8). The white blood cell median nadir was between 2,700 and 3,600 cells/μl for cycles one through four (range, 800 to 9,400 cells/μl). One patient experienced an autonomic neuropathy, one a flare of gouty symptoms, five a transient increase in serum creatinine, and one had skin necrosis due to subcutaneous drug infiltration. Two patients with primary bladder cancer had a protocol break, receiving only 15 mg/m² of Adriamycin. Of note, not all patients tolerated the planned chemotherapy on days 15 and 22. The percentage who did not varied between 58% and 81% on day 15 and between 72% and 75% on day 22; yet, 95% of patients did receive the full M-VAC dose at the start of each cycle. Delay in recycling was caused primarily by surgical restaging and, to some extent, by scheduling of hospital admission. The actual median intervals between cycles were 34 to 36 days (range, 27–63).

DISCUSSION

This pilot neoadjuvant M-VAC study finds that significant downstaging can occur by cystoscopic criteria in 63% of patients, by cytologic criteria in 62%, by all noninvasive T procedures in 24%, and by P staging in 36% (Table 11–9). Of more importance, the study has illustrated the difficulties in evaluating response in a neoadjuvant setting. Using T staging by TURB alone is inadequate and can lead to significant clinical understaging (T < P). In addition, noninvasive procedures can be confusing and produce clinical overstaging (T > P). Although the higher incidence of post–M-VAC T_0 status for initial T_2 lesions could be attributed to a greater chemotherapeutic effect on minimal disease, the higher rate may simply be the result of an aggressive surgical procedure after an initially observed major reduction in tumor size from T_4 to T_2, thereby rendering the patient disease free (T_0) at the next cystoscopy. In essence, such patients are being treated *adjuvantly* rather than neoadjuvantly.

M-VAC does not appear to be effective against nontransitional cell components, existing T_{is}, or in preventing the development of new T_{is} and invasive tumors elsewhere in the urothelium. Of note, three patients were observed to have a nontransitional cell histology in the post–M-VAC surgical specimen without evidence of such pathology in the initial lesion.

TABLE 11–8.
Dose Administration and Hematologic Toxicity of Neoadjuvant M-VAC*

	Cycle			
	1 (n = 57)	2 (n = 51)	3 (n = 32)	4 (n = 28)
WBC nadir (10^3 cells/μl)				
Median	3.0	3.6	2.9	3.3
Range	1.1–7.5	1.0–7.3	1.2–7.0	0.8–9.4
Platelet nadir (10^3 cells/μl)				
Median	260	289	280	221
Range	70–528	22–370	112–699	82–801
Percent receiving 100% dose				
Days 1 and 2	97	95	94	96
Day 15	72	66	56	70
Day 22	82	73	75	84
Cycle interval (Days)				
Median	34	35	36	
Range	27–63	28–57	27–68	

*M-VAC = methotrexate, vincristine, Adriamycin, cisplatin; WBC = white blood cells.

TABLE 11–9.
CR Rates With Neoadjuvant M-VAC*

Response by	CR (%)
All T staging	24
Cytology	62
TURB	
T_0	54
T_0 and T_{is}	63
Surgery	
P_0	28
P_0 and P_{is}	36

*CR = complete remission; M-VAC = methotrexate, vinblastine, Adriamycin, cisplatin; TURB = transurethral resection of the bladder.

Such findings may simply be a sampling error or possibly due to post-therapy "tumor conversion."

Although the present M-VAC data suggest that more than three cycles will induce a higher P_0 incidence, as stated previously, aggressive surgical resection of residual disease after significant tumor regression by M-VAC may also have affected the response rate. Future trials will have to consider the extent of surgical resection prior to protocol entry and stratify for this patient-selection factor. In fact, another trial could evaluate the effect of radical TURB (Hall et al. 1984) prior to initiating neoadjuvant/adjuvant chemotherapy.

M-VAC is toxic, but not too toxic for a neoadjuvant regimen for patients with high-stage, high-grade lesions, considering that, without it, more than half will die in 5 years. While M-VAC may make disease more readily resectable, the ultimate challenge is whether this or other chemotherapeutic regimens will increase the disease-free interval and the 5-year survival rates of patients with urothelial cancers.

Acknowledgment

The author gratefully acknowledges the editorial assistance of Ms Martha Gold.

REFERENCES

1. Hall RR, Newling DWW, Ramsden PD, et al. 1984. Treatment of invasive bladder cancer by local resection and high dose methotrexate. *Br J Urol* 56:668–672.
2. Richie JP, Shipley WU, Yagoda A. 1985. Cancer of the bladder, in DeVita VT Jr, Hellman S, Rosenberg SA (eds): *Cancer: Principles and Practice of Oncology,* ed 2. Philadelphia, JB Lippincott Co, pp 915–928.
3. Scher HI, Yagoda A, Herr HW, et al. 1988a. Neoadjuvant M-VAC (methotrexate, vinblastine, doxorubicin and cisplatin) effect on the primary bladder lesion. *J Urol* 139:470–474.
4. Scher HI, Yagoda A, Herr HW, et al. 1988b. Neoadjuvant M-VAC (methotrexate, vinblastine, doxorubicin and cisplatin) for extravesical urinary tract tumors. *J Urol* 139:475–477.
5. Skinner DG, Lieskovsky G. 1988. Management of invasive and high grade bladder cancer, in Skinner DG, Lieskovsky G (eds): *Diagnosis and Management of Genitourinary Cancer.* Philadelphia, WB Saunders Co, pp 295–312.
6. Smith JA, Whitmore WF. 1981. Regional lymph node metastasis from bladder cancer. *J Urol* 126:591–593.
7. Sternberg CN, Yagoda A, Scher HI, et al. 1988. M-VAC (methotrexate, vinblastine, doxorubicin and cisplatin) for advanced transitional cell carcinoma of the urothelium. *J Urol* 139:461–469.
8. Sternberg CN, Yagoda A, Scher HI, et al. 1985. Preliminary results of M-VAC (methotrexate, vinblastine, doxorubicin, and cisplatin) for transitional cell carcinoma of the urothelium. *J Urol* 133:402–407.
9. Van Oosterom AT, Akaza H, Hall R, et al. 1986. Response criteria phase II/phase III invasive bladder, in Denis L, Niijima T, Prout G, et al (eds): *Proceedings of the First International Development Conference on Guidelines for Clinical Research in Bladder Cancer,* New York, Alan R. Liss, pp 301–310.
10. Yagoda A. 1985. Progress in the treatment of advanced urothelial tract tumors. *J Clin Oncol* 3:1448–1450.

Chapter 12

Treatment of Advanced Transitional Cell Carcinoma of the Renal Pelvis and Ureter

Clayton D. K. Chong, M.D.

Christopher J. Logothetis, M.D.

Transitional cell carcinoma (TCC) of the upper urinary tract (renal pelvis and ureter) is a rare tumor, constituting less than 5% of all urothelial tumors. Because of its rarity, few studies have been reported, and accrued populations are usually small. In general, these reports indicate that survival is dependent on tumor grade and stage (Batata et al. 1975; Babaian and Johnson 1980; Heney et al. 1981; Johnson 1982; Nocks et al. 1982; Mills and Vaughn 1983; Davis et al. 1987). Surgery (nephroureterectomy) can confer a prolonged disease-free survival on patients with early-stage and low-grade disease (stages O and A, grade 1) (Cummings 1980; Murphy et al. 1981), but for those with invasive (stages B or C) and high-grade tumors (grade 2–3), the outcome is poor—5-year survival rates in the range of 20% to 40%. Advanced disease (stage D) is nearly universally fatal: several authors report 0% to 5% 2-year survival rates for patients with stage D tumors.

Information on chemotherapy responses of upper urinary tract TCC is scarce and usually anecdotal. An initial study done at The University of Texas M. D. Anderson Cancer Center, which included seven patients, reported two partial responses and one transient complete response, yielding a mean survival time of only 8 months (Trindade et al. 1981).

With the development of combination chemotherapy programs such as M-VAC (methotrexate, vinblastine, doxorubicin [Adriamycin], cisplatin), CMV (cisplatin, methotrexate, vinblastine), and CISCA (cisplatin, cyclophosphamide, Adriamycin), significant durable responses have been achieved in advanced urothelial cancers of the bladder (Logothetis et al. 1985a,b; Yagoda 1987). Similar responses in the upper urinary tract are anticipated. However, because of the rarity of this tumor, no recent studies have so indicated. In this chapter, we review our experience in the treatment of advanced TCC of the upper urinary tracts.

THE UNIVERSITY OF TEXAS M. D. ANDERSON CANCER CENTER STUDY

Patients

From 1981 through 1986, 24 patients with advanced metastatic TCC of the upper urinary tract were referred to UT M. D. Anderson Cancer Center for therapy. None had previously received chemotherapy, but four patients had received postoperative adjuvant radiation therapy. Sixteen tumors originated in the renal pelvis and eight in the ureter. Tumors occurred in a male-female distribution of 2:1, and the mean age of this population was 61 years. Pathologic diagnosis was confirmed by the Department of Pathology after reviewing accessible cytologic or biopsy-derived material. The neoplasms were graded according to the guidelines proposed by the World Health Organization (Mostofi et al. 1973) and were assigned a stage classification based on that proposed by Batata and associates (1975).

Patient characteristics are summarized in Table 12–1. These patients are best reviewed when separated into two major groups: group 1, patients with local-regional metastatic disease and group 2, patients with distant metastatic disease. In this chapter we also present a third group of nine patients (the multimodality therapy group). These patients received postoperative chemotherapy following nephroureterectomy for high-grade, high-stage disease without evidence of metastasis. These three groups will be analyzed separately, then summarized collectively.

TABLE 12–1.
Stage D Transitional Cell Carcinoma of the Upper Urinary Tract: Patient Characteristics

		Metastatic Site	
Characteristic	No. of Patients (n = 24)	Regional (n = 9)	Distant (n = 15)
Sex			
Male	19	6	13
Female	5	3	2
Histologic type			
TCC*	21	8	13
TCC + adenocarcinoma	2	—	2
TCC + squamous cell carcinoma	1	1	—
Grade			
2	2	1	1
3	22	8	14
Origin			
Renal pelvis	17	7	10
Ureter	7	2	5
Stage at diagnosis			
A	1	—	1
B	1	—	1
C	9	3	6
D	13	6	7
Prior treatment			
Nephroureterectomy	15	6	9
Partial nephrectomy and ureterectomy	1	1	—
Segmental ureterectomy	1	—	1
Radiotherapy	4	1	3
Chemotherapy	0	0	0

*TCC = transitional cell carcinoma.

Treatment

Local-Regional Disease

Nine patients presented with locally recurrent or regional metastatic disease. Eight tumors were TCC, and one was TCC with a squamous cell transformation; eight patients had grade 3 tumors, and one had a grade 2 tumor. Prior treatments included nephroureterectomies in 6 patients, adjuvant radiation in 1 patient, and a partial cystectomy and ureterectomy in 1 patient.

Five patients were treated with CISCA and two with M-VAC. One patient was treated with cyclophosphamide alone, and one patient received 5-fluorouracil (5-FU) and mitomycin C. Three complete responses (CR) were achieved, one of which is recent and still ongoing at 36+ weeks (Table 12–2). Two patients who achieved a CR have relapsed after responses lasting 24 and 108 weeks. One of these patients died at 168 weeks, and the other is alive with disease at 158+ weeks. One partial response (PR) lasted 82 weeks. Five patients failed to respond to systemic therapy; their mean survival was 51 weeks (20–110 weeks).

Toxicity was comparable to that described for treatment of bladder TCC. We observed a slightly increased incidence of renal insufficiency in a few patients receiving chemotherapy who had a solitary kidney. These patients, however, were able to receive chemotherapy without major dosage adjustments.

Distant Metastatic Disease

Fifteen patients without previous chemotherapy exposure and with distant metastatic disease were referred for therapy. Thirteen patients had pure TCC, and two had adenocarcinoma transformation. All tumors were moderate to high grade (grade 2, 2; grade 3, 13). Nine patients had undergone nephroureterectomies, 1 a segmental ureterectomy, and 3 patients had received adjuvant radiation therapy (see Table 12–1).

All patients were treated with combination chemotherapy. Five received CISCA, 6 received M-VAC, and 4 patients received other chemotherapy combinations, including 5-FU and mitomycin C or cyclophosphamide plus cisplatin, with or without radiation.

One CR was achieved, and the patient is alive without disease at 80+ weeks (see Table 12–2). Four PRs were achieved, and 10 patients did not respond (NR). The mean survival duration of the 4 patients achieving a PR was 93 weeks; the 10 nonresponding patients survived a mean of 64 weeks. No significant differences in response were noted between patients treated with CISCA and M-VAC. None of the patients receiving alternate programs responded to chemotherapy. Toxicity was comparable to that described for patients with local-regional disease.

TABLE 12–2.
Stage D Upper Urinary Tract TCC*: Chemotherapy Responses (1980–1986)

Responses†	Patients (n = 24)		Metastatic Site	
	No.	%	Regional (n = 9)	Distant (n = 15)
Complete	4	17	3	1
Partial	5	21	1	4
All responses	9	38	4	5
No response	15	62	5	10

*TCC = transitional cell carcinoma.
†Responses measured by standard criteria.

Discussion

Metastatic TCC of the upper urinary tract is aggressive and carries an unfavorable prognosis. However, like urothelial tumors of bladder origin, it is responsive to chemotherapy. Four CRs and five PRs among 24 evaluable patients yielded an overall response rate of 38%. Two patients who achieved CR have subsequently relapsed, one at 24 weeks and the other at 108 weeks. Four of 9 patients (44%) with local-regional disease responded (three CRs, one PR), and 5 of 15 patients (33%) with widely disseminated disease achieved an objective response, one of which was complete (see Table 12–2). Although the numbers are small, our data suggest that regional disease is more responsive to systemic chemotherapy than widely metastatic disease. This trend is similar to that noted with urothelial cancers of the lower urinary tract where, although objective responses are seen at all sites of disease, a higher frequency of durable CRs occurs in regional-nodal metastatic disease (Logothetis et al. 1985b; Yagoda 1987).

Historically, studies have shown that survival with metastatic upper-tract TCC beyond 3 years is virtually nonexistent (Batata et al. 1975; Heney et al. 1981; Johnson 1982; Davis et al. 1987). Table 12–3 summarizes 3-year survival results from several studies: none of the patients with metastatic TCC of the upper tract lived beyond 3 years. Because our study has had such a short follow-up, we cannot assess accurately the effect of chemotherapy responses on overall survival. However, a trend suggests that patients who achieve an objective response have longer survivals than nonresponders (Table 12–4), a mean of 100 weeks vs. a mean of only 62 weeks.

TABLE 12–3.
Stage D Upper-Tract TCC: 3-Year Survival Results*

Study (yr)		No. of Patients	Survival (3 yr)
NBCCG	(1982)	20	0
Mayo	(1981)	66	0
MSKCC	(1975)	9	0
MDACC	(1980)	4	0

*TCC = transitional cell carcinoma; NBCCG = National Bladder Cancer Collaborative Group; MSKCC = Memorial Sloan-Kettering Cancer Center; MDACC = UT M.D. Anderson Cancer Center.

TABLE 12–4.
Survival Durations: Stage D Upper Tract TCC* (1980–1986)

Response	Patients (n = 24)	Survival Duration (wk)	
		Mean	Range
Objective response	9	100	28–168
Partial response	5	85	
Complete response	4	110	
No response	15	62	16–148

*TCC = transitional cell carcinoma.

Little has been reported in the literature about chemotherapeutic responses of upper-tract TCC. Our results clearly show that these tumors are responsive to combination therapy including cisplatin with or without methotrexate. The usually advanced disseminated presentation at entry into this study may account for response rates that are lower than those recently reported for bladder cancer. A larger population of patients is needed to evaluate fully the responsiveness of these upper-tract tumors to the systemic combination chemotherapy programs that are now being used to treat metastatic urothelial tumors of the bladder (CISCA, CMV, M-VAC).

PRIMARY MULTIMODAL THERAPY

In a cancer that has a high likelihood of disseminating despite its localized clinical presentation, early treatment with systemic therapy is justified. Our experience with lower-tract TCC has shown a survival benefit and possible improved cure fraction when postoperative chemotherapy is given to patients with high-grade invasive bladder cancer (Logothetis et al. 1985a). At UT M. D. Anderson Cancer Center, we believe that the same survival benefit can be achieved for those with upper-tract TCC. Accordingly, we have administered chemotherapy postoperatively to patients with high-grade invasive TCC of the upper urinary tract. Patients who had a grade 3 tumor of any stage, a stage B tumor with lymphatic or vascular permeation, or a stage C or D tumor are candidates for postoperative chemotherapy.

We have treated nine patients with combined surgery and postoperative chemotherapy. All nine presented with stage C disease. The predominant grade was grade 3 in 7 patients and grade 2 in 2 patients. Histologic types were TCC in 6 patients, TCC plus adenocarcinoma in 2, and TCC plus squamous cell carcinoma in 1. All 9 patients had undergone a radical nephroureterectomy, and 1 patient had received postoperative radiation therapy. Five courses of CISCA chemotherapy were planned to be delivered. Eight patients received all 5 courses and one patient received 4 courses. Toxicity was similar to that reported for patients with bladder cancer. No major complications were encountered. The characteristics of the patients and survival statistics are summarized in Table 12–5.

The single patient treated with postoperative chemotherapy following radiation therapy is alive without evidence of recurrent disease at 90 + weeks. Of the 8 patients who received only CISCA chemotherapy, 4 have subsequently developed recurrent disease; their mean disease-free interval was 67 weeks, and the mean actuarial survival duration is 110 weeks. Four patients are currently without evidence of recurrent disease after a mean disease-free interval of 126 weeks (range, 60–216 weeks). A larger study with a longer follow-up is needed before any definite survival benefit can be determined.

Several investigators have reported improved local control and a possible survival benefit using postoperative radiation for high-risk patients (disease > stage B and grade 2) (Babaian et al. 1980; Brookland and Richter 1985), although the majority of those patients have ultimately relapsed with systemic disease. However, because systemic chemotherapy is active in upper-tract TCC, as in bladder TCC, it should broaden the benefit of treatment when used postoperatively. Since systemic disease, rather than regionally recurrent tumors, is the major threat to survival, chemotherapy is the most reasonable form of postoperative therapy. Systemic postoperative chemotherapy, as demonstrated in our study, is tolerated well and can be delivered safely without significant morbidity. This combined multimodal approach promises to improve survival.

TABLE 12–5.
Multimodality Therapy for Transitional Cell Carcinoma of the Upper
Urinary Tract (1982–1986)*

Characteristic	Patients (n = 9)	Survival (Wk) Mean	Range
Histologic type			
TCC	6		
TCC + adenocarcinoma	2		
TCC + squamous cell carcinoma	1		
Grade			
3	7		
2	2		
Stage at diagnosis			
C	9		
Survival duration			
CISCA			
Disease-free	4	126	60–216
Recurrence	4	DFS 67	13–108
		Actuarial 110	66–206
CISCA + radiation			
Disease-free	1	90+	

*TCC = transitional cell carcinoma; CISCA = cisplatin, cyclophosphamide, Adriamycin; DFS = disease-free survival.

CONCLUSION

Metastatic transitional cell carcinoma of the upper tract is, historically, universally fatal. By using the aggressive combination chemotherapy effective in its lower-tract counterpart, responses, complete and partial, can be achieved. However, because of the rarity of this tumor, this study can only suggest a definite survival advantage on the basis of the few patients who responded to chemotherapy. Larger studies are indicated. Because of the unfavorable prognosis for patients with metastatic disease, earlier treatment with a combined approach of aggressive surgical intervention (nephroureterectomy) plus postoperative chemotherapy is justified. The UT M. D. Anderson Cancer Center group recommends aggressive use of combination chemotherapy for metastatic disease and combined multimodal treatment (surgery and postoperative chemotherapy) for high-grade, invasive TCC of the renal pelvis and ureter.

REFERENCES

1. Babaian RJ, Johnson DE. 1980. Primary carcinoma of the ureter. *J Urol* 123:357–359.
2. Babaian RJ, Johnson DE, Chan RC. 1980. Combination nephroureterctomy and postoperative radiotherapy for infiltrative ureteral carcinoma. *Int J Radiat Oncol Biol Phys* 6:1229–1232.
3. Batata MA, Whitmore WF Jr, Hilaris BS, et al. 1975. Primary carcinoma of the ureter: A prognostic study. *Cancer* 35:1626–1632.
4. Brookland RK, Richter MP. 1985. The postoperative irradiation of transitional cell carcinoma of the renal pelvis and ureter. *J Urol* 133:952–955.
5. Cummings KB. 1980. Nephroureterctomy: Rationale in the management of transitional cell carcinoma of the upper urinary tract. *Urol Clin North Am* 7:569–578.

6. Davis BW, Hough AS, Gardner WA. 1987. Renal pelvic carcinoma: Morphological correlates of metastatic behavior. *J Urol* 137:857–861.
7. Heney MG, Nocks BN, Daly JJ, et al. 1981. Prognostic factors in carcinoma of the ureter. *J Urol* 125:632–636.
8. Johnson DE. 1982. Renal pelvic and ureteral tumors, in Johnson DE, Boileau MA (eds): *Genitourinary Tumors: Fundamental Principles and Surgical Techniques.* New York, Grune & Stratton, pp 353–370.
9. Logothetis CJ, Samuels ML, Ogden S, et al. 1985a. Adjuvant chemotherapy for invasive bladder carcinoma: A preliminary report (abstract). *Proc Am Soc Clin Oncol* 4:108.
10. Logothetis CJ, Samuels ML, Ogden S, et al. 1985b. Cyclophosphamide, doxorubicin and cisplatin chemotherapy for patients with locally advanced urothelial tumors with or without nodal metastases. *J Urol* 134:460–464.
11. Mills C, Vaughan ED Jr. 1983. Carcinoma of the ureter: Natural history, management and 5-year survival. *J Urol* 129:275–277.
12. Mostofi FK, Sobin LH, Torloni H. 1973. *Histological Typing of Urinary Bladder Tumours. International Histological Classification of Tumours, No. 10.* Geneva, World Health Organization.
13. Murphy DM, Zincke H, Furlow WL. 1981. Management of high grade transitional cell cancer of the upper urinary tract. *J Urol* 125:25–29.
14. Nocks BN, Heney NM, Daly JJ, et al. 1982. Transitional cell carcinoma of renal pelvis. *Urology* 19:472–477.
15. Trindade A, Samuels ML, Logothetis CJ. 1981. Chemotherapy of carcinoma of the renal pelvis: Preliminary report. *Urology* 18:54–59.
16. Yagoda A. 1987. Chemotherapy of urothelial tract tumors. *Cancer* 60:464–472.

Chapter 13

Urinary Tract Tumors: Commentary

Douglas E. Johnson, M.D.

Christopher J. Logothetis, M.D.

Andrew C. von Eschenbach, M.D.

SUPERFICIAL BLADDER CARCINOMA

In the quarter of a century since Jones and Swinney (1961) and Veenema and colleagues (1962) first emphasized the value of intravesical chemotherapy in treating and preventing superficial bladder carcinoma, only three drugs—thiotepa, mitomycin, and bacille Calmette-Guérin (BCG)—have withstood the scrutiny of clinical use. Excellent reviews of intravesical therapy for superficial bladder tumors by Soloway (1985) and Herr et al. (1987) have pointed out the two major problems facing the clinician today, namely, (1) identifying the patients who are most likely to benefit from intravesical therapy, and (2) selecting the best agent with the least side effects. Cost must also be considered as a factor.

Soloway (Chapter 2) addresses the first of these problems. He suggests that all patients in whom the tumor is confined to the urothelium (T_a or T_{is}) or lamina propria (T_1) and is not amenable to endoscopic ablation or who have either multiple or recurrent tumors (placing them at high risk for further recurrences) are candidates for intravesical therapy. Although intravesical chemotherapy is usually well tolerated and poses few risks to the patient, it is inconvenient, invasive, and expensive. Consequently, we tend to be more selective than Soloway in recommending intravesical chemotherapy and use guidelines similar to those suggested by Herr et al. (1987). They reserve intravesical therapy for patients who are at the highest risk for tumor recurrence or progression. They include patients with stage T_1 papillary tumors (especially multiple), multifocal papillary stage T_a tumors (grades 2 or 3), multifocal T_{is} (three or more discrete lesions or 25% or greater mucosal surface involved), symptomatic T_{is}, and persistently positive urine cytologic results after a transurethral resection.

Which drug is the best to use initially remains an enigma. A prospective randomized study reported by Heney (1985) comparing the efficacy and toxicity of thiotepa and mitomycin in patients with transitional cell carcinoma of the bladder showed mitomycin to be slightly more effective in achieving an overall complete response (39% vs. 27%, respectively), although Zincke and associates (Chapter 4) have shown both drugs to be equally effective in reducing bladder tumor recurrences. Since studies reported by the National Bladder Cancer Group (Koontz et al. 1985) have demonstrated that intravesical mitomycin has a significant ablative effect in patients who have failed intravesical thiotepa therapy, and in view of the tremendous price differential, we have generally reserved mitomycin for patients who failed to respond to thiotepa or could not tolerate the drug because of allergy or myelosuppression.

Currently, however, as discussed by Soloway (Chapter 2) and Herr (Chapter 3), BCG is being recommended with increasing frequency, both for therapy and for prophylaxis. Although its use must still be considered investigational (Cole 1987) and lacks official approval from the United States Food and Drug Administration (FDA), it is readily available and should be considered the agent of choice for treating carcinoma in situ.

INVASIVE BLADDER CANCER

Since the introduction of cisplatin as treatment for patients with metastatic bladder carcinoma over a decade ago, the survival rate has been slowly but definitely improving. A review of our patients at The University of Texas M. D. Anderson Cancer Center with stage D bladder carcinoma for the years 1974 and 1975 showed a median survival of only 3 months (Samuels et al. 1979). Today, using combination chemotherapy, Yagoda and colleagues (Chapter 11) suggest these same patients would achieve a median survival in excess of 3 years, with some patients obtaining much longer complete remissions.

Currently, a number of active combination chemotherapy programs are under investigation, but the two most widely employed have been CISCA (cisplatin, cyclophosphamide, and doxorubicin [Adriamycin] and M-VAC (methotrexate, vinblastine, Adriamycin, and cisplatin). Although there are no published prospective randomized studies comparing these programs, preliminary results (Logothetis unpublished data, 1988) from a recently completed study at UT M. D. Anderson Cancer Center suggest little differences in overall activity. In analyzing complete responses, Logothetis reports 39% of the patients with disseminated transitional cell carcinoma achieved a complete response using CISCA (Chapter 5). Yagoda and associates (Chapter 11) report a 37% complete-response rate in patients with advanced urothelial tumors treated with M-VAC. Similarly, Lo et al. (Chapter 7) report a 35% complete-response rate for patients treated with CMV (cisplatin, methotrexate, vinblastine). As a result of these gains in treating advanced presentations, emphasis is being directed at introducing systemic chemotherapy at an earlier stage. Consequently, our treatment of patients with invasive bladder cancer has undergone major changes in the last few years.

Less than a decade ago the preferred treatment for invasive bladder carcinoma was an integrated combination of preoperative radiotherapy and radical cystectomy plus urinary diversion. Today, radiotherapy is seldom used, and the primary treatment consists of a radical cystectomy and pelvic lymph node dissection. Although radical cystectomy provides local tumor control in over 90% of patients, more than 40% die from disseminated disease. In an attempt to improve survival rates, systemic chemotherapy, administered either before (neoadjuvant) or after (adjuvant) surgery, has been introduced. When chemotherapy was administered postoperatively to patients who were at high risk for developing subsequent metastasis (extravesical extension of local disease; invasion of contiguous pelvic organs; vascular invasion; or lymph node metastasis), the disease-free survival rate increased from 31% to 62% (Logothetis Chapter 9). Survival data from neoadjuvant trials are currently lacking, but the pilot neoadjuvant M-VAC study reported by Yagoda and associates (Chapter 11) has shown that tumors can be significantly downstaged in over 60% of patients, and it is expected that this will be translated into improved 5-year survival rates for patients who have transitional cell carcinoma of the bladder.

Although neither CISCA nor M-VAC appears to be as effective against nontransitional cell components, we have recently demonstrated a survival advantage for patients who have mixed tumors (Logothetis Chapter 9). Whether this advantage could be improved by using different delivery systems as discussed by Montie et al. (Chapter 8) or employing different combination chemotherapeutic agents remains to be evaluated.

Initially, there was great concern as to whether the usually elderly patient with invasive bladder cancer could tolerate both radical surgery and systemic chemotherapy. In early studies when radiation, surgery, and chemotherapy were combined in various integrated approaches, patient compliance was extremely poor. Raghavan (Chapter 10) reports that high-dose intravenous cisplatin can be safely administered preemptively to elderly patients with impaired renal function, provided that meticulous and experienced medical and nursing supervision is available. In addition, numerous recent studies attest to the fact that chemotherapy and radical surgery can be safely combined with acceptable morbidity and a high patient-compliance rate. Over 75% of the patients in our adjuvant chemotherapy program received the full five courses, and another 15% received four courses. Similarly, Yagoda and associates reported from their neoadjuvant trial (Chapter 6) that 95% of their patients received the full M-VAC dosage, and although the program was toxic, it was "not too toxic for a neoadjuvant regimen."

UPPER-TRACT UROTHELIAL TUMORS

The favorable experiences garnered from employing combination chemotherapy for advanced bladder cancer have led to trials for the similar management of upper-tract tumors. As a result of our encouraging but admittedly preliminary experience using adjuvant chemotherapy (Chong and Logothetis Chapter 12) and the fact that current drug programs depend largely on nephrotoxic drugs for their tumoricidal activity, we have restructured our approach to the management of upper-tract tumors.

Patients who present with radiographic evidence suggesting invasive renal pelvic, infundibular, calyceal, or midureteral or upper-ureteral invasive disease receive several courses of neoadjuvant chemotherapy before undergoing radical nephroureterectomy. Patients who present with invasive distal-ureteral carcinoma and who have no evidence of multifocal disease beyond the lower ureter receive neoadjuvant therapy before undergoing distal ureterectomy and reimplantation (Johnson 1982). Adjuvant chemotherapy is used whenever surgical-pathologic findings demonstrate invasive disease or regional metastatic spread.

CONCLUSIONS

Tremendous strides have been made over the past 5 to 7 years in the treatment of patients presenting with advanced urothelial carcinoma. Combination chemotherapy programs containing cisplatin, methotrexate, and Adriamycin are capable of eradicating metastatic urothelial tumors. This success has spurred a number of investigators to employ systemic therapy earlier, either before (neoadjuvant) or after (adjuvant) radical surgery, and preliminary results suggest these approaches are translating into improved survival rates. As our successes increase, we will need to explore ways to reduce the morbidity of therapy and to eliminate the need for organ-sacrificing surgery and its attendant changes in the patient's body image and life style.

REFERENCES

1. Cole HM. 1987. Bacillus Calmette-Guérin immunotherapy in bladder cancer. *JAMA* 257:1238–1240.
2. Heney NM. 1985. First-line chemotherapy of superficial bladder cancer: Mitomycin vs thiotepa. *Urology* 26(suppl):27–29.
3. Herr HW, Laudone VP, Whitmore WF Jr. 1987. An overview of intravesical therapy for superficial bladder tumors. *J Urol* 138:1363–1368.
4. Johnson DE. 1982. Distal ureterectomy and direct ureteroneocystostomy facilitated by the psoas-bladder hitch procedure, in Johnson DE, Boileau MA (eds): *Genitourinary Tumors: Fundamental Principles and Surgical Techniques.* New York, Grune & Stratton, pp 385–392.
5. Jones HC, Swinney J. 1961. Thio-TEPA in the treatment of tumours of the bladder. *Lancet* 2:615–618.
6. Koontz WW Jr, Heney NM, Soloway MS, et al. 1985. Mitomycin for patients who have failed on thiotepa. *Urology* 26(suppl):30–35.
7. Samuels ML, Moran ME, Johnson DE, et al. 1979. CISCA combination chemotherapy for metastatic carcinoma of the bladder, in Johnson DE, Samuels ML (eds): *Cancer of the Genitourinary Tract.* New York, Raven Press, pp 101–106.
8. Soloway MS. 1985. Overview of treatment of superficial bladder cancer. *Urology* 26(suppl):18–26.
9. Veenema RJ, Dean AL Jr, Roberts M, et al. 1962. Bladder carcinoma treated by direct instillation of thio-TEPA. *J Urol* 88:60–63.

_____

Chapter 14

Renal Cell Carcinoma: Clinically Relevant Advances

David A. Swanson, M.D.

A. Kevin Raymond, M.D.

The management of advanced renal cell carcinoma remains one of our most challenging problems in genitourinary oncology. There is still no available drug or combination of drugs that is consistently effective for patients who have metastatic renal cell carcinoma. Some promise is offered by advances in biologic therapy, however.

The high relapse rate of patients with locoregional tumors (stages I–III) who undergo radical nephrectomy contributes to the frustrations of managing this disease. Even the ability to identify the ultimate clinical behavior of any given tumor would be a major advance. In this area, application of techniques such as flow cytometry to renal tumors has demonstrated better correlation between tumor ploidy and biologic behavior than was seen previously with nuclear grade. Investigators are also using monoclonal antibodies to define renal cell tumor phenotypes that may correlate with prognosis. In this chapter, we review briefly those recent advances that have potential clinical relevance.

PROGNOSTIC INDICATORS

Staging

Historically, the pathologist's role in the management of renal cell carcinoma has been largely restricted to evaluating the surgical specimen, the description of which forms the basis for various staging classifications. The classification system of Robson has been the most popular and clearly offers crude prognostic information (Robson et al. 1969). Recognizing certain histologic subtypes like oncocytoma and sarcomatoid renal cell carcinoma—tumors with predictably very good and very poor clinical courses, respectively—also helps define prognosis, but only in a limited number of patients because these subtypes are very rare (Lieber et al. 1981; Tomera et al. 1983a; Ro et al. 1987). However, stage as a prognostic variable is not sufficient by itself for our needs because tumors within any given stage, even stage I or stage IV, exhibit diverse patterns of behavior and widely different long-term results.

Histologic Grading

Although clinicians and pathologists have long recognized that histologic grade, whatever the grading system, correlates somewhat with clinical behavior (Arner et al. 1965; Skinner et al. 1971; Syrjanen and Hjelt 1978), they have relatively recently realized that nuclear grade may be a more sensitive predictor of tumor behavior, or at least a variable that can refine a prediction based on stage (Fuhrman et al. 1982; Tomera et al. 1983b; Tosi et al. 1986). Our own review of 55 patients who had stage I renal cell carcinomas reveals that increasing nuclear grade (1 to 4), corresponding to increasing nuclear size and complexity (angularity of the nuclear membrane, presence and characteristics of nucleoli, and frequency of mitoses), clearly correlated with virulence of clinical behavior when grade 1 and grade 4 neoplasms were compared (Green et al. in press). However, in our study, grades 2 and 3 tumors were the majority and exhibited no distinct patterns of behavior. In this respect, even histologic grading appears to be too crude a criterion to predict clinical behavior accurately except, perhaps, at the extremes of the grading spectrum.

Cytometric Findings

Flow cytometry has added another tool for the evaluation of renal cell carcinoma (Bennington and Mayall 1983; Schwabe et al. 1983; Otto et al. 1984). Although this technique could originally be used only on fresh tissue, recent advances allow the use of paraffin-embedded tissue (Roos et al. 1986). This permits archival material to be studied in a "prospective" fashion and then correlated with follow-up clinical information. A number of investigators have demonstrated that ploidy and DNA content correlate with nuclear grade and stage (Klöppel et al. 1986; Ljungberg et al. 1986a; Rainwater et al. 1987). Abnormal ploidy tends to correlate with increasing grade and stage, although this relationship is not absolute. Furthermore, although the tumor's ploidy does not predict the outcome for any given patient, Ljungberg et al. (1986a) noted that among 55 patients presenting with non-metastatic renal cell carcinoma, 32 of 33 survivors had diploid neoplasms, but all 22 patients who had aneuploid tumors died of disease.

The relationship between ploidy and biologic behavior is complex. For one thing, even among grade 1 oncocytic tumors—tumors known to be associated with an excellent prognosis—11% of tumors in one series demonstrated a distinct aneuploid peak on the DNA histogram; the aneuploid peak was present in 24% of grade 2 oncocytic tumors (Rainwater et al. 1986). Ljungberg and his colleagues have shown a similar heterogeneity with respect to DNA content in both primary and metastatic tumors, although there was generally concordance in any one patient between tumors in the primary and metastatic site (Ljungberg et al. 1985, 1986c; Ljungberg 1986). When the two lesions did not have the same DNA content, however, these investigators report that the clinical course of the patient was more dependent on the DNA content of the metastatic lesion than that of the primary tumor (Ljungberg et al. 1986b). Among 7 patients whose metastatic tumors contained diploid or near-diploid DNA content, 1 died, 2 were alive with disease, and 4 were free of disease after excision of a solitary metastasis, whereas all 7 patients with aneuploid metastases—even if solitary—died quickly (Ljungberg et al. 1986c).

The data to date suggest that cytometry provides information that may be complementary to grade and stage and may help predict the clinical behavior of tumors previously "lumped" in a middle category by other variables (Tribukait 1987). Some investigators have attempted to integrate DNA content into a "malignancy index," incorporating histologic pattern, nuclear grade, pathologic stage, DNA index, and cell-cycle phase (Baisch et al. 1986). The "corrected" index was 91% predictive of biologic behavior.

Monoclonal Antibodies

Hybridoma technology permits the production of monoclonal antibodies, which can be used as molecular probes to characterize the antigenic profile of tumors by immunohisto-chemical techniques. It is hoped that information obtained at the molecular level will be more precise and potentially more useful than information at only the cytostructural level. Investigators in several laboratories have produced a large number of monoclonal antibodies to kidney antigens (Bander 1987). The presence or absence of these antigens on a given cell defines an antigenic phenotype and, using antigenic phenotypes of normal kidney cells as a reference, can characterize renal cancers.

Many renal cancers do not express a full complement of normal antigens, and some express antigens found only on some renal cancers and not on normal kidney sections (Bander 1987; Schärfe et al. 1985). Antigenic expression has already identified several molecular subtypes of renal cancer, and one phenotype has been identified already that correlates with clinical behavior (Bander 1987). Other investigators have approached this relationship from a slightly different direction, studying the expression of 15 cellular oncogenes in fresh renal cancers; the c-*onc* genes were variably expressed in nine tumors examined (Slamon et al. 1984). Investigations into the clinical relevance of these various phenotypes continue, but it seems reasonable to expect that, based on known results in other tumors, this type of information should prove prognostically useful.

Other applications for monoclonal antibodies in diagnosing renal cell carcinoma are still speculative. Nonetheless, only a small extrapolation from proved technology seems necessary to imagine that monoclonal antibodies might some day have a role in diagnosis and staging through radioimmunoscintigraphy, particularly when metastases are the result of a clinically occult neoplasm. In addition, using a reliable tumor marker based on a monoclonal antibody might greatly enhance surveillance after definitive therapy. Immunohistochemical techniques might also be combined with cytofluorometric techniques to refine further our knowledge of a given tumor and to predict more accurately its clinical behavior.

BIOLOGIC THERAPY

Although clinical trials of new cytotoxic drugs and combinations have not been completely abandoned, the thrust of research to find effective systemic therapy for renal cell carcinoma today has moved away from such traditional studies with their generally barren results. Investigators have long suspected that renal cell carcinoma is susceptible to immunologic manipulation and have conducted a variety of innovative experiments. Despite occasional reports of excellent results (Tallberg et al. 1985), however, prospective randomized trials have not confirmed consistent efficacy for so-called immunologic therapy (McKune 1983; deKernion 1984).

Nonetheless, advances in molecular biology and recombinant DNA technology have stimulated massive research efforts with biologic response modifiers, which represent an approach to therapy based on the stimulation of host antitumor responses. Broadly speaking, biologic response modifiers comprise immunomodulators, cytokines (lymphokines and monokines), and monoclonal antibodies, of which the last two categories have demonstrated relevance for renal cell carcinoma.

Lymphokines and monokines (produced by lymphocytes and monocytes, respectively) are hormone-like molecules produced by normal cells in response to specific stimuli; they serve as messengers—modulating immune functions and regulating production of other biologic response modifiers—although they may have direct cytotoxic effects on the tumor as well. Lymphokines include the interferons and interleukin 2 (IL-2), whereas tumor-necrosis factor, interleukin 1, and colony-stimulating factor are monokines. Adequate quantities of these agents, in the form of cloned molecules produced by recombinant DNA technology, are now available for clinical testing.

Hybridoma technology, first reported in 1975 by Koehler and Milstein, permits a veritable factory to be set up to produce unlimited quantities of a specific (monoclonal) antibody. Because they can be used to regulate growth factors or to block cell-surface receptors for molecules regulating tumor growth or attachment, monoclonal antibodies are also considered biologic response modifiers. Their specificity for tumor-associated antigens or surface receptors means that monoclonal antibodies may also have therapeutic potential in combination with radionuclides, cytotoxic drugs, or even other biologic response modifiers.

Lymphokines

Interferon

Clinical trials of interferon in the late 1970s demonstrated its antitumor activity in a variety of tumors, and we began to treat patients with metastatic renal cell carcinoma in early 1980. The initial trial with partially purified human leukocyte (alpha) interferon (IFN-α) produced a complete response (CR) in 3 of 50 patients (6%), a partial response (PR) in 10 patients (20%), and some evidence of biologic response to the drug in an additional 11 patients (22%), confirming interferon's antitumor effect against renal cell cancer (Quesada et al. 1983, 1985). Subsequent trials at The University of Texas M. D. Anderson Cancer Center with recombinant alpha interferon (rIFN-α) and recombinant interferon gamma (rIFN-γ) and their combination confirmed the activity of various interferons against renal cell carcinoma at doses accompanied by acceptable toxicity (Swanson and Quesada 1988). Other investigators have confirmed our findings, and it is now clear that the response rates for interferon exceed those reported for standard cytotoxic chemotherapy (Neidhart 1986; Umeda and Niijima 1986; Muss et al. 1987). So far, however, combinations of interferons or of interferon plus other biologic response modifiers or chemotherapeutic agents have not proved superior to single-agent interferon in clinical trials, although such potentially synergistic combinations continue to be tested enthusiastically.

Interleukin 2

Another lymphokine with clinical relevance is IL-2. Since the initial dramatic report of a "possible new approach to the treatment of cancer" only 4 years ago (Rosenberg et al. 1985), additional clinical testing has confirmed both the efficacy and morbidity of IL-2, with and without lymphokine-activated killer (LAK) cells, for patients with renal cell carcinoma (Rosenberg et al. 1986a), although the morbidity of IL-2 may be decreased by constant infusion (West et al. 1987). In fact, among 57 evaluable patients with metastatic renal cell cancer, 21 of whom received IL-2 alone and 36 IL-2 plus LAK cells, 13 patients (23%) achieved a CR or PR (Rosenberg et al. 1987). A recent update showed that among 34 patients who received high-dose IL-2 after nephrectomy, 13 (38%) achieved a CR or PR. Initially it appeared that the patients receiving IL-2 plus LAK cells had a higher objective response rate than those who received IL-2 alone, but preliminary results of a randomized trial using only high-dose IL-2 in nephrectomized patients do not confirm this difference (W. M. Linehan, personal communication, 1987). Further research in the field of adoptive transfer has identified tumor-infiltrating lymphocytes (TIL), which, in mice, appear to be 50 to 100 times more effective in their therapeutic potency than LAK cells (Rosenberg et al. 1986b). They can also mediate antitumor effects in the absence of IL-2, although low doses of IL-2 enhance the effects of TIL. This raises the hope that comparable effects might be achieved in humans with less toxicity than is produced now by high doses of IL-2.

Monoclonal Antibodies

Several general strategies for cancer treatment by monoclonal antibodies have been proposed: (1) immunologic destruction of tumor cells, (2) targeting to molecules that are critical for growth or differentiation of tumor cells, and (3) delivery of antitumor agents (Scheinberg and Houghton 1987). The latter is one of the most appealing strategies, perhaps the so-called magic bullet dreamed of by German bacteriologist Paul Ehrlich in the early 1900s. Monoclonal antibody activity has been studied in very few solid tumors, but early clinical trials are under way for some, particularly melanoma and colorectal and renal cancers (Bander 1987).

For renal cell carcinoma, many different monoclonal antibodies have been identified that appear to react specifically with renal tissues, renal carcinoma, or both (Schärfe et al. 1985; Bander 1987; Hashimura et al. 1987). Bander and his colleagues were able to use radionuclide-labeled monoclonal antibodies to localize human renal cancer xenografts in mice (Bander 1984). Lange et al. (1985) used ^{131}I-mAb A6H to treat nude mice growing human renal cancer xenografts; the result included a decrease in tumor size and a survival rate statistically better than that of control groups. In an on-going trial, Bander et al. (1987) have noted several objective measurable tumor regressions in patients with metastatic renal cell cancer undergoing monoclonal antibody therapy with one of several antibodies approved for clinical trials. One of 9 patients receiving unlabeled mAb F23 achieved a PR, and two mixed responses occurred among the 20 patients who received ^{131}I-mAb F23 (Real et al. 1987). Thus, although many technical problems in immunoreactivity and pharmacokinetics remain, many investigators believe that monoclonal antibodies almost certainly will achieve a prominent role in clinical medicine in the next few years.

CONCLUSION

Most of the recent advances that have demonstrated, or at least potential, relevance for the management of advanced renal cell carcinoma are technological. Flow cytometry permits determination of the DNA content of cells, and data already show that ploidy may be a more sensitive predictor of clinical behavior than earlier pathologic variables like stage and histologic grade. Hybridoma technology is the basis for production of monoclonal antibodies. Using monoclonal antibodies as molecular probes, we can delineate antigenic profiles that possibly define clinical phenotypes. Our goal is to understand better the biologic potential for aggressiveness in any given tumor and to predict more accurately its clinical behavior. Until systemic therapy for this disease becomes consistently effective, knowing in advance which tumors may subsequently metastasize and which tumors may respond (or fail to respond) to therapy could be clinically very important.

Our hope, however, is to develop therapy so effective that it renders moot the question of subsequent clinical behavior. Again, technology has provided us the tools to understand tumors and their response to host antitumor mechanisms at the molecular level. Some agents of biologic therapy, such as interferons and interleukin 2, have already demonstrated that they can induce more objective responses than can standard therapy, although their high toxicity still limits routine clinical use. Other forms of biologic therapy, such as monoclonal antibody-based therapy, are largely unproved, if not untested. To date, clinical relevance of biologic therapy has only been suggested, not confirmed, but based on the early results and the technology behind such therapy, many investigators are optimistic that we are closer than ever to having effective systemic therapy for renal cell carcinoma.

REFERENCES

1. Arner O, Blanck C, von Schreeb T. 1965. Renal adenocarcinoma: Morphology, grading of malignancy, prognosis. A study of 197 cases. *Acta Chir Scand [Suppl]* 346:1–50.
2. Baisch H, Otto U, Klöppel G. 1986. Malignancy index based on flow cytometry and histology for renal cell carcinoma and its correlation to prognosis. *Cytometry* 7:200–204.
3. Bander NH. 1987. Monoclonal antibodies in urologic oncology. *Cancer* 60:658–667.
4. Bander NH, Welt S, Houghton AN. 1984. Radionuclide imaging of human renal cancer with labeled monoclonal antibodies. *Am Coll Surg Bull* 35:652–655.
5. Bennington JL, Mayall BH. 1983. DNA cytometry on four-micrometer sections of paraffin-embedded human renal adenocarcinoma and adenomas. *Cytometry* 4:31–39.
6. deKernion JB. 1984. Immunotherapy of renal cell carcinoma, in Kurth KH, Debruyne FMJ, Schroeder FH, et al (eds): *Progress and Controversies in Oncological Urology*. European Organization for Research on the Treatment of Cancer: Genitourinary Group, Monograph no. 1. New York, Alan R. Liss, pp 409–421.
7. Fuhrman SA, Lasky LC, Limas C. 1982. Prognostic significance of morphologic parameters in renal cell carcinoma. *Am J Surg Pathol* 6:655–663.
7a. Green LK, Ayala AG, Ro JY, et al. In press. The role of nuclear grading in stage I renal cell carcinoma. *Urology*.
8. Hashimura T, Caulfield MJ, Tubbs R, et al. 1987. Novel monoclonal antibodies (mAbs) reactive with renal carcinoma (RC) cells (abstract). *Proc Am Soc Clin Oncol* 6:245.
9. Klöppel G, Knofel WT, Baisch H, et al. 1986. Prognosis of renal cell carcinoma related to nuclear grade, DNA content and Robson stage. *Eur Urol* 12:426–431.
10. Lange PH, Vessella RL, Chiou RK, et al. 1985. Monoclonal antibodies in human renal cell carcinoma and their use in radioimmune localization and therapy of tumor xenografts. *Surgery* 98:143–149.
11. Lieber MM, Tomera KM, Farrow GM. 1981. Renal oncocytoma. *J Urol* 125:481–485.
12. Ljungberg B. 1986. DNA content in renal cell carcinoma: A clinical study with special reference to tumor heterogeneity and prognosis. *Scand J Urol Nephrol [Suppl]* 161:1–47.
13. Ljungberg B, Forsslund G, Stenling R, et al. 1986a. Prognostic significance of the DNA content in renal cell carcinoma. *J Urol* 135:422–426.
14. Ljungberg B, Stenling R, Roos G. 1986b. DNA content and prognosis in renal cell carcinoma: A comparison between primary tumors and metastases. *Cancer* 57:2346–2350.
15. Ljungberg B, Stenling R, Roos G. 1985. DNA content in renal cell carcinoma with reference to tumor heterogeneity. *Cancer* 56:503–508.
16. Ljungberg B, Stenling R, Roos G. 1986c. Prognostic value of deoxyribonucleic acid content in metastatic renal cell carcinoma. *J Urol* 136:801–804.
17. McCune CS. 1983. Immunologic therapies of kidney carcinoma. *Semin Oncol* 10:431–436.
18. Muss HB, Costanzi JJ, Leavitt R, et al. 1987. Recombinant alfa interferon in renal cell carcinoma: A randomized trial of two routes of administration. *J Clin Oncol* 5:286–291.
19. Neidhart JA. 1986. Interferon therapy for the treatment of renal cancer. *Cancer* 57:1696–1699.
20. Otto U, Baisch H, Huland H, et al. 1984. Tumor cell deoxyribonucleic acid content and prognosis in human renal cell carcinoma. *J Urol* 132:237–239.
21. Quesada JR, Swanson DA, Gutterman JU. 1985. Phase II study of interferon alpha in metastatic renal-cell carcinoma: A progress report. *J Clin Oncol* 3:1086–1092.
22. Quesada JR, Swanson DA, Trindade A, et al. 1983. Renal cell carcinoma: Antitumor effects of leukocyte interferon. *Cancer Res* 43:940–947.

23. Rainwater LM, Farrow GM, Lieber MM. 1986. Flow cytometry of renal oncocytoma: Common occurrence of deoxyribonucleic acid polyploidy and aneuploidy. *J Urol* 135:1167–1172.

24. Rainwater LM, Hosaka Y, Farrow GM, et al. 1987. Well differentiated clear cell renal carcinoma: Significance of nuclear deoxyribonucleic acid patterns studied by flow cytometry. *J Urol* 137:15–20.

25. Real FX, Bander NH, Yeh S, et al. 1987. Monoclonal antibody F23: Radiolocalization and phase I study in patients with renal cell carcinoma (abstract). *Proc Am Soc Clin Oncol* 6:240.

26. Ro JY, Ayala AG, Sella A, et al. 1987. Sarcomatoid renal cell carcinoma: Clinicopathologic. A study of 42 cases. *Cancer* 59:516–526.

27. Robson CJ, Churchill BM, Anderson W. 1969. The results of radical nephrectomy for renal cell carcinoma. *J Urol* 101:297–301.

28. Roos G, Stenling R, Ljungberg B. 1986. DNA content in renal cell carcinoma: A comparison between flow and static cytometric methods. *Scand J Urol Nephrol* 20:295–300.

29. Rosenberg SA, Lotze MT, Muul LM, et al. 1986a. A new approach to the therapy of cancer based on the systemic administration of autologous lymphokine-activated killer cells and recombinant interleukin-2. *Surgery* 100:262–270.

30. Rosenberg SA, Lotze MT, Muul LM, et al. 1985. Observations on the systemic administration of autologous lymphokine-activated killer cells and recombinant interleukin-2 to patients with metastatic cancer. *N Engl J Med* 313:1485–1492.

31. Rosenberg SA, Lotze MT, Muul LM, et al. 1987. A progress report on the treatment of 157 patients with advanced cancer using lymphokine-activated killer cells and interleukin-2 or high-dose interleukin-2 alone. *N Engl J Med* 316:889–897.

32. Rosenberg SA, Spiess P, Lafreniere R. 1986b. A new approach to the adoptive immunotherapy of cancer with tumor-infiltrating lymphocytes. *Science* 233:1318–1321.

33. Schärfe T, Becht E, Kaltwasser R, et al. 1985. Tumor-specific monoclonal antibodies for renal cell carcinoma. *Eur Urol* 11:117–120.

34. Scheinberg DA, Houghton AN. 1987. Current status of antitumor therapy with monoclonal antibodies. *Oncology* 1:31–37.

35. Schwabe HW, Adolphs HD, Vogel J. 1983. Flow-cytophotometric studies in renal carcinoma. *Urol Res* 11:121–125.

36. Skinner DG, Colvin RB, Vermillion CD, et al. 1971. Diagnosis and management of renal cell carcinoma: A clinical and pathologic study of 309 cases. *Cancer* 28:1165–1177.

37. Slamon DJ, deKernion JB, Verma IM, et al. 1984. Expression of cellular oncogenes in human malignancies. *Science* 224:256–262.

38. Swanson DA, Quesada JR. 1988. Interferon therapy for metastatic renal cell carcinoma. *Semin Surg Oncol.* 4:174–177.

39. Syrjanen K, Hjelt L. 1978. Grading of human renal adenocarcinoma. *Scand J Urol Nephrol* 12:49–55.

40. Tallberg T, Tykka H, Mahlberg K, et al. 1985. Active specific immunotherapy with supportive measures in the treatment of palliatively nephrectomized, renal adenocarcinoma patients: A thirteen-year follow-up study. *Eur Urol* 11:233–243.

41. Tomera KM, Farrow GM, Lieber MM. 1983a. Sarcomatoid renal carcinoma. *J Urol* 130:657–659.

42. Tomera KM, Farrow GM, Lieber MM. 1983b. Well differentiated (grade I) clear cell renal carcinoma. *J Urol* 129:933–938.

43. Tosi P, Luzi P, Baak JPA, et al. 1986. Nuclear morphometry as an important prognostic factor in stage I renal cell carcinoma. *Cancer* 58:2512–2518.

44. Tribukait B. 1987. Flow cytometry in assessing the clinical aggressiveness of genito-urinary neoplasms. *World J Urol* 5:108–122.

45. Umeda T, Niijima T. 1986. Phase II study of alpha interferon on renal cell carcinoma: Summary of three collaborative trials. *Cancer* 58:1231–1235.

46. West WH, Tauer KW, Yannelli JR, et al. 1987. Constant-infusion recombinant interleukin-2 in adoptive immunotherapy of advanced cancer. *N Engl J Med* 316:898–905.

Chapter 15

New Cytotoxic Single-Agent Therapy for Renal Cell Carcinoma*

Alan Yagoda, M.D.

Adenocarcinoma of the kidney has been and still remains insensitive to cytotoxic agents. Single agents and combination-drug regimens used prior to 1983 have been reviewed (Hrushesky and Murphy 1977; Harris 1983), and the data show complete remission (CR) or partial remission (PR) in only 0% to 2% to 7% to 10% of patients, an incidence that may represent "background noise." So-called "spontaneous" regression has been observed in 0.5% to 24% of cases (Oliver 1987) a prospective study of 69 patients with bidimensionally measurable metastases noted 7% who showed spontaneous tumor regression. In this series, there were three CRs and two PRs lasting 6 to 48 months. The long list of older agents includes dactinomycin (actinomycin D), carmustine (BCNU), chlorozotocin, lomustine (CCNU), semustine (methyl-CCNU), etoposide (VP-16-213), methotrexate, triazinate (Baker's antifol), vinblastine, and vindesine.

Similarly, objective tumor regression following hormonal manipulation has been insignificant, 0% to 2% to 5% to 7%, when large numbers of clinical studies are evaluated. In the review by Harris (1983), there were 43 responses (9%) among 477 patients given progestins, 9 (8%) among 115 treated with androgens, and 10 (6%) among 162 receiving antiandrogens. For 1,011 patients entered into 38 single-agent trials, the overall response rate was 9% (92 patients), and for 20 combination trials enrolling 406 patients, the response rate was 17% (69 patients). Yet, many of these trials are older studies that employed differing, generally less strict, response criteria. Even newer hormonal agents such as flutamide (Ahmed et al. 1984) and high-dose medroxyprogesterone acetate (Kjaer and Frederiksen 1986) have induced remission in less than 5% of patients. Not only does the clinical, but also laboratory, evidence suggest no role for hormonal manipulation (Ronchi et al. 1984; Ahmed et al. 1984). Steroid hormone receptors do not appear to be increased preferentially in human renal cell carcinoma cells; in fact, levels seem to be less than those found in the normal renal tissue.

Although higher response rates have been reported when investigators use the response categories of minor response (MR) and stabilization of disease (STAB: <25% change or <25% decrease and 50% increase in tumor size), the "true" (objective) response rates (CR + PR) are significantly lower.

*This study was supported in part by the Isidore Komanoff/Solid Tumor Service Funds.

Patient selection, undoubtedly, has been a critical silent statistician in evaluating the antitumor activity of agents tested against renal cell cancer. Not infrequently, initial studies suggest efficacy in a limited number of patients; however, after more extensive study, such agents, singly and in combination, prove ineffective. Patients with a good performance status and minimal disease in lung and lymph nodes seem to be more responsive than those presenting with extensive disease in lung, lymph nodes, liver, bone, and abdominal/visceral sites. In many trials with interferon or interleukin 2, with or without lymphokine-activated cells, higher remission rates have been noted in patients with minimal pulmonary and nodal disease (Krown 1985), despite the fact that the primary tumor either failed to respond or even progressed (mixed response). Prior nephrectomy may be another variable. Biologic-agent trials have recorded better response rates in nephrectomized than in nonnephrectomized patients, although data from chemotherapy trials have been less impressive. While studies by Schornagel et al. (1987) and Neidhart et al. (1987) have found no difference in response, Marshall et al. (1987) described remission in 14 of 31 nephrectomized vs. none of 14 non-nephrectomized patients. Thus, some single-agent phase II disease-site pilot studies in patients with minimal measurable disease may achieve better results because of these patient-selection factors. Large cooperative group studies that permit a more varied patient entry generally have been unable to confirm significant antitumor activity.

Most studies require that, to be entered, patients must have never received cytotoxic agents, or even hormones, irradiation, or immunologic therapies, yet there is little evidence to indicate that previously treated patients should be excluded from phase II studies. However, of note is the recent report of Fojo et al. (1987), who described expression of a human multidrug-resistant gene, mdr-1 mRNA, in renal cell carcinoma, suggesting that these tumors may be inherently drug resistant and that other therapeutic maneuvers will be needed to reverse this resistance.

The older drug trials indicate that vinblastine and the nitrosoureas have marginal anti-tumor activity, with response rates in the range of 5% to 10% at best. Interferon, which induces reponse in 10% to 15% or 20% of patients, particularly in those with minimal pulmonary and lymph-nodal involvement, seems to be minimally better. Recent trials combining a cytotoxic agent with interferon produce results statistically similar to those using interferon alone (Tables 15–1 and 15–2), although one study suggests that cytotoxic agents administered *after* interferon therapy may be more effective (Dexeus et al. 1987).

A review of phase II trials in this disease since 1983 (Tables 15–1 and 15–2) also uncovers little evidence of significant antitumor activity. Most remission rates remain at the "background noise" level and perhaps, in fact, can be explained by an effect on the patient's immunologic status. While the initial report of Marshall et al. (1987) on coumarin and cimetidine, a regimen believed to affect immunologic parameters, is interesting, further trials are needed to confirm its efficacy.

Future studies will probably evaluate monoclonal antibodies, alone or conjugated with cytotoxic agents, and interleukin 2, with or without lymphokine-activated killer cells, combined with cytotoxic chemotherapy. Present alternatives for therapy of renal cell carcinoma are so ineffective that medical oncologists should have no hesitancy in offering an investigational or experimental approach as initial treatment.

Acknowledgment

The author gratefully acknowledges the editorial assistance of Ms Martha Gold.

TABLE 15–1.
New Single Agents for Renal Cell Carcinoma

Drug	Entered Into Study	Adequately Treated	CR + PR	Unpretreated*	Regimen†
Amsacrine					
Schneider et al. 1980	21	21	0	16	90–180 mg/m² q3w
Van Echo et al. 1980	16	16	0	14	120–150 mg/m² q3w
Amrein et al. 1983	42	42	1	11	120–160 mg/m² q3w
Earhart et al. 1983	66	61	1	20	90–120 mg/m² q4w
Diaziquone (AZQ)					
Nichols et al. 1982	20	20	0	18	20–27.5 mg/kg q4w
Hansens et al. 1984	33	29	1	25	27 mg/m² q4w
Decker et al. 1986	22	15	0	15	20 mg/m²/w × 4w
Stephens et al. 1986	57	55	1	30	30–40 mg/m² q3w
Bisantrene					
Scher et al. 1982	27	26	0	16	260—300 mg/m² q3w
Myers et al. 1982	42	37	2	33	260–280 mg/m² q3w
Evans et al. 1985	24	20	1	19	180 mg/m²/w × 3w q6w
Elson et al. 1987	33	26	3	19	260 mg/m² q4w
Coumarin + cimetidine					
Marshall et al. 1987	45	42	14	43	100 mg po + 1200 mg po qd
10-Deaza-aminopterin (10-DAAM)					
Scher et al. 1984	14	12	0	10	30–37.5 mg/m² qw
4′ Demethoxydaunorubicin (idarubicin)					
Scher et al. 1985	21	19	0	14	12.5–17.5 mg/m² q3w
4′ Deoxydoxorubicin (esorubicin)					
Van Oosterom et al. 1986	33	27	0	27	30 mg/m² q3w
Kish et al. 1986	15	15	1	15	25–30 mg/m² q3–4w
Williams et al. 1986	23	21	0	21	30 mg/m² q3w
Braich et al. 1986	13	12	1	7	25–30 mg/m² q3w
Carlson et al. 1987	25	24	0	24	30 mg/m² q3w
Dibromodulcitol (1,6-dibromo-1,6-dideoxy-D-galactitol)					
Mischler et al. 1981	13	13	1	0	135–200 mg/m²/d × 10d q4w
Brubaker et al. 1986a	31	31	3	31	180 mg/m²/d × 10d po q4w
Elliptinium					
Sternberg et al. 1985	14	8	0	10	800–1000 mg/m²/d × 5d q4w
Caille et al. 1985	40	38	5	25	800–1000 mg/m²/d × 5d q4w
4′ Epiadriamycin (epirubicin)					
Benedetto et al. 1983	20	19	0	12	85–110 mg/m² q3w
Fludarabine					
Balducci et al. 1987	36	30	0	30	25 mg/m²/d × 5d q4w
Floxuridine (FUDR) continuous infusion (5′-deoxy-5-fluorouridine)					
Hrushesky et al. 1987	19	18	6	8	0.15–0.25 mg/kg/d × 14d q4w
Gallium nitrate					
Schwartz et al. 1984	12	10	0	7	100–200 mg/m²/d × 7d continuous infusion
Vugrin et al. 1987	35	25	0	25	700 mg/m² bolus q2w
ICRF-187 (1,4,4′[(1-methyl-1,2-ethanediyl)-2,6-piperazinedione])					
Brubaker et al. 1986b	40	40	0	23	2,600–3,800 mg/m²/w × 4w
Ifosfamide with Mesna					
Fossa et al. 1980	15	11	1	11	50–60 mg/kg/d × 5d q4w
De Forges et al. 1987	19	16	1	12	3,000 mg/m²/d × 2d q4w
Interferon + cyclophosphamide					
Wadler et al. 1987	25	21	1	6	10 MU/m² tiw SC + 25 mg bid po

(Continued.)

TABLE 15–1 (cont.).
New Single Agents for Renal Cell Carcinoma

Drug	Entered Into Study	Adequately Treated	CR + PR	Unpretreated*	Regimen[†]
Interferon + doxorubicin					
Muss et al. 1985	17	15	0	13	10 MIU/m² SC and IV + 20 mg/m² qw
Interferon + vinblastine					
Figlin et al. 1985	24	23	3	23	3 MIU/d × 5d + 0.15 mg/kg qw
Fossa et al. 1986	20	16	5	13	36 MU tiw IM + 0.10–0.15 mg/kg q2–3w
Schornagel et al. 1987	66	57	9	57	18 MIU tiw + 0.1 mg/kg q3w
Neidhart et al. 1987	82	82	9	82	3–20 MU/m²/d × 5d q2w + 5–10 mg/m² q4wk
Lonidamine					
Weinerman et al. 1986	33	25	2	23	450 mg po qd
Misonidazole + cyclophosphamide					
Glover et al. 1986	38	31	1	26	5,000 mg po + 1,000–1,200 mg/m² q3w
Metronidazole + mitomycin C					
Stewart et al. 1987	15	12	3	12	6,000 mg po + 14–20 mg/m² q7w
Mitoguazone (MGBG; methylglyoxal-*bis*-guanylhydrazone)					
Todd et al. 1980	20	18	4	?	500–900 mg/m² qw
Zeffren et al. 1981	33	31	0	19	400–700 mg/m² qw
Fuks et al. 1981	14	14	0	7	500–600 mg/m²qw
Child et al. 1982	45	30	3	25	500 mg/m² qw
Knight et al. 1983	95	87	4	62	600 mg/m² qw
Mitoxantrone					
Taylor et al. 1984	53	49	0	31	12 mg/m² q3w
Gams et al. 1986	58	48	0	31	5 mg/m² qw
Van Oosterom et al. 1984	33	27	0	0	30 mg/m² q3w
Oliver et al. 1987	13	13	1	?	?
NMF (n-methylformamide)					
Sternberg et al. 1986	18	16	0	13	800–1,000 mg/m²/d × 5d q4w
Silva et al. 1986	14	11	0	11	800–1,000 mg/m²/d × 5d q4w
PALA (phosphoro-N-acetyl-L-aspartic acid)					
Natale et al. 1982	15	15	0	7	3,750–4,500 mg/m² qw
Earhart et al. 1983	52	51	2	23	1,500 mg/m²/d × 5d q3w
PCNU (1-([2-chloroethyl])-3([2,6-dioxo-1-piperidyl])nitrosourea)					
Harvey et al. 1984	37	34	1	17	75–100 mg/m² q6w
Elson et al. 1987	47	45	0	33	75–100 mg/m² q6w
Spirogermanium					
Schulman et al. 1984	36	36	0	18	80 mg/m² tiw × 2w
Saiers et al. 1987	32	26	0	9	80–120 mg/m² tiw
Streptozocin					
Licht et al. 1987	20	18	1	15	500 mg/m²/d × 5d q4w
Teniposide (VM-26)					
Hire et al. 1979	13	12	0	8	30 mg/m²/d × 5d q3w
Pfeifle et al. 1986	34	32	3	?	60 mg/m²/d × 5d q3-4w
Oishi et al. 1987	59	51	1	16	100 mg/m²/w × 4w

(Continued.)

TABLE 15–1 (cont.).
New Single Agents for Renal Cell Carcinoma

| Drug | No. of Patients | | | | |
	Entered Into Study	Adequately Treated	CR + PR	Unpretreated*	Regimen[†]
TGU (1,2,4-triglycidylurazol)					
Bruntsch et al. 1986	18	14	0	18	600–800 mg/m² q4w
Wagner et al. 1987	16	16	0	16	600 mg/m² q4w
Vinblastine by continuous infusion					
Zefferen et al. 1984	10	10	0	?	0.75–2 mg/m²/d × 5d q3–4w
Kuebler et al. 1984	19	19	3	14	1.5–1.9 mg/m²/d × 5d q4w
Tannock et al. 1985	14	14	0	12	1.5–1.7 mg/m²/d × 5d q3w
Crivellari et al. 1987	25	21	2	20	1.4–1.6 mg/m²/d × 5d q3w

*Numbers of unpretreated (no prior cytotoxic chemotherapy) patients are not always clearly delineated; some numbers have been estimated from available data.
[†]Some doses and schedules vary, and each article should be reviewed.

TABLE 15–2.
Summary of Response Rates With 31 New Agents

Agents	No. of Patients Evaluable	CR + PR (%)
Alkylating agents	327	3
Diaziquone (AZQ)	119	2
Dibromodulcitol	44	9
Ifosfamide with Mesna	27	7
ICRF-187	40	0
PCNU	79	1
Streptozocin	18	6
Amsacrine	140	1
Anthracyclines	137	2
4' Epiadriamycin	19	0
4' Demethoxydaunorubicin	19	0
4' Deoxydoxorubicin	99	2
Coumarin + cimetidine	42	33
10-Deaza-aminopterin	12	0
Elliptinium	46	11
Fludarabine	30	0
Floxuridine (FUDR) by infusion	18	33
Gallium nitrate	35	0
Interferon + chemotherapy	214	13
+ Cyclophosphamide	21	5
+ Doxorubicin	15	0
+ Vinblastine	178	15
Lonidamine	25	8
Mitoquazone (MG-BG)	180	6
Anthracenediones	246	3
Mitoxantrone	137	1
Bisantrene	109	6
NMF (n-methylformamide)	27	0
PALA (n-[phosphonoacetyl]-1-aspartate)	66	3
Radiation sensitizers + chemotherapy	43	9
Misonidazole + cyclophosphamide	31	3
Metronidazole + mitomycin C	12	25
Spirogermanium	62	0
TGU (1,2,4-triglycidylurazol)	30	0
Teniposide (VM-26)	95	4
Vinblastine by infusion	64	8

REFERENCES

1. Ahmed T, Benedetto P, Yagoda A, et al. 1984. Estrogen, progesterone, and androgen-binding sites in renal cell carcinoma: Observations obtained in phase II trial of flutamide. *Cancer* 54:477–481.

2. Amrein PC, Coleman M, Richards F II, et al. 1983. Phase II study of amsacrine in metastatic renal cell carcinoma: A Cancer and Leukemia Group B study. *Cancer Treat Rep* 67:1043–1044.

3. Balducci L, Blumenstein B, Von Hoff DD, et al. 1987. Evaluation of fludarabine phosphate in renal cell carcinoma: A Southwest Oncology Group study. *Cancer Treat Rep* 71:543–544.

4. Benedetto P, Ahmed T, Needles B, et al. 1983. Phase II trial of 4'epi-adriamycin for advanced hypernephroma. *Am J Clin Oncol* 6:553–554.

5. Braich TA, Salmon SE, Robertone A, et al. 1986. Phase II trial of esorubicin (4'deoxydoxorubicin) in cancers of the breast, colon, kidney, lung and melanoma. *Invest New Drugs* 4:269–274.

6. Brubaker LH, Nelson MO Jr, Birch R, et al. 1986a. Treatment of advanced adenocarcinoma of the kidney with mitolactol: A Southeastern Cancer Study Group Trial. *Cancer Treat Rep* 70:305–306.

7. Brubaker LH, Vogel CL, Einhorn LH, et al. 1986b. Treatment of advanced adenocarcinoma of the kidney with ICRF-187: A Southeastern Cancer Study Group Trial. *Cancer Treat Rep* 70:915–916.

8. Bruntsch U, Dodion P, Ten Bokkel Huinink WW, et al. 1986. Primary resistance of renal adenocarcinoma to 1,2,4-triglycidylurazol (TGU, NSC 332488), a new triexpoxide cytostatic agent: A phase II study of the EORTC early clinical trials group. *Eur J Cancer Clin Oncol* 22:697–699.

9. Caille P, Mondesir JM, Droz JP, et al. 1985. Phase II trial of elliptinium in advanced renal cell carcinoma. *Cancer Treat Rep* 69:901–902.

10. Carlson RW, Williams RD, Billingham ME, et al. 1987. Phase II trial of esorubicin in the treatment of metastatic carcinoma of the kidney: A study of the Northern California Oncology Group. *Cancer Treat Rep* 71:767–768.

11. Child JA, Bono AV, Fossa SD, et al. 1982. An EORTC phase II study of methyl-glyoxal *bis*-guanylhydrazone in advanced renal cell cancer. *Eur J Cancer Clin Oncol* 18:85–87.

12. Crivellari D, Tumolo S, Frustaci S, et al. 1987. Phase II study of five-day continuous infusion of vinblastine in patient with metastatic renal-cell carcinoma. *Am J Clin Oncol* 10:231–233.

13. Decker DA, Kish J, Al-Sarraf M, et al. 1986. Phase II clinical evaluation of AZQ in renal cell carcinoma. *Am J Clin Oncol* 9:126–128.

14. De Forges A, Droz JP, Ghosen M, et al. 1987. Phase II trial of ifosfamide/mesna in metastatic adult renal carcinoma. *Cancer Treat Rep* 71:1103–1105.

15. Dexeus FH, Logothethis CJ, Quesada J, et al. 1987. Potential increase in efficacy of chemotherapy after treatment of patients (Pts) with metastatic renal cell carcinoma (RCC) with interferon (IFN) (abstract). *Proc Am Soc Clin Oncol* 6:100.

16. Earhart RH, Elson PJ, Rosenthal SN, et al. 1983. PALA and AMSA in advanced renal cell carcinoma. *Am J Clin Oncol* 6:555–560.

17. Elson PJ, Earhart RH, Kvols LK, et al. 1987. Phase II studies of PCNU and bisantrene in advanced renal cell carcinoma. *Cancer Treat Rep* 71:331–332.

18. Evans WK, Shepherd FA, Blackstein ME, et al. 1985. Phase II evaluation of bisantrene in patients with advanced renal cell carcinoma. *Cancer Treat Rep* 69:727–728.

19. Figlin RA, deKernion JB, Maldazys J, et al. 1985. Treatment of renal cell carcinoma with alpha (human leucocyte) interferon and vinblastine in combination: A phase I-II trial. *Cancer Treat Rep* 69:263–267.

20. Fojo AT, Shen DW, Mickley LA, et al. 1987. Intrinsic drug resistance in human kidney cancer is associated with expression of a human multidrug-resistance gene. *J Clin Oncol* 5:1922–1927.

21. Fossa SD, Talle K. 1980. Treatment of metastatic renal cell carcinoma with ifosfamide and mesnum with and without irradiation. *Cancer Treat Rep* 64:1103–1108.

22. Fossa SD, de Garis ST, Heier MS, et al. 1986. Recombinant interferon alfa-2a with or without vinblastine in metastatic renal cell carcinoma. *Cancer* 57(suppl):1700–1704.

23. Fuks JZ, Van Echo DA, Aisner J, et al. 1981. Phase II trial of methyl-G (methylglyoxal *bis*-guanylhydrazone) in patients with metastatic renal cell carcinoma. *Cancer Clin Trials* 4:411–414.

24. Gams RA, Nelson O, Birch R. 1986. Phase II evaluation of mitoxantrone in advanced renal cell carcinoma: A Southeastern Cancer Study Group Trial. *Cancer Treat Rep* 70:921–922.

25. Glover D, Trump D, Kvols L, et al. 1986. Phase II trial of misonidazole (MISO) and cyclophosphamide (CYC) in metastatic renal cell carcinoma. *Int J Radiat Oncol Biol Phys* 12:1405–1408.

26. Hansens M, Gallmeier WM, Vermorken J, et al. 1984. Phase II trial of diaziquone in advanced renal adenocarcinoma. *Cancer Treat Rep* 68:1055–1056.

27. Harris DT. 1983. Hormonal therapy and chemotherapy for renal-cell carcinoma. *Semin Oncol* 10:422–430.

28. Harvey JH, Smith FP, Bowers MW, et al. 1984. Phase II trial of PCNU in advanced renal cell carcinoma and malignant melanoma. *Cancer Treat Rep* 68:1049–1050.

29. Hire EA, Samson MK, Fraile RJ, et al. 1979. Use of VM-26 as a single agent in the treatment of renal carcinoma. *Cancer Clin Trials* 2:293–295.

30. Hrushesky WJ, Murphy GP. 1977. Current status of the therapy of advanced renal cell carcinoma. *J Surg Oncol* 9:277–288.

31. Hrushesky WJM, Roemeling R, Rabatin J, et al. 1987. Continuous FUDR infusion is effective in progressive renal cell cancer (RCC) (abstract). *Proc Am Soc Clin Oncol* 6:108.

32. Kish J, Ensley J, Tapazoglou E, et al. 1986. Phase II evaluation of deoxydoxorubicin for patients with advanced and recurrent renal cell cancer (abstract). *Proc Am Soc Clin Oncol* 5:106.

33. Kjaer M, Frederiksen PL. 1986. High-dose medroxyprogesterone acetate in patients with renal adenocarcinoma and measurable lung metastases: A phase II study. *Cancer Treat Rep* 70:431–432.

34. Knight WA III, Drehlichman A, Fabian C, et al. 1983. Mitoguazone in advanced renal carcinoma: A phase II trial of the Southwest Oncology Group. *Cancer Treat Rep* 67:1139–1140.

35. Krown SE. 1985. Therapeutic options in renal-cell carcinoma. *Semin Oncol* 12(suppl 5):13–17.

36. Kuebler JP, Hogan TF, Trump DL, et al. 1984. Phase II study of continuous 5-day vinblastine infusion in renal adenocarcinoma. *Cancer Treat Rep* 68:925–926.

37. Licht JD, Garnick MC. 1987. Phase II trial of streptozocin in the treatment of advanced renal cell carcinoma. *Cancer Treat Rep* 71:97–98.

38. Marshall ME, Mendelsohn L, Butler K, et al. 1987. Treatment of metastatic renal cell carcinoma with coumarin (1,2-benzopyrone) and cimetidine: A pilot study. *J Clin Oncol* 5:862–866.

39. Mischler NE, Tormey DC, Klotz J, et al. 1981. Phase II study of dibromodulcitol in colorectal, kidney, and other carcinomas. *Cancer Clin Trials* 4:407–410.

40. Muss HB, Welander C, Caponera M, et al. 1985. Interferon and doxorubicin in renal cell carcinoma. *Cancer Treat Rep* 69:721–722.

41. Myers JW, Von Hoff DD, Coltman CA Jr, et al. 1982. Phase II evaluation of bisantrene in patients with renal cell carcinoma. *Cancer Treat Rep* 66:1869–1871.

42. Natale RB, Yagoda A, Kelsen DP, et al. 1982. Phase II trial of PALA in hypernephroma and urinary bladder cancer. *Cancer Treat Rep* 66:2091–2092.

43. Neidhart J, Harris J, Tuttle R. 1987. A randomized study of Wellferon (WFN) with or without vinblastine (Vbl) in advanced renal cancer (abstract). *Proc Am Soc Clin Oncol* 6:239.

44. Nichols WC, Kvols LK, Richardson RL, et al. 1982. A phase II study of aziridinylbenzoquinone (AZQ) in advanced genitourinary (GU) cancer (abstract). *Proc Am Soc Clin Oncol* 1:117.

45. Oishi N, Berenberg J, Blumenstein BA, et al. 1987. Teniposide in metastatic renal and bladder cancer: A Southwest Oncology Group study. *Cancer Treat Rep* 71:1307–1308.

46. Oliver RTD. 1987. Unexplained "spontaneous" regression and its relevance to the clinical behavior of renal cell carcinoma and its response to interferon (abstract). *Proc Am Soc Clin Oncol* 6:98.

47. Pfeifle D, Renter N, Hahn R, et al. 1984. Phase II trial of VM-26 in advanced measurable renal cell carcinoma (abstract). *Proc Am Soc Clin Oncol* 3:162.

48. Ronchi E, Pizzocaro G, Miodini P, et al. 1984. Steroid hormone receptors in normal and malignant human renal tissue: Relationship with progestin therapy. *J Steroid Biochem* 21:329–335.

49. Saiers JH, Slavik M, Stephens RL, et al. 1987. Therapy for advanced renal cell cancer with spirogermanium: A Southwest Oncology Group Study. *Cancer Treat Rep* 71:207–208.

50. Scher HI, Schwartz S, Yagoda A, et al. 1982. Phase II trial of bisantrene for advanced hypernephroma. *Cancer Treat Rep* 66:1653–1655.

51. Scher HI, Yagoda A, Ahmed T, et al. 1984. Phase II trial of 10-deazaaminopterin for advanced hypernephroma. *Anticancer Res* 4:409–410.
52. Scher HI, Yagoda A, Ahmed T, et al. 1985. Phase II trial of 5-demethoxydaunorubicin (DMDR) for advanced hypernephroma. *Cancer Chemother Pharmacol* 14:79–80.
53. Schneider RJ, Woodcock TM, Yagoda A. 1980. Phase II trial of 4'-(9-acridinylamino)methanesulfon-m-anisidide (AMSA) in patients with metastatic hypernephroma. *Cancer Treat Rep* 64:183–185.
54. Schornagel J, Verwey J, Huinink TB, et al. 1987. Phase II study of recombinant interferon alpha-2 (IFN) and vinblastine (Vbl) in advanced renal carcinoma (RCC) (abstract). *Proc Am Soc Clin Oncol* 6:106.
55. Schulman P, Davis RB, Rafla S, et al. 1984. Phase II trial of spirogermanium in advanced renal cell carcinoma: A Cancer and Leukemia Group B study. *Cancer Treat Rep* 68:1305–1306.
56. Schwartz S, Yagoda A. 1984. Phase I-II trial of gallium nitrate for advanced hypernephroma. *Anticancer Res* 4:317–318.
57. Silva H, Abrams J, Olver I, et al. 1986. Phase II trial of n-methylformamide (NMF) in patients with unresectable or recurrent renal cell carcinoma (abstract). *Proc Am Soc Clin Oncol* 5:107.
58. Stephens RL, Kirby R, Crawford ED, et al. 1986. High dose AZQ in renal cancer: A Southwest Oncology Group phase II study. *Invest New Drugs* 4:57–59.
59. Sternberg CN, Yagoda A, Casper E, et al. 1985. Phase II trial of elliptinium in advanced renal cell carcinoma and carcinoma of the breast. *Anticancer Res* 5:415–417.
60. Sternberg C, Yagoda A, Scher HI. 1986. Phase II trial of N-methylformamide in renal cell carcinoma. *Cancer Treat Rep* 70:681–682.
61. Stewart DJ, Futter N, Irvine A, et al. 1987. Mitomycin-C and metronidazole in the treatment of advanced renal-cell carcinoma. *Am J Clin Oncol* 10:520–522.
62. Tannock IF, Evans WK. 1985. Failure of 5-day infusion in the treatment of patients with renal cell carcinoma. *Cancer Treat Rep* 69:227–228.
63. Taylor SA, Von Hoff DD, Baker LH, et al. 1984. Phase II clinical trial of mitoxantrone in patients with advanced renal cell carcinoma: A Southwest Oncology Group study. *Cancer Treat Rep* 68:919–920.
64. Todd RF, Garnick MB, Canellos GP 1980. Chemotherapy of advanced renal adenocarcinoma with methylglyoxal *bis*-guanylhydrazone (methyl-GAG) (abstract). *Proc Am Assoc Cancer Res Am Soc Clin Oncol* 21:340.
65. Van Echo DA, Markus S, Aisner J, et al. 1980. Phase II trial of 4'-(9-acridinylamino)methanesulfon-m-anisidide (AMSA) in patients with metastatic renal cell carcinoma. *Cancer Treat Rep* 64:1009–1010.
66. Van Oosterom AT, Bono AV, Kaye SB, et al. 1986. 4' Deoxydoxorubicin in advanced renal cancer: A phase II study in previously untreated patients from the EORTC Genito-Urinary Tract Cancer Cooperative Group (letter). *Eur J Cancer Clin Oncol* 22:1531–1532.
67. Van Oosterom AT, Fossa SD, Pizzocaro G, et al. 1984. Mitoxantrone in advanced renal cancer: A phase II study in previously untreated patients from the EORTC Genito-Urinary Tract Cancer Cooperative Group. *Eur J Cancer Clin Oncol* 20:1239–1241.
68. Vugrin D, Einhorn LH, Birch R. 1987. Phase II trial of gallium nitrate in patients with metastatic renal carcinoma (abstract). *Proc Am Assoc Cancer Res* 28:203.
69. Wadler S, Einzig A, Dutcher JP, et al. 1987. Phase II trial of recombinant alpha 2b interferon (IFN) and low dose cyclophosphamide (CY) in advanced melanoma and renal cell carcinoma (abstract). *Proc Am Soc Clin Oncol* 6:246.
70. Wagner H, Possinger K, Bremer K, et al. 1987. Phase II trial of 1,2,4-triglycidylurazol in patients with metastasized renal cell carcinoma. *Cancer Treat Rep* 71:209–210.
71. Weinerman BH, Eisenhauer EA, Besner JG, et al. 1986. Phase II study of lonidamine in patients with metastatic renal cell carcinoma: A National Cancer Institute of Canada Clinical Trials Group Study. *Cancer Treat Rep* 70:751–754.
72. Williams RD, Torti FM, Carlson RW, et al. 1986. A phase II trial of 4'deoxydoxorubicin (DxDx) in metastatic carcinoma of the kidney: A study of the Northern California Oncology Group (abstract). *Proc Am Soc Clin Oncol* 5:109.
73. Zeffren J, Yagoda A, Kelsen D, et al. 1984. Phase I-II trial of a 5-day continuous infusion of vinblastine sulfate. *Anticancer Res* 4:411–413.
74. Zeffren J, Yagoda A, Watson RC, et al. 1981. Phase II trial of methyl-GAG in advanced renal cancer. *Cancer Treat Rep* 65:525–527.

Chapter 16

Treatment of Metastatic Renal Cell Carcinoma With Interferons

Jorge R. Quesada, M.D.

Approximately 20,000 new cases of renal cell carcinoma are diagnosed in the United States every year. Unfortunately, close to 80% of the patients have either regional or metastatic disease at the time of diagnosis. Survival expectancy remains dismal: 50% of the patients die within the first 12 months from diagnosis. There is no effective systemic treatment for metastatic renal cell carcinoma. Recent reviews (Hrushesky and Murphy 1977; Harris 1983) summarizing results of clinical studies that used present conventional methods of tumor-response assessment revealed low response rates for hormonotherapy and chemotherapy. More than 400 patients treated with either female or male hormones since 1971 achieved an objective response rate of only 2% (Harris 1983).

Similarly, no chemotherapeutic agent or regimen has demonstrated clear effect against metastatic renal cell cancer (Hrushesky and Murphy 1977; Harris 1983). Response rates to traditional chemotherapeutic agents used individually are mostly 10% or less. Similar response rates have been obtained with newer chemotherapeutic agents, including epidoxorubicin, dianhydrogalactitol, methylglyoxal-bis-guanylhydrazone (methyl GAG), phosphoro-N-acetyl-L-aspartic acid (PALA), amsacrine (AMSA), and others. Vinblastine has often been regarded as the most active single agent against renal cell carcinoma, but randomized studies that have included vinblastine have failed to demonstrate antitumor activity superior to that of other chemotherapeutic agents. Combination chemotherapy has not improved the efficacy of single agents (Hrushesky and Murphy 1977; Harris 1983).

Renal cell carcinoma is the malignant tumor most often associated with spontaneous regression. Freed and collaborators (1977) published a review containing 51 well-documented cases. An immune-mediated phenomenon is favored as an explanation for this rare event (estimated incidence <1%), but this hypothesis has not yet been substantiated. Diverse in vitro models have demonstrated tumor-specific immune cell-mediated cytotoxicity toward malignant renal carcinoma cells (Hersh et al. 1979). The immunocompetence of patients with advanced disease is progressively impaired, and their prognosis seemingly correlates with the functional status of the immune system. These observations led to the use of diverse methods aimed to enhance the host's immune defenses. Objective tumor responses to non-specific immunotherapy (bacillus Calmette-Guerin, *Corynebacterium parvum*) and active specific immunotherapy (tumor vaccines) have been reported. Attempts to transfer tumor-specific cell-mediated immunity led to the use of impurified cellular products, including immune RNA and transfer factor, which resulted in occasional transient tumor responses (Hersh et al. 1979).

The lack of effective therapy and the immunologic findings suggesting that renal cell carcinoma is amenable to biologic control prompted us at The University of Texas M. D. Anderson Cancer Center in 1981 to explore the antitumor activity of partially purified alpha interferon (IFN-α) in metastatic renal cell cancer. The broad spectrum of biologic activities displayed by interferons had aroused considerable interest in them as potential therapeutic agents against malignant disease. Distinct clinical activity has now been demonstrated against hairy cell leukemia, chronic myelocytic leukemia, and other human tumors (Quesada and Gutterman 1987). Interferons are potent cell-growth inhibitors, but the biochemical events that mediate this activity are poorly understood. Evidence is growing that cellular proliferation may be regulated by opposing actions between growth-promoting factors and interferons. Additionally, interferons are known to be potent immunostimulants, activating predominantly cytotoxic effector cells (Quesada and Gutterman 1987).

ALPHA INTERFERONS

Activity Against Renal Cell Carcinoma

Our original study reported on the activity of partially purified IFN-α (State Serum Institute, Finnish Red Cross Center) in 19 selected patients, who received a dose of 3 million units (MU) per day by intramuscular injection (Quesada et al. 1983). Five patients (26%) showed partial responses in the lungs or mediastinum. In addition, two other patients had a minor response, and in three patients, we saw mixed effects (decrease in the size of some lesions with simultaneous increase in numbers of existing lesions). These findings were subsequently confirmed in a larger series of patients (Quesada et al. 1985b) and were supported by work from other investigators who used other types or sources of IFN-α and diverse treatment designs (deKernion et al. 1983; Edsmyr et al. 1985; Kirkwood et al. 1985).

Subsequently, we confirmed these results using a highly purified recombinant DNA-derived IFN-α (rIFN-α) (Quesada et al. 1985a). Twenty-nine percent of 41 patients treated with rIFN-α at doses ranging from 10 to 20 MU/m^2 achieved remission. However, none of the 15 patients who received 2 MU/m^2 responded to this treatment. The reasons for the requirement for larger doses of the rIFN-α as compared with the partially purified preparation are unclear. Perhaps the partially purified IFN-α contained additional subspecies of IFN-α or substances other than interferon that contributed to its antitumor effects.

Selection of patients influences the response rate. In our series, most of the responding patients were men with a good performance status whose primary tumor had been resected, whose metastases were confined to the chest, and whose overall tumor load was small. The response rate of patients with metastases confined to the lung or mediastinum can be as high as 40%. The impact of dose and patient selection is shown in Table 16–1. Our data and those of other investigators (Mass et al. 1983; Sarna et al. 1987) suggest that for recombinant alpha interferons, doses greater than 10 MU/m^2 produce higher response rates, but that response rate remains poor for patients with poor prognostic factors, including unresected primary tumor, recurrent tumors, and retroperitoneal, brain, or liver metastases.

Although all interferons are immunogenic, we found that an unusually high incidence (30%) of neutralizing antibodies developed against rIFN-α-2a. It is still unclear whether these antibodies adversely affected the outcome of responsive patients, but we found that tumor

TABLE 16–1.
Recombinant Alpha Interferons in Renal Cell Carcinoma

Dose (MU)	No. of Patients	Responses (CR/PR) (%)	Patients With Poor Prognostic Factors (%)	Reference
10–20/m²	41	29	20	Quesada et al. 1985a
3–36	24	26	32	Sarna et al. 1987
2/m²	15	0	33	Quesada et al. 1985a
2/m²	46	10	60	Muss et al. 1987

*CR = complete response; PR = partial response.

relapse was coincidental with the appearance of antibodies and that responses in most of the patients who developed antibodies were short (<2 months) (Quesada et al. 1985a).

Human lymphoblastoid interferon, which is derived from a transformed lymphoid cell line, contains a mixture of eight species of IFN-α. Several phase II studies of this interferon have been conducted with renal cell carcinoma, achieving responses as high as 38% in previously untreated patients who had favorable clinical characteristics (Neidhart et al. 1984). Minimal activity was reported in other studies characterized by patients with an unfavorable tumor burden and distribution of metastases (Vugrin et al. 1985; 1986).

Toxicity

The diversity of biologic effects of interferons results in a multiplicity of adverse physiologic functions. The acute influenza-like syndrome has been well described and is prevalent regardless of the type of interferon. Some variation in quality and severity exists according to the type of interferon, route of administration, schedule, and dose. Fatigue and asthenia have been identified as the most prevalent nonacute symptoms and perhaps the most frequent dose-limiting toxicities. In general, with daily doses of 1 to 9 MU IFN-α, tolerance and compliance are good. Doses between 18 and 36 MU two to three times per week are reasonably well tolerated, but doses above 50 MU are rarely tolerable beyond 4 weeks. At such doses, interferons can be very toxic, inducing perturbances of the central nervous system and gastrointestinal tract and, rarely, renal and cardiac toxicity. Most severe symptoms can be effectively ameliorated pharmacologically or by modifying the dose or frequency of administration (Quesada et al. 1986).

BETA AND GAMMA INTERFERONS

Investigators have accumulated considerably less experience using beta interferon (IFN-β) or gamma interferon (IFN-γ) in renal cell carcinoma. In a phase I-II study of recombinant IFN-β at various dose levels (0.01 to 150 MU/m² given intravenously twice weekly), three partial remissions (20%) were observed among 15 patients with renal cell tumors (Rinehart et al. 1986a).

Recently we have published the results of two sequential phase II studies of rIFN-γ in 33 patients with metastatic renal cell carcinoma (Quesada et al. 1987). The response rate was 7% when the agent was delivered by either daily intramuscular injection or intravenously by continuous infusion. Similar results have been published by other investigators (Rinehart et al. 1986b), suggesting that the antitumor activity of rIFN-γ against renal cell cancer is inferior to that of alpha-interferons. The differences observed between IFN-α and IFN-γ may be related to the biologic and molecular characteristics of these molecules, but clinical variables in the populations studied cannot be ruled out.

INTERFERON COMBINATIONS

We initiated several pilot studies combining IFN-α with other biologic response modifiers in an effort to increase the response rate, the incidence of complete responses, or the duration of responses. All of these studies were based on laboratory observations that had demonstrated synergism between the agents used. Combinations of alpha and gamma interferons or alpha interferon with double-stranded RNA or difluoromethylornithine have not improved response rates over the results obtained with alpha interferons alone. Combinations of alpha interferons with chemotherapeutic agents have also failed to show clinical additive or synergistic effects, whereas toxicity has been enhanced in these studies (Figlin et al. 1985; Muss et al. 1985).

More recently, Dexeus and colleagues (1987) at UT M. D. Anderson Cancer Center observed four partial remissions and three minor responses among 12 patients treated with FAMP (5-fluorouracil, hydroxyrubicin, mitomycin C, and cisplatin). All patients had in common a history of prior exposure to diverse interferon programs. Although anecdotal in nature, our results have prompted us to conduct a randomized clinical study comparing FAMP alone with IFN-α followed by FAMP. The contention is that the apparently increased sensitivity to the chemotherapy may be the result of the prior exposure to IFN-α, which somehow modified the biologic characteristics of otherwise resistant malignant cells.

CONCLUSIONS AND PROSPECTS

The use of interferons represents a modest advance in the treatment of metastatic renal cell carcinoma. A small selected proportion of patients can obtain temporary benefit from treatment. Further studies are required to establish optimal doses and schedules of administration. More important, however, the reaction of renal cell carcinoma to interferons has further confirmed the sensitivity of this tumor to biologic response modifiers, something that had already been suspected from preliminary work with immunotherapeutic agents. Conceivably, the responses observed in those early trials might have been associated with the induction of cytokines such as IFN-α. Newer biologic agents, including tumor necrosis factor (TNF) and interleukin 2 (IL-2) are promising. A recent study administering high doses of IL-2 and activated autologous killer cells has reported activity against renal cell carcinoma (Rosenberg et al. 1987). Overall, these data indicate a role for biologic agents among the therapeutic options against renal cell cancer; as a consequence, new clinical studies should be enthusiastically pursued.

REFERENCES

1. deKernion JB, Sarna G, Figlin R, et al. 1983. The treatment of renal cell carcinoma with human leukocyte alpha interferon. *J Urol* 130:1063–1066.
2. Dexeus FH, Logothetis CJ, Quesada J, et al. 1987. Potential increase in efficacy of chemotherapy after treatment of patients with metastatic renal cell carcinoma with interferon (abstract). *Proc Am Soc Clin Oncol* 6:245.
3. Edsmyr F, Esposti PL, Andersson L, et al. 1985. Interferon therapy in disseminated renal cell carcinoma. *Radiother Oncol* 4:21–26.

4. Figlin RA, deKernion JB, Maldazys J, et al. 1985. Treatment of renal cell carcinoma with α (human-leukocyte) interferon and vinblastine in combination: A phase I-II trial. *Cancer Treat Rep* 69:263–267.

5. Freed SZ, Halperin JP, Gordon M. 1977. Idiopathic regression of metastases from renal cell carcinoma. *J Urol* 118:538–542.

6. Harris DT. 1983. Hormonal therapy and chemotherapy of renal cell carcinoma. *Semin Oncol* 10:422–430.

7. Hersh EM, Wallace S, Johnson DE, et al. 1979. Immunological studies in human urological cancer, in Johnson DE, Samuels ML (eds): *Cancer of the Genitourinary Tract*. New York, Raven Press, pp 47–56.

8. Hrushesky WJ, Murphy GP. 1977. Current status of the therapy of advanced renal carcinoma. *J Surg Oncol* 9:277–278.

9. Kirkwood JM, Harris JE, Vera R, et al. 1985. A randomized study of low and high doses of leukocyte α-interferon in metastatic renal cell carcinoma: The American Cancer Society Collaborative Trial. *Cancer Res* 45:863–871.

10. Muss HB, Costanzi JJ, Leavitt R, et al. 1987. Recombinant alfa interferon in renal cell carcinoma: A randomized trial of two routes of administration. *J Clin Oncol* 5:286–291.

11. Muss HB, Welander C, Caponera M, et al. 1985. Interferon and doxorubicin in renal cell carcinoma. *Cancer Treat Rep* 69:721–722.

12. Neidhart JA, Gagen MM, Young D, et al. 1984. Interferon-α therapy of renal cancer. *Cancer Res* 44:4140–4143.

13. Quesada JR, Gutterman JU. 1987. Interferons in the treatment of human neoplasms. *J Interferon Res* 7:575–581.

14. Quesada JR, Kurzrock R, Sherwin SA, et al. 1987. Phase II studies of recombinant human interferon gamma in metastatic renal cell carcinoma. *J Biol Response Mod* 6:20–27.

15. Quesada JR, Rios A, Swanson DA, et al. 1985a. Antitumor activity of recombinant-derived interferon alpha in metastatic renal cell carcinoma. *J Clin Oncol* 3:1522–1528.

16. Quesada JR, Swanson DA, Gutterman JU. 1985b. Phase II study of interferon alpha in metastatic renal cell carcinoma: A progress report. *J Clin Oncol* 3:1086–1092.

17. Quesada JR, Swanson DA, Trindade A, et al. 1983. Renal cell carcinoma: Antitumor effects of leukocyte interferon. *Cancer Res* 43:940–947.

18. Quesada JR, Talpaz M, Rios A, et al. 1986. Clinical toxicity of interferons in cancer patients: A review. *J Clin Oncol* 4:234–243.

19. Rinehart J, Malspeis L, Young D, et al. 1986a. Phase I/II trial of human recombinant β-interferon serine in patients with renal cell carcinoma. *Cancer Res* 46:5364–5367.

20. Rinehart JJ, Malspeis L, Young D, et al. 1986b. Phase I/II trial of human recombinant interferon gamma in renal cell carcinoma. *J Biol Response Mod* 5:300–308.

21. Rosenberg SA, Lotze MT, Muul LM, et al. 1987. A progress report on the treatment of 157 patients with advanced cancer using lymphokine activated killer cells and interleukin 2 or high dose interleukin 2 alone. *N Engl J Med* 316:889–897.

22. Sarna G, Riglin R, deKernion J. 1987. Interferon in renal cell carcinoma: The UCLA experience. *Cancer* 59:610–612.

23. Vugrin D, Hood L, Laszlo J. 1986. A phase II trial of high-dose human lymphoblastoid alpha interferon in patients with advanced renal carcinoma. *J Biol Response Mod* 5:309–312.

24. Vugrin D, Hood L, Taylor W, et al. 1985. Phase II study of human lymphoblastoid interferon in patients with advanced renal carcinoma. *Cancer Treat Rep* 69:817–820.

Chapter 17

The Human Tumor Clonogenic Assay: Clinical Applications for Interferon Therapy

David R. Strayer, M.D.

William A. Carter, M.D.

Isadore Brodsky, M.D., Ph.D.

Numerous laboratory studies and clinical trials have indicated that interferons (IFNs) possess antiproliferative activity against a variety of human malignancies. Most trials to date have used natural or recombinant alpha interferon (IFN-α) preparations. More recently, beta interferon (IFN-β), gamma interferon (IFN-γ), and combinations of interferons have also begun to be assessed in the clinic. Knowledge of the relative in vitro sensitivity of human malignancies to these interferons may be useful for orienting clinical trials and directing therapy on an individualized basis.

In 1977, Hamburger and Salmon developed an in vitro technique for cloning human tumor stem cells, a method that is being used increasingly to evaluate the antiproliferative potential of new chemical and biologic agents against a wide variety of human tumors. The technique is based on an earlier clonogenic assay for myeloma stem cells, originally developed for murine studies by McCulloch and his co-workers (Park et al. 1971).

THE HUMAN TUMOR CLONOGENIC ASSAY

The human tumor clonogenic assay requires the careful preparation of a single-cell suspension from fresh tumor biopsy material, using DNAse and collagenase, gentle mechanical agitation, or both to free the tumor cells from the matrix. The tumor cells were plated in a two-layer semisolid agar system containing tissue culture medium supplemented by fetal bovine and horse serum, insulin, and vitamin C as described previously (Strayer et al. 1986a). The number of tumor cell colonies (>40 cells per colony) was determined with an inverted-phase contrast microscope after 10 to 20 days by manual counting. For adequate evaluation of drug sensitivity, at least 30 colonies must grow from an inoculum of 5×10^5 tumor cells per culture plate.

The clonogenicity of different histologic types of human tumors is variable. For example, we obtain adequate growth with over 70% of renal cell carcinoma specimens, but with only 50% to 60% of breast carcinoma specimens. Astrocytomas present a special problem: we have been unable to clone tumor cells from 5 patients with low-grade (1–2) disease, but have had an 83% success rate with tumor cells from 6 others with high-grade (3–4) disease (Strayer et al. 1987b).

TUMOR CELL SENSITIVITY TO INTERFERONS IN THE CLONOGENIC ASSAY

The antiproliferative activity of interferon against clonogenic tumor cells was assessed by adding the interferons to the culture medium. In the case of IFN-α, which has a half-life of 10 to 12 days, this equated with a continuous exposure of the clonogenic tumor cells to the drug. In the case of IFN-β, which has a half-life of less than 1 day, drug exposure was brief. Thus, direct comparison of the antiproliferative activity of interferons with different half-lives is difficult. However, the relative sensitivities of different histologic tumor types to each interferon can be determined. Sensitivity to interferons in the clonogenic assay was defined as a 60% reduction of colony formation following exposure to 1,000 units/ml.

Different histologic tumor categories vary in their sensitivity not only to the various species of interferons but even to different subspecies of IFN-α (Salmon et al. 1983; Strayer et al. 1984b). Table 17–1 shows the relative rank of tumor types based on assay of at least four tumors (adapted from Durie and Strayer 1985). Comparison of the relative rank of several tumor types to different IFN-αs showed that the most sensitive solid tumor to the leukocyte alpha interferon (IFN-α[Le]), renal cell carcinoma, is ranked sixth to IFN-α-2a and shows no sensitivity to DNA-derived alpha interferon (IFN-α-D). It is of interest that Quesada reported that approximately 10 times more IFN-α-2a (20 mU/m² daily) than of IFN-α(Le) (3 mU daily) was required to achieve similar response rates (29% and 26%, respectively) in renal cell carcinoma (Quesada et al. 1985a, b). Moreover, the median duration of response for IFN-α(Le) therapy was 6 months, or twice that achieved for IFN-α-2a. These data suggest that IFN-α(Le) may have greater activity against renal cell carcinoma than some of the recombinant formulations. Colon carcinoma is ranked last with all three IFN-αs and has not been a responsive tumor in clinical trials.

TABLE 17–1.
Relative Rank by Sensitivity of Some Solid Tumors to Alpha Interferons in the Clonogenic Assay

Relative Rank	% Inhibition of Tumor Colony Formation					
	IFN-α(Le)*		IFN-α-2a[†]		IFN-α-D[‡]	
	Tumor	% Inhibition	Tumor	% Inhibition	Tumor	% Inhibition
1	Renal cell	36	Melanoma	52	Sarcoma	25
2	Breast	33	Lung	50	Lung	22
3	Ovarian	33	Ovarian	34	Melanoma	11
4	Melanoma	31	Sarcoma	33	Ovarian	11
5	Sarcoma	20	Breast	28	Breast	0
6	Lung	20	Renal cell	23	Renal cell	0
7	Colon	0	Colon	17	Colon	0

*≥60% inhibition, using 1,000 units IFN-α(Le)/ml.
[†]≥50% inhibition, using 800 units IFN-α-2a/ml.
[‡]≥50% inhibition, using 20 units IFN-α-D/ml.

CORRELATION WITH THERAPEUTIC RESPONSE

Therapy began with 3 million units (MU) IFN-α(Le) intramuscularly or 0.5 MU IFN-β intravenously 5 days a week and was then maintained with the same dose thrice weekly. These regimens were well tolerated and permitted patients to pursue their normal activities. Ten of 13 patients who had tumors that showed significant sensitivity (≥60% tumor colony reduction) in the clonogenic assay have had partial (46%) or minor (31%) responses (Table 17–2). Both partial and minor responses to IFN-α(Le) therapy appear clinically significant because the median time to progression was 16 and 6.5 months, respectively. Lung metastases stabilized in two patients with renal cell carcinoma whose disease was progressing prior to interferon therapy. All five patients with renal cell carcinoma that showed resistance to IFN-α(Le) (<60% tumor colony reduction) had progressive disease. Indeed, one patient, whose tumor showed significant stimulation of tumor colony formation following exposure to IFN-α(Le) in vitro, was treated with IFN-α(Le) before the in vitro results were obtained. This patient had rapidly progressing tumor growth and died within 2 months. Stimulation of colony formation by IFN-α preparations has been seen in 18% to 26% of tumors studied (Ludwig et al. 1983; Strayer et al. 1984b). Thus, interferon therapy may enhance tumor growth in a subset of patients. We and others (Durie and Strayer 1985) have seen patients who had significant stimulation of tumor colony formation in the clonogenic assay and exacerbation of disease with interferon therapy. Thus, assessing the response of tumors to interferons in the clonogenic assay before initiating treatment may be useful, not only to identify patients likely to respond clinically, but also to identify those who may be at risk for exacerbation of disease during therapy.

We have recloned tumor biopsy specimens from several patients repeatedly during the course of IFN-α(Le) or IFN-β therapy. In one patient with renal cell carcinoma, lung metastases regressed completely during IFN-α(Le) therapy, but a brain mass persisted. The brain metastasis was surgically excised and found to be resistant to the IFN-α(Le). In another patient with a metastatic rectal carcinoid tumor, multiple superficial liver metastases regressed during IFN-β therapy (Strayer et al. 1984a). Prior to IFN-β therapy, a liver metastasis showed sensitivity to both IFN-β and IFN-α(Le) in the clonogenic assay. A small residual tumor remaining after therapy with IFN-β was biopsied and found to be resistant to IFN-β and IFN-α(Le). We do not know whether the tumor had been resistant originally or whether it had developed resistance during the course of IFN-β therapy.

TABLE 17–2.
Correlation of Clinical Responses to IFN With Tumor Sensitivity* in the Clonogenic Assay

Tumor Type	No. of Patients			
	Partial Response[†]	Minor Response[‡]	Stablization	Progression
	IFN-α(Le)			
Renal cell carcinoma	3	3	2	1
Breast carcinoma	2	0	0	0
Sarcoma	0	1	0	0
	IFN-β			
Carcinoid	1	0	0	0
Total patients	6 (46%)	4 (31%)	2 (15%)	1 (8%)

*60% tumor colony reduction (1,000 units/ml).
[†]Partial response, >50% tumor regression.
[‡]Minor response, >25% regression of tumor.

COMBINATION STUDIES OF LEUKOCYTE ALPHA INTERFERON AND MISMATCHED DOUBLE-STRANDED RNA

The clonogenic assay has been used to study synergy between IFN-α(Le) and mismatched double-stranded RNA (dsRNA). Mismatched dsRNA (Ampligen) is an analogue of poly-I:poly-C, which retains the IFN-inducing and antiproliferative properties while triggering much less toxicity (Strayer et al. 1982; Brodsky et al. 1985).

Mismatched dsRNA has demonstrated antiproliferative activity against a variety of fresh human tumor samples in the clonogenic assay. Tumors showing sensitivity included glioblastoma (4/4), melanoma (5/13), carcinoid tumor (3/6), and lung (2/3), breast (5/14), ovarian (4/11), and colorectal (1/8) carcinoma. Overall, 42% of the human tumors studied in vitro showed sensitivity (>50% decrease in colony formation) to mismatched dsRNA (250 μg/ml) (Strayer et al. 1986a). Patients with metastatic cancer have been treated in a phase I study of mismatched dsRNA. The clinical results indicate dose-related antitumor effects (10–40 mg, 0/10; 80–120 mg, 3/12; 200–500 mg, 4/10), including complete regression of a mediastinal mass in a patient with adenocarcinoma of the lung (100-mg dose level), complete remission of multiple pulmonary nodules in a patient with renal cell carcinoma at the 200-mg dose level, and a complete response at 300 mg in a patient with melanoma (Strayer et al. 1987a). No clinically significant side effects have been seen in over 2,000 patient-treatment-weeks within the dosage range (10–500 mg twice weekly).

Recent studies of combination treatment using IFN-α(Le) and mismatched dsRNA demonstrate synergistic antiproliferative effects against fresh human tumor cells (Strayer et al. 1986b). The antiproliferative activity of mismatched dsRNA and IFN-α(Le) were studied individually and in combination on fresh human solid tumor biopsy samples using the clonogenic assay. Tumor cells were plated in soft agar in the presence of IFN-α(Le), mismatched dsRNA, neither, or both, and colonies were counted at 15 to 20 days. Colony formation adequate to evaluate IFN-α(Le)/mismatched dsRNA sensitivity (>30 colonies per plate) was obtained in 53 cases. A synergistic antitumor effect of the combined IFN-α(Le) (1,000 units/ml) and mismatched dsRNA (250 μg/ml) treatment was seen in 2 of 6 breast carcinomas (33%), 2 of 5 ovarian carcinomas (40%), 4 of 8 melanomas (50%), and 20 of 34 renal cell carcinomas (59%). The antiproliferative effect of IFN-α(Le) against renal cell carcinoma was potentiated more than 20-fold (mean) by the synergistic interaction with mismatched dsRNA. A majority (65%) of renal tumors (22/34) were sensitive (>60% decrease in colony formation) to the combination treatment, whereas the sensitivity to IFN-α(Le) (24%) and mismatched dsRNA (21%) individually was low. These results indicate that IFN-α(Le) and mismatched dsRNA in combination may be more effective at exerting an antiproliferative effect than either agent alone.

These observations have encouraged us to initiate phase I-II clinical trials using IFN-α in combination with mismatched dsRNA. These studies represent an important test of the ability of this assay system to predict for the effects of combination therapy. We hope that the use of in vitro–directed combination therapy will eventually improve the response rate and the ultimate survival of patients with cancer.

REFERENCES

1. Brodsky I, Strayer DR, Krueger LJ, et al. 1985. Clinical studies with Ampligen (mismatched double-stranded RNA). *J Biol Response Mod* 4:669–675.
2. Durie BGM, Strayer DR. 1985. Studies with interferons in the human tumor assay system. *Interferon Letter II* 3:1–3.

3. Hamburger AW, Salmon SE. 1977. Primary bioassay of human tumor cells. *Science* 197:461–463.
4. Ludwig CU, Durie BGM, Salmon SE, et al. 1983. Tumor growth stimulation in vitro by interferons. *Eur J Cancer Clin Oncol* 19:1625–1632.
5. Park CH, Bergsagel DE, McCulloch EA. 1971. Mouse myeloma tumor stem cells: A primary cell culture assay. *JNCI* 46:411–422.
6. Quesada JR, Rios A, Swanson D, et al. 1985a. Antitumor activity of recombinant-derived interferon alpha in metastatic renal cell carcinoma. *J Clin Oncol* 3:1522–1528.
7. Quesada JR, Swanson DA, Gutterman JU. 1985b. Phase II study of interferon alpha in metastatic renal-cell carcinoma: A progress report. *J Clin Oncol* 3:1086–1092.
8. Salmon SE, Durie BGM, Young L, et al. 1983. Effects of cloned human leukocyte interferons in the human tumor stem cell assay. *J Clin Oncol* 1:217–225.
9. Strayer DR, Carter WA, Brodsky I, et al. 1984a. Carcinoid tumor response to fibroblast interferon. *JAMA* 251:1682–1683.
10. Strayer DR, Carter WA, Brodsky I, et al. 1982. Clinical studies with mismatched double-stranded RNA, in: *Texas Reports on Biology and Medicine, The Interferon System: A Review to 1982,* vol 41, pt 2. Galveston, The University of Texas Medical Branch, pp 663–671.
11. Strayer DR, Carter WA, Crilley P, et al. 1987a. Complete responses in solid tumor patients without side effects or toxicity using mismatched double-stranded RNA (Ampligen) (abstract). *Proc Am Soc Clin Oncol* 6:240.
12. Strayer DR, Watson P, Carter WA, et al. 1986a. Antiproliferative effect of mismatched double-stranded RNA on fresh human tumor cells analyzed in a clonogenic assay. *J Interferon Res* 6:373–379.
13. Strayer DR, Watson P, Mayberry S, et al. 1986b. Synergistic antitumor effect of interferon-α and mismatched double-stranded RNA against fresh human tumor cells (abstract). *J Cell Biochem* (suppl)10C:246.
14. Strayer DR, Weisband J, Carter WA, et al. 1987b. Growth of astrocytomas in the human tumor clonogenic assay and sensitivity to mismatched dsRNA and interferons. *Am J Clin Oncol* 10:281–284.
15. Strayer DR, Weisband J, Carter WA, et al. 1984b. Sensitivity of renal cell carcinoma to leukocyte interferon in the human tumor clonogenic assay, in Salmon SE, Trent JM (eds): *Human Tumor Cloning.* New York, Grune & Stratton, pp 585–593.

Chapter 18

The Biologic Heterogeneity of Metastatic Renal Cell Carcinoma

Isaiah J. Fidler, D.V.M., Ph.D.

Seiji Naito, Ph.D.

Andrew C. von Eschenbach, M.D.

Human renal cell carcinoma (HRCC) is a relatively uncommon type of cancer. The prognosis of this cancer is usually poor because no effective therapy has been established for its advanced stages. This is because, by the time of diagnosis in the majority of patients, renal cell carcinoma has already metastasized to visceral organs. Since metastases can be located in different organs and in different regions within the same organ, it is not surprising that the response of metastatic tumor cells to therapy varies and the efficiency of delivering therapeutic agents to destroy tumor cells without producing undesirable toxic effects is relatively low. The major obstacle to treating metastasis, however, is that tumor cells in primary neoplasms and in metastases are biologically heterogeneous: they contain multiple cell populations exhibiting diversity in variables such as growth rate, cell-surface properties, antigenicity, karyotypes, marker enzymes, sensitivity to cytotoxic drugs, and invasive and metastatic capacities (Fidler and Poste 1985; Fidler and Balch 1987).

Short of preventing renal cell carcinoma, the urologist's most important goal is to understand the mechanisms responsible for the development of biologic heterogeneity in neoplasms (and in their metastases) and the process by which tumor cells can invade and spread to grow in distant organs. Only a better understanding of these biologic processes will allow significant improvements in how we deal with the problem of cancer metastasis and the design of better therapies for malignant disease. Developing a suitable model for in vivo studies of the biology and therapy of renal cell cancer is mandatory if these goals are to be reached. In this chapter, we review some recent data from our laboratories that deal with basic concepts of cancer metastasis, using HRCC as a primary example, and with the development of a suitable athymic nude mouse model for in vivo studies of this cancer.

PATHOGENESIS OF CANCER METASTASIS

The process of cancer metastasis comprises a large series of interrelated steps. To produce a clinically relevant lesion, metastatic cells must survive all the steps of the process. The outcome of this process depends on the intrinsic properties of both the tumor cells and host factors (Fidler et al. 1978; Poste and Fidler 1979; Fidler and Hart 1982; Poste 1982; Fidler 1984; Weiss 1985; Poste 1986; Fidler and Balch 1987). The major steps in the formation of a metastasis are as follows: (1) After the initial transforming event, either unicellular or multicellular, neoplastic cells must grow progressively, with nutrients for the expanding tumor mass initially supplied by simple diffusion. (2) Extensive vascularization must occur if a tumor mass is to exceed 1 or 2 mm in diameter. The synthesis and secretion of tumor angiogenesis factor probably plays a key role in establishing a neocapillary network from the surrounding host tissue (Folkman and Klagsburn 1987). (3) Local invasion of the host stroma by some tumor cells can occur by several nonmutually exclusive mechanisms (Mareel 1983; Liotta 1986). (4) Thin-walled venules, like lymphatic channels, offer very little resistance to penetration by tumor cells and provide the most common pathways for tumor cells to enter the circulation. Although clinical observations have suggested that carcinomas frequently metastasize and grow via the lymphatic system and malignant tumors of mesenchymal origin more often spread by the hematogenous route, the presence of numerous venolymphatic anastomoses invalidates this concept. (5) Next, small tumor cell aggregates become detached and embolize while the vast majority of circulating tumor cells are being rapidly destroyed. (6) Once the tumor cells have survived the circulation, they must arrest in the capillary beds of organs by adhering either to capillary endothelial cells or to the subendothelial basement membrane, which may be exposed. (7) Extravasation occurs next, probably by the same mechanisms that influence initial invasion. (8) Proliferation within the organ parenchyma completes the metastatic process. To continue growing, the micrometastases must develop a vascular network and continue to evade the host immune system. Once established, the cells from the new growth can invade, penetrate blood vessels, and enter the circulation to produce additional metastases (Fidler and Balch 1987).

LYMPHATIC VS. HEMATOGENOUS METASTASIS

Although early clinical observations led to the impression that carcinomas spread mainly by the lymphatic route and mesenchymal tumors spread mainly by means of the bloodstream, we now know that the lymphatic and vascular systems have numerous connections (del Regato 1977) and that disseminating tumor cells may pass from one system to the other (Carr 1983). For these reasons, the division of metastasis into lymphatic spread and hematogenous spread is arbitrary. During invasion, tumor cells can easily penetrate small lymphatic vessels and be passively transported in the lymph. Tumor emboli may arrest in the first lymph node encountered on their route, or they may bypass regional-draining lymph nodes to form distant nodal metastases ("skip metastasis"). Although this phenomenon was recognized in the late 1800s (Paget 1889), its implications for treatment were frequently ignored in the development of surgical approaches to cancer treatment (Weiss 1985; Fidler and Balch 1987).

The circulating tumor cells themselves do not constitute metastasis, since most tumor cells released into the bloodstream are rapidly destroyed (Fidler 1970; Weiss 1986). Using radiolabeled tumor cells, we found that by 24 hours after the cells enter the circulation, less than 1% are still viable, and less than 0.1% of tumor cells placed into the circulation eventually survive to produce metastases (Fidler 1970). Nevertheless, the greater the number of cells released by a primary tumor, the greater the probability that some cells will survive to form metastases (Price et al. 1986). The number of tumor emboli in the circulation appears to correlate well with the size and clinical duration of the primary tumor (Fidler 1973a, b), and the development of necrotic and hemorrhagic areas in large tumors facilitates metastasis by providing tumor cells easy access to the circulation (Weiss 1985).

Once metastatic cells reach the microcirculation, they interact with cells of the vascular endothelium. These interactions include nonspecific mechanical lodgement of tumor cell emboli as well as formation of stable adhesions between tumor cells and small-vessel endothelial cells. The organ distribution of metastatic foci is believed to depend, in part, on the ability of blood-borne malignant cells to adhere to specific endothelium and produce endothelial cell retraction (Nicolson 1982a, b).

Extravasation of arrested tumor cells is believed to operate by mechanisms similar to those responsible for local invasion (Nicolson et al. 1985). In addition, the invasion, survival, and growth of malignant cells at particular secondary sites involves their responses to tissue or organ factors. Tumor cells can recognize tissue-specific motility factors that direct their movement and invasion (Pauli et al. 1983). After they invade organ parenchyma, they must also respond to organ-specific factors that influence their growth.

Clearly only a few of the tumor cells that enter the circulation can produce metastases. The development of metastases could represent the fortuitous survival of a few tumor cells or the selection from the parent tumor of a subpopulation of metastatic cells endowed with properties that enhance their survival (Fidler 1973b; Fidler and Kripke 1977). Most recent data prove that neoplasms are indeed biologically heterogeneous and that metastasis is indeed a selective process (Talmadge and Fidler 1982).

METASTATIC HETEROGENEITY OF PRIMARY NEOPLASMS AND METASTASES

The concept that neoplasms are heterogeneous is not new. Almost a century ago, Paget (1889) analyzed 735 autopsy records of patients with breast cancer and concluded that the pattern of metastasis was nonrandom and therefore not due to chance, but rather that some tumor cells ("seeds") had affinity for growth in the environment provided by a certain organ ("soil"). Only when the "seed and soil" were matched did metastases develop. This hypothesis has recently received considerable support. Organ-specific metastasis occurs from many transplantable experimental tumors (Fidler 1973b; Fidler and Nicolson 1976; Hart and Fidler 1980; Tarin and Price 1981; Hart 1982; Nicolson 1982a, b; Tarin 1982; Poste 1982, 1986) and was reported recently for autochthonous human tumor in patients with peritoneovenous shunts (Tarin et al. 1984a, b).

The first experimental proof of metastatic heterogeneity of neoplasms was provided by Fidler and Kripke in 1977 working with the murine B16 melanoma. Using the modified fluctuation assay of Luria and Delbruck (1943), we showed that different tumor cell clones, each derived from an individual cell isolated from the parent tumor, varied significantly in their ability to produce lung metastases following inoculation into syngeneic mice. Control subcloning procedures demonstrated that the observed diversity was not a consequence of the cloning procedure (Fidler and Kripke 1977). That preexisting tumor cell subpopulations proliferating in the same tumor exhibit heterogeneous metastatic potential has since been confirmed in many laboratories on a wide range of experimental animal tumors of different histories and histologic origins (reviewed in Fidler and Poste, 1985).

GROWTH AND METASTASIS OF TUMOR CELLS ISOLATED FROM HUMAN RENAL CELL CARCINOMA

Most of the data on metastatic heterogeneity and biologic behavior of neoplasms have been derived from studies in rodent systems. Until recently, relatively few data have been available on the in vivo behavior of human cancer cells isolated from surgical specimens. To some extent this has been due to the lack of suitable models for isolating metastatic and nonmetastatic tumor cells and the lack of a suitable laboratory model for the in vivo testing of human tumor cells. The development of the athymic nude mouse (Rygaard and Povlsen 1969) and its use for studies of metastasis (reviewed in Fidler 1986) has proved valuable in studying many aspects of human neoplasms. Although several investigators have reported the successful transplantation of HRCC cells into nude mice (Katsuoka et al. 1976; Hoehn and Schroeder 1978; Otto et al. 1981, 1984a, b; Naito et al. 1982; Clayman et al. 1985), the usefulness of this model has been limited. Like other human tumor cells, HRCC cells transplanted into the skin rarely metastasize in nude mice, regardless of their malignancy in the patient (Hanna 1980; Pollack and Fidler 1982; Sharkey and Fogh 1984; Fidler 1986).

Recent reports from our laboratory have shown that the site of tumor growth can influence the production of metastasis (Fidler 1986). The intrasplenic injection of human tumor cells derived from several well-established cell lines, such as colon carcinoma or prostatic carcinoma (Kozlowski et al. 1984), or freshly isolated from human colorectal carcinomas (Giavazzi et al. 1986a, b) allowed the expression of metastatic potential, whereas implantation of the same cells into the subcutis did not. One notable exception was an established HRCC line in which cells grown in the spleen did not produce metastases in the liver or lung.

We wished to determine whether the methods for isolating cells from a surgical specimen of HRCC influenced the biologic behavior of the cancer cells (Naito et al. 1986). The tumor tissue was obtained from a primary renal tumor subsequent to a radical nephrectomy in a 43-year-old man. The tumor was diagnosed as a renal cell carcinoma that extensively invaded perinephric fat. Tumor tissue was dissociated enzymatically with collagenase (type 1, 200 units/ml) and deoxyribonuclease (DNase) (270 units/ml). The procedure yielded a suspension of highly viable single tumor cells or very small clumps of cells. The cell suspension was divided into three aliquots. One aliquot was used to produce a tissue culture line. The second was injected subcutaneously in the lateral aspect of the anterior thoracic wall; 2 months later, one subcutaneous tumor was excised and dissociated enzymatically, and the cells were established in culture. The third aliquot of the original HRCC cell suspension was injected directly into the kidneys of nude mice. The mice were killed 2 months later. In 2 mice the kidney tumor exceeded 2 cm in diameter, and in 1 mouse we found a grossly visible tumor nodule in the liver. Moreover, the peritoneum was full of ascites fluid. Tumor cells isolated from the kidney tumor and the liver nodule by enzymatic dissociation were established as individual cell lines in culture. A cell line was also established from the ascitic cells. The cells from these five lines grew on plastic as monolayer cultures that had a similar morphology. The human origin of all the lines was ascertained by detailed karyotypic analysis and by isoenzyme determinations. No contamination with mouse cells was found. For details and designation of the various lines see Figure 18–1.

Because the five HRCC cell lines were derived from five different isolation conditions (culture, subcutaneous tumor, renal tumor, liver metastasis from the renal tumor, ascites from the renal tumor), we asked whether the cell lines exhibited biologic heterogeneity, including differences in metastatic potential, and whether different implantation sites in nude

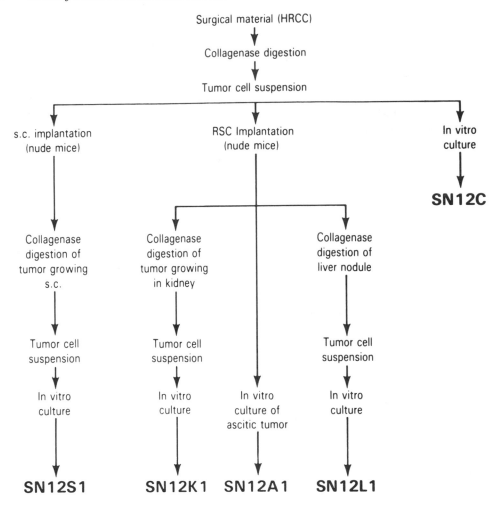

FIG 18–1.
The procedures used to isolate five different cell lines from a surgical specimen of renal cell carcinoma. *HRCC* = human renal cell carcinoma; *s.c.* = subcutaneous; *RSC* = renal subcapsule.

mice would influence metastatic behavior. Cells from each line were injected subcutaneously, intraperitoneally, intravenously, intrasplenically, and beneath the renal capsule of nude mice. All the lines were tumorigenic after subcutaneous or renal subcapsule injection, although the rate of tumor growth varied among the five lines. The metastatic behavior of the HRCC cells was influenced by both the nature of the tumor cells and the route of injection. The biologic behaviors of HRCC cells isolated by direct culture technique (SN12C) and those isolated from HRCC tumors and grown first in the nude mice and then established in culture differed (Table 18–1). This difference raises a question about which method should be routinely employed if human tumor cell lines are to be isolated either for biologic studies or for analysis of sensitivity to therapeutic agents.

Cell lines derived from HRCC tumors produced by the original HRCC cells injected into the skin (SN12S1) or into the kidney (SN12K1) of nude mice also differed in their biologic properties. Cell lines derived from a liver metastasis (SN12L1) and ascites (SN12A1) also exhibited unique biologic properties. These findings raise a second question: which organ site of nude mice should be used for transplanting freshly isolated HRCC cells?

TABLE 18–1.
Local Growth and Metastasis of Human Renal Cell Carcinoma After Implantation of 1×10^6 Cells Into the Spleen or Renal Subcapsule of Nude Mice

Cell Line	Spleen			Renal Subcapsule		
	Local Growth*	Lung Metastases[†]		Local Growth	Lung Metastases[†]	
		Incidence	Median (Range)		Incidence	Median (Range)
SN12C	5/6	0/6	0 (0)	6/6	5/6	7 (0–21)
SN12S1	4/8	3/8	0 (0–37)	5/5	4/5	13 (0–158)
SN12K1	4/6	1/6	0 (0–3)	5/5	5/5	4 (2–61)
SN12L1	1/6	2/6	0 (0–1)	6/6	6/6	32 (17–64)
SN12A1	0/5	1/5	0 (0–1)	8/8	3/8	0 (0–7)

*Number of positive mice/number of mice injected.
[†]Lung tumor colonies, each exceeding 0.1 mm in diameter.

The growth rate of cells from the five lines varied under both in vitro and in vivo (subcutaneous or kidney implantation) conditions (Tables 18–1 and 18–2). There was no direct correlation between growth rates in vitro, at a subcutaneous site, or in the kidney. The growth rate of tumor cells in vitro can be regulated by manipulation of the environment (serum, media, temperature). Similarly, different organ environments influence the growth of some, although not all, tumor cells, as was predicted by the original "seed and soil" hypothesis of Paget (Poste and Fidler 1979; Morrissey et al. 1980; Hart and Fidler 1980; Tarin and Price 1981; Hart 1982; Tarin 1982; Kozlowski et al. 1984; Tarin et al. 1984a, b).

The growth of the HRCC in the skin, kidney, and liver metastasis and in the ascites form in nude mice must have selected for cells with different biologic properties. This conclusion is based on the following data. First, the highly malignant SN12L1 cells exhibited invasive and metastatic properties regardless of the organ site of implantation, whereas cells of the SN12A1 line were relatively nonmetastatic. Second, in nude mice, the metastatic properties of the cells were stable despite the 8-week-long assay. Third, the highest incidence of metastasis from most cell lines was produced subsequent to growth in the kidneys. In particular, cells of the highly metastatic SN12L1 line produced metastases to liver, lung, and lymph nodes. These results reemphasize that both tumor-cell properties and host factors determine the outcome of metastasis.

TABLE 18–2.
The Growth and Spread of HRCC Cells After Subcutaneous, Intravenous, or Intraperitoneal Implantation Into Nude Mice

Cell Line	Subcutaneous Injection			Intravenous Injection		Intraperitoneal Injection		
	Incidence of Tumors*	Lung Metastasis[†]		Experimental Lung Metastasis[†]		Incidence of Ascites	Lung Metastasis[†]	
		Incidence	Median (Range)	Incidence	Median (Range)		Incidence	Median (Range)
SN12C	5/6	4/5	7 (0–40)	1/6	0 (0–2)	2/6	1/6	0 (0–8)
SN12S1	5/6	5/5	28 (6–99)	6/6	1 (1–2)	4/6	2/6	0 (0–12)
SN12K1	5/6	3/5	4 (0–21)	4/6	2 (0–13)	3/5	4/5	2 (0–21)
SN12L1	7/7	6/7	5 (0–14)	4/5	4 (0-12)	2/6	1/6	0 (0–2)
SN12A1	5/6	4/5	1 (0–19)	0/6	0 (0)	5/6	2/6	0 (0–3)

*Number of positive mice/number of mice injected. Cell inoculum was 1×10^6 cells.
[†]Number of lung tumor colonies, each exceeding 0.1 mm in diameter.

TABLE 18–3.
Metastatic Behavior of Human Renal Cell Carcinoma Cells in Athymic Nude Mice

Cell Line	Route of Implantation*	Wk of Autopsy	No. of Lung Metastases, Median (Range)	Tumor Growth in Peritoneal Organs[†]
SN12C	SC	12	7 (1–74)	None
	RSC	8	27 (4–49)	6/7 diaphragm, 5/7 lymph nodes, 4/7 liver, ascites
SN12L1	IV	8	4 (0–12)	None
	SC	8	5 (0–14)	None
	IP	8	0 (0–2)	6/6 pancreas, diaphragm, lymph nodes, 4/6 seminal vesicles, 2/6 ascites, kidney
	Spleen	8	0 (0–1)	8/8 lymph nodes
	RSC	5	32[‡] (17–64)	6/6 pancreas, diaphragm, lymph nodes, 5/6 seminal vesicles, ascites, 4/6 liver

*SC = subcutaneous; RSC = renal subcapsule; IV = intravenous; IP = intraperitoneal.
[†]Number of mice with tumors/total number of mice injected.
[‡]The number of lung tumor colonies differed significantly from other groups injected with SN12L1 cells ($P<.005$).

DIFFERENT BEHAVIORS OF HUMAN RENAL CELL CARCINOMAS IMPLANTED INTO THE SKIN AND KIDNEY OF NUDE MICE

The injection of HRCC cells into the subcutis or renal subcapsule produced tumors in all the mice. The tumors in the kidney, however, grew more rapidly than did the subcutaneous tumors (Table 18–3). For this reason, nude mice injected with cells into the kidney became moribund well before mice injected subcutaneously. The difference in the sizes of tumors growing in the kidney or the skin was also significant (Naito 1987a, b).

Two weeks after tumor cells were injected subcutaneously, the nude mice exhibited small well-vascularized tumor nodules with areas of central necrosis surrounded by a thick fibrous capsule. At this time, the tumors in the injected kidney were localized in either the renal parenchyma or the capsule with prominent areas of invasive growth into the renal parenchyma. The kidney tumors were free of necrosis and were not encapsulated.

By 6 weeks after injection, the subcutaneous tumors exceeded 10 mm in diameter. They were well circumscribed and encapsulated by a fibrous connective tissue. Greater than 70% of the tumor was necrotic, and yet the periphery of the tumor mass was well vascularized. Some invasion into the muscle occurred. At this time, tumors in the kidney were larger and infiltrative. Most of the renal parenchyma was destroyed by the growing tumor, leaving only a part of the renal medulla uninvolved. The tumor adhered to the liver and peritoneum, and the diaphragm and mesenteric and omental lymph nodes contained growing cancer. Grossly apparent pulmonary metastases were also found in the mice (Naito et al. 1987a).

Tumor cell implantation into the kidney has been used to propagate human xenografts in nude mice and to detect responsiveness to drug therapy (Bogden et al. 1978; Bogden and Hoff 1984). However, growth in the kidney does not assure that metastasis will occur. For example, we have observed that although human colorectal carcinoma cells readily proliferate in the spleen and kidney of nude mice and frequently metastasize from the spleen, they do not metastasize from the kidney (Giavazzi et al. 1986b). Clinical observations have suggested that the response of human cancer metastases to anticancer drugs is also influenced by the anatomical location of the lesions. With few exceptions, metastases in lymph nodes and skin of women with breast carcinoma responded better than their skeletal or pulmonary metastases. Similar differential responses to various cytotoxic drugs have also been reported for metastatic lesions in different organs. Subcutaneously transplanted mouse neoplasms were sensitive to three cytotoxic agents, whereas the same tumor cells implanted intracerebrally were not. Although it is tempting to attribute the difference in chemotherapy response to heterogeneity in cell populations, the influence of the organ environment must not be ignored.

The viability and growth of tumor cells depend on an adequate source of nutrients. The degree of tumor vascularity can control the delivery of nutrients, clearance of metabolites, and the delivery of cytotoxic drugs to a lesion. Measurements of blood flow in subcutaneous tumors of rats reveal a lack of autoregulation in response to infusions of angiotensin II. Thus, the injection of angiotensin II should lead to contraction of normal blood vessels and could enhance chemotherapeutic drug delivery to tumors where the vessels are dilated. Finally, the extent of tumor angiogenesis, a host response to a growing neoplasm, differs among different organs, which obviously could contribute to a differential response of metastases to anticancer drugs.

CONCLUSIONS

The process of cancer metastasis is sequential and selective, and some of its events contain stochastic elements (Price et al. 1986). Metastatic growth constitutes the end point of many lethal events that few tumor cells can survive. Primary tumors have heterogeneous metastatic properties, and the outcome of metastasis depends on the interplay of tumor cells with various host factors. This concept is more optimistic than that of metastasis as a random process. A selective biologic process is regulated by the interaction of tumor cells with their host, and these complex interactions can be studied and manipulated.

Human neoplasms are biologically heterogeneous. The extensive cellular diversity found in malignant neoplasms is generated by the rapid emergence of clonal subpopulations of tumor cells with different properties that include invasion, metastasis, and responsiveness to treatment. By the time metastases are diagnosed, the lesion can be 1 cm^3 in size, thus containing greater than 10^9 cells. The destruction of 99.9% of the cells still leaves 10^6 cells to proliferate and rapidly generate biologic diversity, including those treatment-resistant variants that are the major obstacle to treating disseminated cancer (Fidler and Balch 1987).

The heterogeneous nature of metastatic human neoplasms can now be studied under defined conditions in athymic nude mice. Several methods for studying the biology of HRCC in the nude mouse have been described, as have techniques to assure the success of these studies. The data show that the young nude mouse can be a useful in vivo model for ascertaining the metastatic potential of HRCC and for selecting and maintaining cell variants of high metastatic potential from heterogeneous human tumors. The design of new therapeutic approaches to metastasis must be based on sound biologic principles. This model for HRCC permits a better understanding of the complexity of the processes of tumor evolution, progression, and metastasis—new knowledge that should lead to meaningful gains in the treatment of disseminated cancer.

REFERENCES

1. Bogden AE, Hoff DD. 1984. Comparison of the human tumor cloning and subrenal capsule assays. *Cancer Res* 44:1087–1090.
2. Bogden AE, Ketton DE, Cobb WR, et al. 1978. A rapid screening method for testing chemotherapeutic agents against human tumor xenografts, in Houchens DP, Ovejera AA (eds): *Proceedings of the Symposium on the Use of Athymic (Nude) Mice in Cancer Research.* New York, Gustav Fisher, pp 231–250.

3. Carr I. 1983. Lymphatic metastasis. *Cancer Metastasis Rev* 22:307–319.
4. Clayman RV, Figenshaw RS, Bear A, et al. 1985. Transplantation of human renal carcinomas into athymic mice. *Cancer Res* 45:2650–2656.
5. del Regato JA. 1977. Pathways of metastatic spread of malignant tumors. *Semin Oncol* 4:33–38.
6. Fidler IJ. 1984. The evolution of biological heterogeneity in metastatic neoplasm, in Nicolson GL, Milas L (eds): *Cancer Invasion and Metastasis: Biologic and Therapeutic Aspects.* New York, Raven Press, pp 5–30.
7. Fidler IJ. 1970. Metastasis: Quantitative analysis of distribution and fate of tumor emboli labeled with ^{125}I-5-iodo-2'-deoxyuridine. *JNCI* 45:773–782.
8. Fidler IJ. 1986. Rationale and methods for the use of nude mice to study the biology and therapy of human cancer metastasis. *Cancer Metastasis Rev* 5:29–49.
9. Fidler IJ. 1973a. The relationship of embolic homogeneity, number, size and viability to the incidence of experimental metastasis. *Eur J Cancer* 9:223–229.
10. Fidler IJ. 1973b. Selection of successive tumor lines for metastasis. *Nature (New Biol)* 242:148–149.
11. Fidler IJ, Balch CM. 1987. The biology of cancer metastasis and implications for therapy. *Curr Probl Surg* 24:129–209.
12. Fidler IJ, Hart IR. 1982. Biological diversity in metastatic neoplasms: Origins and implications. *Science* 217:998–1003.
13. Fidler IJ, Kripke ML. 1977. Metastasis results from pre-existing variant cells within a malignant tumor. *Science* 197:893–895.
14. Fidler IJ, Nicolson GL. 1976. Organ selectivity for implantation, survival, and growth of B16 melanoma variant tumor lines. *JNCI* 57:1199–1202.
15. Fidler IJ, Poste G. 1985. The cellular heterogeneity of malignant neoplasms: Implications for adjuvant chemotherapy. *Semin Oncol* 12:207–221.
16. Fidler IJ, Gersten DM, Hart IR. 1978. The biology of cancer invasion and metastasis. *Adv Cancer Res* 28:149–250.
17. Folkman J, Klagsburn M. 1987. Angiogenic factors. *Science* 235:444–447.
18. Giavazzi R, Campbell DE, Jessup JM, et al. 1986a. Metastatic behavior of tumor cells isolated from primary and metastatic human colorectal carcinomas implanted into different sites in nude mice. *Cancer Res* 46:1928–1933.
19. Giavazzi R, Jessup JM, Campbell DE, et al. 1986b. Experimental nude mouse model of human colorectal cancer liver metastases. *JNCI* 77:1303–1308.
20. Hanna N. 1980. Expression of metastatic potential of tumor cells in young nude mice is correlated with low levels of natural killer cell-mediated cytotoxicity. *Int J Cancer* 26:675–680.
21. Hart IR. 1982. "Seed and soil" revisited: Mechanisms of site-specific metastasis. *Cancer Metastasis Rev* 1:5–17.
22. Hart IR, Fidler IJ. 1980. Role of organ selectivity in the determination of metastatic patterns of B16 melanoma. *Cancer Res* 40:2281–2287.
23. Hoehn WA, Schroeder FH. 1978. Renal cell carcinoma: Two new cell lines and a serially transplantable nude mouse tumor (NC 65). *Invest Urol* 16:106–112.
24. Katsuoka Y, Baba S, Hata M, et al. 1976. Transplantation of human renal cell carcinoma to the nude mice: As an intermediate of in vivo and in vitro studies. *J Urol* 115:373–376.
25. Kozlowski JM, Fidler IJ, Campbell D, et al. 1984. Metastatic behavior of human tumor cell lines grown in the nude mouse. *Cancer Res* 44:3522–3529.
26. Liotta LA. 1986. Tumor invasion and metastases: Role of the extracellular matrix. Rhoads Memorial Award Lecture. *Cancer Res* 46:1–7.
27. Luria SE, Delbruck M. 1943. Mutations of bacteria from virus sensitivity to virus resistance. *Genetics* 28:491-511.
28. Mareel MM. 1983. Invasion in vitro: Methods of analysis. *Cancer Metastasis Rev* 2:201–219.
29. Morrissey LW, Sidky YA, Auerbach R. 1980. Regional differences in the growth of tumor cells injected intraperitoneally into syngeneic mice. *Cancer Res* 40:2197–2201.
30. Naito S, Giavazzi R, Walker SM, et al. 1987a. Growth and metastatic behavior of human tumor cells implanted into nude mice. *Clin Exp Metastasis* 5:135–146.

31. Naito S, Kanamuri T, Hisano S, et al. 1982. Human renal cell carcinoma: Establishment and characterization of two new cell lines. *J Urol* 128:1117–1122.

32. Naito S, von Eschenbach AC, Fidler IJ. 1987b. Different growth pattern and biologic behavior of human renal cell carcinoma implanted into different organs of nude mice. *JNCI* 78:377–385.

33. Naito S, von Eschenbach AC, Giavazzi R, et al. 1986. Growth and metastasis of tumor cells isolated from a human renal cell carcinoma implanted into different organs of nude mice. *Cancer Res* 46:4109–4115.

34. Nicolson GL. 1982a. Metastatic tumor cell attachment and invasion assay utilizing vascular endothelial cell monolayer. *J Histochem Cytochem* 30:214–220.

35. Nicolson GL. 1982b. Cancer metastasis: Organ colonization and the cell-surface properties of malignant cells. *Biochim Biophys Acta* 695:113–176.

36. Nicolson GL, Dulski K, Basson C, et al. 1985. Preferential organ attachment and invasion in vitro by B16 melanoma cells selected for differing metastatic colonization and invasive properties. *Invasion Metastasis* 5:144–158.

37. Otto U, Huland H, Baisch H, et al. 1984a. Transplantation of human renal cell carcinoma into NMRI nu/nu mice. II. Evaluation of response to vinblastine sulfate monotherapy. *J Urol* 131:134–138.

38. Otto U, Kloppel G, Baisch H. 1984b. Transplantation of human renal cell carcinoma into NMRI nu/nu mice. I. Reliability of an experimental tumor model. *J Urol* 131:130–133.

39. Otto U, Kollerman MW, Kloppel W, et al. 1981. Transplantation von menschlichem Nierenadenokarzinomgewebe auf die nackte Maus. *Urol Int* 36:110–116.

40. Paget S. 1889. The distribution of secondary growths in cancer of the breast. *Lancet* 1:571–573.

41. Pauli BU, Schwartz DE, Thonar EJ, et al. 1983. Tumor invasion and host extracellular matrix. *Cancer Metastasis Rev* 2:129–152.

42. Pollack VA, Fidler IJ. 1982. Use of young nude mice to select subpopulations of tumor cells with increased metastatic potential from nonsyngeneic neoplasms. *JNCI* 69:137–141.

43. Poste G. 1982. Experimental systems for analysis of the malignant phenotype. *Cancer Metastasis Rev* 1:141–199.

44. Poste G. 1986. Pathogenesis of metastatic disease: Implications for current therapy and for the development of new therapeutic strategies. *Cancer Treat Rep* 70:183–199.

45. Poste G, Fidler IJ. 1979. The pathogenesis of cancer metastasis. *Nature* 283:139–146.

46. Price JE, Aukerman SL, Fidler IJ. 1986. Evidence that the process of murine melanoma metastasis is sequential and selective and contains stochastic elements. *Cancer Res* 46:5172-5178.

47. Rygaard J, Povlsen CO. 1969. Heterotransplantation of a human malignant tumor to "nude" mice. *Acta Pathol Microbiol Scand* 77:758–760.

48. Sharkey FE, Fogh J. 1984. Considerations in the use of nude mice for cancer research. *Cancer Metastasis Rev* 3:341–360.

49. Talmadge JE, Fidler IJ. 1982. Cancer metastasis is selective or random depending on the parent tumor population. *Nature* 27:593–594.

50. Tarin D. 1982. Investigations of the mechanisms of metastatic spread of naturally occurring neoplasms. *Cancer Metastasis Rev* 1:215–225.

51. Tarin D, Price JE. 1981. Influence of microenvironment and vascular anatomy on "metastatic" colonization potential of mammary tumors. *Cancer Res* 41:3604–3609.

52. Tarin D, Price JE, Kettlewell MGW, et al. 1984a. Clinicopathological observations on metastasis in man studied in patients treated with peritoneovenous shunts. *Br Med J* 288:749–751.

53. Tarin D, Price JE, Kettlewell MGW, et al. 1984b. Mechanisms of human tumor metastasis studied in patients with peritoneovenous shunts. *Cancer Res* 44:3584–3592.

54. Weiss L. 1986. Metastatic inefficiency: Causes and consequences. *Cancer Rev* 3:1–24.

55. Weiss L. 1985. *Principles of Metastasis.* Orlando, Fla, Academic Press.

Chapter 19

Renal Cell Carcinoma: Commentary

Douglas E. Johnson, M.D.

Andrew C. von Eschenbach, M.D.

Christopher J. Logothetis, M.D.

No malignancy has proved more resistant and unyielding to cellular alteration and destruction by systemic chemotherapy than renal cell carcinoma. Our disappointments and frustrations have been well chronicled by Yagoda in Chapter 15. Of the myriad drugs that have been tested for activity against metastatic renal cell carcinoma, either alone or in combinations, vinblastine originally appeared to be the most active (Hrushesky and Murphy 1977). Early reports recorded 14 objective regressions induced by vinblastine in 60 patients studied (Talley 1973; Hagan et al. 1974), but continued experience confirmed only marginal antitumor activity.

In the absence of effective chemotherapy, and after animal studies suggested that renal cell carcinoma was hormonally dependent (Kirkman 1959), it was only natural that interest would be directed towards hormonal therapy. Bloom (1973), an early advocate of hormonal therapy, reported a 22% tumor regression rate in patients with metastatic renal cell carcinoma. However, subsequent controlled clinical and laboratory studies failed to support the early enthusiasm. Nevertheless, physicians were slow to abandon its use owing to the lack of serious side effects and the dearth of effective chemotherapeutic agents.

The continued lack of effective drug therapy has led investigators to explore a number of other avenues—renal artery embolization, hyperthermia, and immunotherapy, either active using tumor vaccines or passive using transfer factor. Results with biologic-response modifiers were at first encouraging. Further experience with interferon, however, has shown that only a small, select population of patients appears to benefit from this form of therapy— namely, men whose performance status is good, whose primary tumor has been completely resected, whose metastases are confined to the chest, and whose overall tumor load is small (Quesada, Chapter 16). Although in some instances interferons seem to show promise, on other occasions they unfortunately enhance tumor activity. Consequently, whenever possible, a clonogenic assay as described by Strayer et al. (Chapter 17) should be performed, not only to identify patients likely to respond clinically to therapy, but also to identify patients who may be at risk for exacerbation of their disease as a result of treatment.

Wilms' tumor (Jaffe, Chapter 20) has served for decades as the model of what can be achieved in solid tumors with a multidisciplinary-multimodal approach, but no such inroads have been made in renal cell carcinoma. It may be, as suggested by Fidler (personal communication, 1987), that the effects of systemic chemotherapy directed at renal cell carcinoma are neutralized by the same cellular and biochemical mechanisms that protect the normal proximal renal tubular cells (from which renal cell carcinoma arises) from the effects of the toxins they excrete and secrete. Certainly, further research needs to be focused on these protective cellular mechanisms.

The physician today, as in the past, is left relying on surgical extirpation for curative therapy—be it for local, regional, or distant disease. The precepts suggested by Robson and colleagues (1968) for radical excision have undergone few modifications over the years. Only recently has the routine requirement for removing the ipsilateral adrenal gland along with the kidney, tumor, perirenal fat, and intact Gerota's capsule come under scrutiny. O'Brien and Lynch (1987) found only a 5.5% incidence of adrenal involvement in patients undergoing radical nephrectomy; all of these had upper-pole lesions, and the adrenal involvement was either apparent at surgery or on preoperative imaging studies. Consequently, it would appear that a modified radical nephrectomy, sparing the adrenal gland, is a satisfactory alternative to radical nephrectomy for patients whose tumors are localized to the middle and lower poles and whose preoperative computerized tomographic scans are normal.

There is also little clinical evidence to suggest that a formal ipsilateral retroperitoneal lymphadenectomy significantly increases survival. Nevertheless, the information it provides that relates to prognosis justifies its routine performance in all but the medically poor-risk patient. The presence of lymph node metastases, irrespective of other local-regional findings, reduces 5- and 10-year survival rates to 17% and 5%, respectively (Golimbu et al. 1986). This ominous finding may well alter what is done surgically, especially when a vena caval thrombus, with its added surgical risks, is also present. Tumor debulking, which has been advocated for some patients with other malignancies for which active antitumor drugs are available to use postoperatively, has proved futile for patients with renal cell carcinoma. The absence of currently available effective therapy precludes any consideration at the moment of routinely employing adjuvant therapy.

If we are ever to understand, predict, and control the various biologic behaviors of renal cell carcinoma, much additional information needs to be gathered regarding this tumor. Swanson and Raymond (Chapter 14) have emphasized the importance of assessing nuclear grade, ploidy, and DNA content. Fidler et al. (Chapter 18) have stressed the importance of studying the heterogeneous nature of this tumor under defined conditions. Several methods of investigation using nude mice are available that, in the near future, should provide more knowledge about the complex processes of tumor evolution, progression, and metastasis that in turn should lead to more successful therapy for patients with advanced disease. In the meantime, assessment should include clonogenic assays, especially for all patients in a high-risk category, so that, should metastasis subsequently develop, a tailored therapeutic regimen can be initiated using the drug or drugs most likely to have activity against the specific tumor.

REFERENCES

1. Bloom HJG. 1973. Hormone-induced and spontaneous regression of metastatic renal cancer. *Cancer* 32:1066–1071.
2. Golimbu M, Joshi P, Sperber A, et al. 1986. Renal cell carcinoma: Survival and prognostic factors. *Urology* 27:291–301.
3. Hagan K, Trapp JD, Rhamy RK, et al. 1974. Treatment of metastatic renal cell carcinoma. *South Med J* 67:1175–1178.

4. Hrushesky WJ, Murphy GP. 1977. Current status of the therapy of advanced renal carcinoma. *J Surg Oncol* 9:277–288.
5. Kirkman H. 1959. Estrogen-induced tumors of the kidney in the Syrian hamster. *NCI Monogr* 1:1–139.
6. O'Brien WM, Lynch JH. 1987. Adrenal metastases by renal cell carcinoma: Incidence at nephrectomy. *Urology* 29:605–607.
7. Robson CJ, Churchill BM, Anderson W. 1968. The result of radical nephrectomy for renal cell carcinoma. *Trans Am Assoc Genitourin Surg* 60:122–126.
8. Talley RW. 1973. Chemotherapy of adenocarcinoma of the kidney. *Cancer* 32:1062–1065.

Chapter 20

The Impact of Chemotherapy on Wilms' Tumor

Norman Jaffe, M.D., D.Sc.

Effective treatment for Wilms' tumor involves a rational application of surgery, radiation, and chemotherapy. The integration of these disciplines began after several chemotherapeutic agents were found to be active against the tumor. This discovery was followed by therapeutic investigation to determine optimum schedules and doses for administering the various components. These investigations were influenced by a new understanding of the pathology of Wilms' tumor and by changing concepts in the system of staging developed by individual institutions and two cooperative groups: the National Wilms' Tumor Study Group (NWTS) in the United States and the International Society for Pediatric Oncology (SIOP) in the United Kingdom and Europe. In this chapter, I review the evolution of the therapeutic protocols and the factors that have influenced their design, and outline protocols currently in use at The University of Texas M. D. Anderson Cancer Center.

PATHOLOGIC CONSIDERATIONS

Wilms' tumor is a complex mixed embryonal neoplasm composed of three elements: blastemal, epithelial, and stromal. Histologically, two broad categories have been recognized: favorable and unfavorable (Beckwith 1983). The favorable type is considered to be the "conventional" form and carries a good prognosis. It is characterized by blastemal, epithelial, and stromal elements devoid of atypia or anaplasia. Small areas of sarcomatous elements in the stroma of an otherwise favorable type apparently do not adversely influence the outlook. The unfavorable type is defined by marked enlargement of nuclei, hyperchromatism of the enlarged nuclei, and multipolar mitotic figures. It is composed of areas of anaplasia that may be focal or diffuse and that predict probable high rates of tumor relapse and death.

Nodal or other potentially metastatic sites are usually the most fertile areas in which to search for anaplasia. Anaplasia is extremely uncommon in patients under 2 years of age, and a high index of suspicion and more thorough sampling techniques are appropriate when it is identified in Wilms' tumor in older children. The phenomenon is usually not found once chemotherapy has been administered, and its presence in this circumstance is presumably prognostically significant. Anaplasia limited to skeletal muscle cells, however, does not appear to be associated with an increased incidence of relapse.

Recent studies have shown a remarkable correlation among the DNA content of Wilms' tumor cells, their histologic subtype, and treatment outcome (Douglass et al. 1986). One study also demonstrated that stemlines of both the primary tumor and metastases were in the diploid and low aneuploid (hyperdiploid) range (van Leeuwen et al. 1987). Tumors with a hyperdiploid content are characteristic of the anaplastic (unfavorable) variety of Wilms' tumor, have numerous complex translocations, and respond poorly to chemotherapy (Douglass et al. 1986; van Leeuwen et al. 1987).

Two separate malignant tumors of the kidney, distinctive from Wilms' tumor, have recently also been recognized (Beckwith 1983). They are "clear cell sarcoma" and "rhabdoid tumor." Clear cell sarcoma was apparently first described by Kidd in 1970, and Marsden et al. (1978) subsequently introduced the name "bone-metastasizing renal tumor of childhood" because of its predilection for bone metastases. It is highly malignant: 42% of the children with this disease described in the NWTS reports developed bone metastases. It responds poorly to the chemotherapeutic agents generally used for Wilms' tumor.

Malignant rhabdoid tumor of the kidney usually occurs in infants. It, too, is highly virulent—one of the most lethal neoplasms of early life. A number of cases have been associated with second primary neuroglial tumors in the midline posterior fossa of the skull (Marsden et al. 1978). The tumor is usually of extrarenal origin (Blatt et al. 1956) and is generally not responsive to conventional Wilms' tumor treatment (Bonnin et al. 1984).

Chemotherapy has been specifically designed for the favorable and the unfavorable types of Wilms' tumor; all other types are treated and analyzed separately.

STAGING

The NWTS introduced five stage classifications (D'Angio et al. 1976) (Table 20–1). "Stage" must not be confused with the term "group," which was used in the initial reports. Preliminary experience demonstrated the staging system to be functional and reliable; it was then refined, and the term "group" was replaced with the word "stage" (Farewell et al. 1981). This has now emerged as a universal mechanism of reporting.

CHEMOTHERAPY

The following chemotherapeutic agents have been shown to have various degrees of activity against Wilms' tumor: dactinomycin (actinomycin D) (Farber et al. 1960; Farber 1966), vincristine (Sutow et al. 1963; Sullivan et al. 1967; Sullivan 1968), cyclophosphamide

TABLE 20–1.
Staging of Wilms' Tumor

Stage	Extent of Disease
I	Tumor confined to kidney and completely resected
II	Microscopic residual tumor (penetration through capsule or into perirenal soft tissue)
III	Gross residual tumor confined to abdomen (lymph node involvement or diffuse peritoneal contamination)
IV	Hematogenous metastases (lung, noncontiguous liver, bone, brain)
V	Bilaterial Wilms' tumor

(Sutow 1967; Finkelstein et al. 1969), doxorubicin (Adriamycin) (Wang et al. 1971; Fossati-Bellani et al. 1975), etoposide (VP-16-213) (Chard et al. 1979), teniposide (VM-26) (Bleyer et al. 1979), and *cis*-diamminedichloroplatinum II (Kamalakor et al. 1977; Baum et al. 1981; Pratt et al. 1981).

Dactinomycin (formerly called actinomycin D) was one of the first agents shown to have therapeutic efficacy. Investigations demonstrated that it had three major anticancer properties: it was tumoricidal, it potentiated the action of radiation therapy, and it reactivated its latent effects (D'Angio et al. 1959; D'Angio 1962). These inherent characteristics were exploited to therapeutic advantage by administering it in combination with radiation therapy for metastatic disease. Later, it was used preoperatively with vincristine. Its most extensive use, however, was as adjuvant postoperative chemotherapy, which improved the survival rate of patients with localized and advanced disease (Tan et al. 1959; Farber 1966; Fernbach and Martyn 1966). Initial (collective) investigations demonstrated that the cure rate for patients receiving dactinomycin as adjuvant therapy was escalated to 50% (175/348) as compared with 35% (128/370) for those not receiving this treatment (Sutow 1979).

The demonstration that dactinomycin was effective against Wilms' tumor was followed by efforts to determine an optimum schedule of administration. Preliminary studies revealed that the relapse rate was higher when patients received single courses of therapy (52%) rather than multiple courses (14%); however, salvaging patients with multidisciplinary strategies eventually yielded an ultimate survival rate not significantly different (71% vs. 80%) (Wolff et al. 1968, 1974). The SIOP later also reported no difference in relapse rates (54% vs. 58%) or in overall survival rate (86% vs. 82%) after single or multiple courses of dactinomycin (Lemerle et al. 1976).

Investigations of vincristine for Wilms' tumor commenced almost a decade after the discovery of the efficacy of dactinomycin (Sutow et al. 1963; Sullivan et al. 1967; Sullivan 1968). The ability of vincristine to produce rapid tumor regression in metastatic disease showed it to be highly active. This prompted its extensive use as a preoperative maneuver. During this period, only limited studies were performed to test its efficacy as adjuvant therapy. Later, however, the Medical Research Council of the United Kingdom (MRC) reported that intensive vincristine therapy was superior to an adjuvant dactinomycin schedule administered every 3 months (Medical Research Council Working Party on Embryonal Tumor in Childhood 1978). This demonstrated the need to define an optimum dosage and schedule of adjuvant treatment.

In the beginning of the 1970s, two collaborating institutions in Boston, the Children's Cancer Research Foundation (subsequently designated the Dana-Farber Cancer Institute) and the Children's Hospital and Medical Center, noted that the combination of vincristine and dactinomycin was highly effective in eradicating overt disease (Fig 20–1). Investigations also demonstrated that the combination could be used successfully as postoperative adjuvant treatment. An overall survival rate of 80% was reported for patients treated during various stages of the disease (Cassidy et al. 1973).

The above result was later confirmed for a larger number of patients in a separate study, NWTS-1 (D'Angio et al. 1976). The study concurrently demonstrated that, in an adjuvant setting, the combination of vincristine and dactinomycin was superior to either drug alone. A subsection of the investigation demonstrated that preoperative vincristine did not confer any overall survival advantage for previously untreated patients with stage IV disease and pulmonary metastases.

The demonstration that adjuvant chemotherapy improved survival rates for patients with Wilms' tumor led to concentrated efforts to devise new and more effective regimens (D'Angio et al. 1980). The vincristine and dactinomycin combination was adopted as the yardstick by

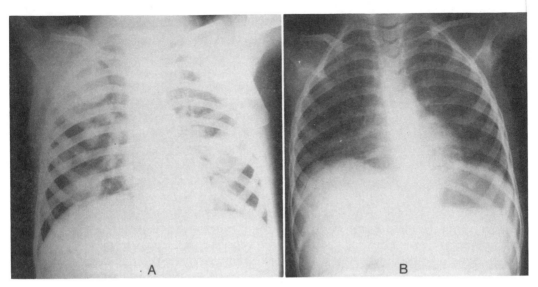

FIG 20–1.
A, chest radiograph demonstrating pulmonary metastases from Wilms' tumor. **B**, 4 weeks later, after treatment with vincristine and dactinomycin (actinomycin D), a dramatic reduction in the number and size of metastases. (From Jaffe N. 1977. Metastasis in malignant childhood tumor: The role of "adjuvant" therapy and the utility of multidisciplinary treatment. *Semin Oncol* 4:119. Used by permission.)

which all subsequent therapeutic protocols were to be measured. The next NWTS study, NWTS-2, attempted to compare its efficacy with that of a three-drug regimen, vincristine, dactinomycin and Adriamycin, in patients with stage II–III disease, some of whom also received postoperative abdominal radiation. The results demonstrated that the relapse-free survival rate for group II–IV, favorable histology, with vincristine and dactinomycin was 63% and with the three-drug regimen was 77%, a difference that was statistically significant ($P = .0004$) (D'Angio et al. 1981).

The addition of Adriamycin to vincristine and dactinomycin as described above did not specifically improve the relapse-free survival rates of patients with stage IV disease or with unfavorable tumors. Further, although the three-drug regimen was found to be superior, researchers considered that the result could possibly also be attributed to a greater dose intensity, inasmuch as the three-drug regimen was delivered more frequently.

During the 1970s, additional forms of combination chemotherapy were shown to be effective against Wilms' tumor. A study of combined vincristine, dactinomycin (actinomycin D), and cyclophosphamide (VAC) in 10 patients yielded a response rate of 100% (6 complete and 4 partial responses) (Ortega et al. 1980). Similarly, a combination of vincristine, dactinomycin, cyclophosphamide, and Adriamycin (DAVE) produced a 100% response (two complete and two partial responses) in four patients with metastatic disease (Dungar et al. 1981). Finally, a combination of vincristine and Adriamycin as adjuvant therapy yielded results similar to those of vincristine and dactinomycin (Camitta et al. 1982).

The improved results achieved with chemotherapy led to additional attempts at modifications and refinements in treatment. Principally these involved studies to determine the feasibility of curtailing the duration of adjuvant chemotherapy. The NWTS-3 investigated the possibility of reducing treatment of stage I disease from 6 months to 3 months. The possibility of eliminating radiation therapy for patients with stage II disease was also studied (D'Angio et al. 1980, 1981). Results of these studies have not been published except in abstract form (D'Angio 1984), and in the interim it would appear prudent to administer treatment to patients with stage I disease for 6 months and to those with more advanced disease for a minimum of 15 months. Preliminary results suggest that radiation therapy is not required for stage II disease.

CHEMOTHERAPY USED AT M. D. ANDERSON CANCER CENTER

Adjuvant Chemotherapy

Adjuvant therapy is based on surgicopathologic staging and incorporates experiences gleaned from individual institutions, the NWTS, and the SIOP. The regimens comprise agents with different mechanisms of action and minimal overlapping toxicities. The tactics and strategies are based on principles established to eradicate cancer (Skipper et al. 1965; Laster et al. 1969; Schabel 1975), which have been extrapolated for use not only against Wilms' tumor but also against other pediatric neoplasms (Jaffe 1977; Jaffe et al. 1977, 1981).

The favorable histologic type is treated with vincristine and actinomycin D (Table 20–2). The unfavorable histologic type is treated with vincristine, Adriamycin, cyclophosphamide, and dactinomycin (A-VAC, Table 20–3). Definitive surgical treatment is performed as soon as feasible, and radiation therapy is individualized according to stage. Chemotherapy commences within 1 week of nephrectomy, as soon as normal bowel mobility is established.

Preoperative Chemotherapy

Preoperative chemotherapy is used for two major categories, inoperable tumors and bilateral Wilms' tumor.

Inoperable Wilms' Tumor

Chemotherapy is administered to all patients who, on admission, have tumors that appear potentially inoperable. Selection is dictated by histologic criteria, frequently established on a specimen obtained by needle biopsy (vide infra). Tumors of favorable histologic type are treated with vincristine and dactinomycin, whereas treatment of the unfavorable variety is with vincristine, Adriamycin, cyclophosphamide, and dactinomycin (see Tables 20–2 and 20–3). Tumors in the unfavorable category are considered to be stage III unless metastases (stage IV) are present.

The experience at UT M. D. Anderson Cancer Center on which this approach is based has been published (Bracken et al. 1982). The inoperable tumors in 16 of 19 patients were rendered operable with preoperative vincristine therapy. A few patients were also treated with radiation and dactinomycin. In the majority, tumor size was gratifyingly reduced, permitting safe surgical procedures. Postoperative treatment generally comprised vincristine and dactinomycin and resulted in cure in 10 of the 19 patients (53%). Similar experiences have been reported by others (Wagget and Koop 1970; Kumar et al. 1975; Wagner and Parresh 1981; Broecker and Perlmutter 1986).

Bilateral Wilms' Tumor

Chemotherapy for bilateral tumors is identical to that employed for inoperable tumors. The hope is that it will render the tumors amenable to surgical extirpation, which may comprise unilateral nephrectomy and contralateral partial nephrectomy or bilateral partial nephrectomies. These maneuvers permit ablation of viable neoplasm and conservation of healthy tissue. The type of surgery is dictated by the extent of tumor and response to

TABLE 20–2.
Treatment of Wilms' Tumor, Favorable Histologic Type

Stage	Chemotherapy*	Radiation	Duration
I	Vincristine Dactinomycin		6 mo
II	Vincristine Dactinomycin		6–12 mo
III	Vincristine Dactinomycin	Abdomen (1,000 cGy)	12–18 mo
IV	Vincristine Dactinomycin	Abdomen, thorax (1,000 cGy each)	18 mo

*Dose and schedule: Vincristine: 1.5 mg/m²/wk × 12 (initially); 1.5 mg/m² days 1 and 5 with dactinomycin (actinomycin D) (every 4 weeks). Dactinomycin: 0.015 mg/kg/day × 5 every 4 weeks (daily dose not to exceed 0.500 mg). Note: Regimen L or K from the National Wilms' Tumor Study III has occasionaly been used.

TABLE 20–3.
Treatment of Wilms' Tumor, Unfavorable Histologic Type (Anaplastic)*

Stage	Chemotherapy[†]	Radiation	Duration
I	Vincristine Dactinomycin		6 mo
II	A-VAC		6–12 mo
III	A-VAC	Abdomen (1,000 cGy)	12–18 mo
IV	A-VAC	Abdomen, thorax (1,000 cGy each)	18 mo

*A-VAC = Adriamycin, vincristine, actinomycin D (dactinomycin), cyclophosphamide.
[†]Dosages and schedules: Stage I, same as for favorable histologic type. Stages II–IV, A-VAC. *Initial phase*: Vincristine, 1.5 mg/m²/wk × 12. Adriamycin, 60 mg/m² by 20 degree infusion every 3 weeks (maximum cumulative dosage 300 mg/m²). Cyclophosphamide, 600 mg/m² by 20 degree infusion every 3 weeks. *VAC phase*: Vincristine, 1.5 mg/m², days 1 and 5. Cyclophosphamide, 300 mg/m²/day × 3–5 every 4 weeks. Actinomycin D, 0.250 mg/m²/day × 5 every 4 weeks (daily dose not to exceed 0.500 mg).

chemotherapy. Postoperatively, chemotherapy and occasionally radiation therapy may also be administered. These therapeutic strategies have yielded survival rates in the vicinity of 60% to 85% (Bishop et al. 1977; Malcolm et al. 1980; Asch et al. 1985). Nonsurgical cure with vincristine and dactinomycin, occasionally supplemented by radiation therapy, has also been reported (Dennicol and Koff 1984; Kay and Tark 1986).

Special Chemotherapy Considerations

Preoperative Chemotherapy to Downstage Tumors

Consecutive trials conducted by the SIOP have demonstrated that a majority of tumors can be downstaged with preoperative radiation therapy and chemotherapy (Tournade et al. 1986). Initial studies also revealed that radiation therapy was effective in preventing abdominal rupture (Lemerle et al. 1976). These studies were followed by the demonstration that preoperative radiation and chemotherapy were equally effective (Lemerle et al. 1983). A recent summary of the SIOP experience revealed that preoperative therapy could escalate the proportion of stage I Wilms' tumors at surgery from 22% to 48%. Further, preoperative treatment with dactinomycin and vincristine permitted 312 of 373 tumors (84%) to be staged as I or II with negative lymph nodes (Voute et al. 1987). This eliminated the need for radiation as a component of local therapy.

Preoperative chemotherapy and radiation therapy are not employed as "routine and standard" treatment for tumors treated initially at UT M. D. Anderson Cancer Center. Such treatment may alter the surgicopathologic staging and invalidate important prognostic variables. It may also inadvertently be administered for benign conditions if the correct diagnosis has not been established.

Salvage Chemotherapy

Patients with favorable tumors may relapse during or following conventional therapy with vincristine and dactinomycin. Such patients can occasionally be salvaged with an alternative treatment. In these circumstances, combination chemotherapy with vincristine and Adriamycin, A-VAC, or VAC is usually attempted (Ortega et al. 1980). An example of the successful application of alternative chemotherapy for relapse in a patient with a favorable tumor is depicted in Figure 20–2. In some instances, radiation therapy may be added to the chemotherapeutic regimen.

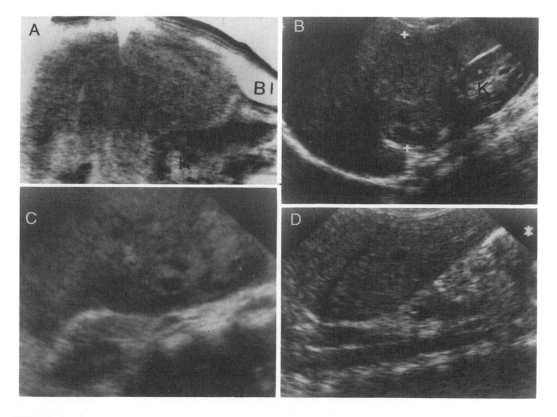

FIG 20–2.
A, abdominal ultrasound demonstrating kidney (*K*), a large Wilms' tumor (*T*), and bladder (*Bl*). **B,** 2 months later, after treatment with vincristine and dactinomycin (actinomycin D), the tumor mass was moderately reduced and the tumor was excised. **C,** 7 months later, recurrent tumor diffusely involved the liver. This was accompanied by hemorrhagic ascites. **D,** interval resolution of hepatic metastases and ascites with dactinomycin and cyclophosphamide. The patient was then treated with cisplatin and etoposide (VP-16-213) as adjuvant therapy.

Several studies have demonstrated that a combination of cisplatin and etoposide is also effective in rescuing a cohort of patients who relapse during or following conventional treatment (Douglass et al. 1987; Loh et al. 1987). This combination is receiving increasing recognition as "retrieval therapy" in view of its initial promising results. Should the preliminary experience be confirmed, consideration may be given to adopting the regimen as front-line treatment, especially for patients in a high-risk (unfavorable histologic type) category.

Chemotherapy-Induced Histologic Changes

Investigations have demonstrated that chemotherapy induces marked changes in the undifferentiated stroma of patients who received it preoperatively. In some instances the blastemous nodules became necrotic and smaller. Differentiated elements including the glomeruloid, tubular, and rhabdomyoblastic components appeared unaffected (Guarda et al. 1984). It is possible that the blastema plays a central role in prognosis because of either its susceptibility to treatment or, if insensitive, its predilection to metastasis (van Leeuwen et al. 1987).

"Maturation" of metastases following chemotherapy and radiation has also been reported (Omar et al. 1986). The mature metastatic nodules were composed of differentiated mesenchymal elements similar to those encountered in the primary tumor. It has been suggested that malignant cells may be induced to revert into phenotypically benign counterparts by selectively destroying the more anaplastic cells.

Chemotherapy for Neoplasms Associated With Wilms' Tumor

Mesoblastic Nephroma.—This is a unique mesodermal neoplasm of the infant kidney that rarely metastasizes (Bolande 1983). One report noted that vincristine and dactinomycin administered to a patient as adjuvant chemotherapy did not prevent metastasis, although metastatic disease in another improved with vincristine, Adriamycin, and cyclophosphamide therapy (Steinfeld et al. 1984).

Nephroblastomatosis.—This term generally refers to the abnormal persistence of embryonal renal tissue that may be associated with the development of Wilms' tumor (Hou and Holman 1961; Huff 1973; Bove and McAdams 1976; Machin 1980a, b; Telander et al. 1980; Heideman et al. 1985). Heideman and his coworkers (1985) suggested that a brief course of relatively nontoxic chemotherapy (vincristine and dactinomycin) might be beneficial by reducing the large volume of the kidneys. It is unknown if chemotherapy can also reduce the instance of subsequent Wilms' tumor. Persistent nodular renal blastoma and associated nephroblastic abnormalities appear to remain in the kidneys of many if not all the treated patients, despite a reduction in renal volume (Heideman et al. 1985). The favorable survival rate and response to chemotherapy of bilateral Wilms' tumor may suggest a strong relationship of the latter to the nodular renal blastema-nephroblastomatosis complex (Kay and Tank 1986).

Toxicity of Chemotherapy

Chemotherapy is generally not well tolerated by children less than 1 year old. For such young children, a reduction of 50% of the recommended dosage is generally advocated (Jones et al. 1984). Adriamycin may cause heart failure (Gillidoga et al. 1976) and is therefore not incorporated into the routine treatment of favorable Wilms' tumor at UT M. D. Anderson Cancer Center. When used for the unfavorable type, the maximum cumulative dose is restricted to 300 mg/m². This reduces the potential for cardiac failure, particularly if pulmonary radiation is also to be administered (Greenwood et al. 1974). Patients with left-sided Wilms' tumor who receive radiation to the tumor bed are possibly at an increased risk of developing heart failure (Pinkel et al. 1982).

Cyclophosphamide may also cause heart failure (Mills and Roberts 1979). Its major complication, however, is hemorrhagic cystitis (Coggins et al. 1959). This is more prone to develop in patients who receive concurrent radiation therapy to the abdomen and pelvis (Jayalakshmamma and Pinkel 1976). In all circumstances, appropriate pretreatment and post-treatment hydration is employed in an effort to prevent the complication. Cyclophosphamide may also cause aspermia (Fairley et al. 1972) and has been linked to the development of leukemia (Tucker et al. 1984).

Vincristine, dactinomycin, Adriamycin, and radiation therapy may prevent compensatory hypertrophy of the liver following a partial hepatectomy (Filler et al. 1969), which may be required for localized metastatic disease. After partial hepatectomy, therefore, chemotherapy (and radiation) should be withheld to permit sufficient time for healing and hepatic regeneration. This generally requires 3 to 4 weeks after the surgical procedure.

Vincristine and dactinomycin, although causing acute toxicity, are generally well tolerated and have not been reported to have permanent delayed sequelae.

DIAGNOSTIC PROCEDURES

New Imaging Techniques

Because of the success achieved with chemotherapy and the availability of sophisticated diagnostic procedures, surgical extirpation is no longer considered an urgent necessity. Ultrasound and computerized axial tomography can define the exact extent of tumor, allowing the physician to implement a planned surgical procedure (De Campo 1986; Reiman et al. 1986). Frequently noninvasive imaging can also help in establishing a therapeutic response. Response in tumors initially considered inoperable usually manifests itself as necrosis and reduced size, although occasionally necrosis alone may be the only indication of response (Shimizu et al. 1987).

Invasion of the vena cava can be demonstrated by ultrasound. This information is critical. It indicates the need for preoperative chemotherapy, which usually causes tumor shrinkage, eradicates the intravascular component, and simplifies the surgical procedure (Kogan et al. 1986). An example of the elimination of tumor in the vena cava with preoperative chemotherapy is shown in Figure 20–3.

Fine-Needle Biopsy

Successful results achieved with chemotherapy have permitted enthusiastic adoption of fine-needle aspiration for diagnostic purposes (Taylor and Nunez 1984; Ducos et al. 1987). This has not been associated with untoward effects, and it is presumed that the procedure, if complicated by microscopic spillage, is rendered safe with effective chemotherapy.

IMPACT OF CHEMOTHERAPY ON PROGNOSTIC FACTORS

A number of prognostic factors have been considered in assessing the outcome of Wilms' tumor. These include patient weight, patient age, tumor extension into the renal vein, epithelial differentiation, and lymph node invasion (Cassidy et al. 1973; D'Angio et al. 1976; Breslow et al. 1986). As a consequence of the efficacy of chemotherapy, the significance of

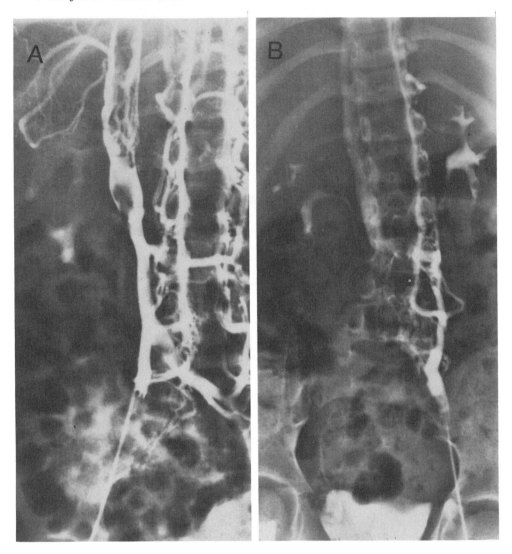

FIG 20–3.
A, inferior vena cavagram demonstrating obstruction by tumor and collateral vessels. **B**, recanalization of inferior vena cava and reduction in collateral circulation after treatment with vincristine and dactinomycin.

many of these factors has been eliminated. Currently, for patients without metastases at diagnosis, only two major factors appear to be independent variables predicting the likelihood of relapse-free survival: tumor histologic type (favorable vs. unfavorable) and regional lymph node invasion (stage III disease) (Breslow et al. 1985). Patients with favorable tumors and metastases at diagnosis have a survival rate comparable to those with stage III (vide infra) (Breslow et al. 1986). For those with unfavorable tumors (anaplastic or sarcomatous), survival expectations are poor regardless of treatment or stage (Breslow et al. 1986).

CURE

Based on reports published by the NWTS, the SIOP, and individual institutions (Cassidy et al. 1973; Lemerle et al. 1983; D'Angio et al. 1984; Allen et al. 1985; Breslow et al. 1985,

1986; Tournade et al. 1986; Green 1987; Voute et al. 1987), patients with favorable histologic types may anticipate the following 3-year survival rates: stage I, 90% to 95%; stages II–III, 80% to 90%; and stage IV, 70% to 80%. All-stage survival is approximately 80% and approaches 100% for the lower stages (Cassidy et al. 1973; Allen et al. 1985). These results, despite occasional late relapses (Kim et al. 1985), are tantamount to cure. Salvage of patients with favorable tumors who relapse while receiving chemotherapy is generally in the vicinity of 30% to 40%. Because of the small numbers evaluated, it is difficult to estimate survival rates for patients with unfavorable tumors. However, for those with stage I disease it is probably 70% to 90%; survival expectation for the other stages is extremely poor.

LATE EFFECTS

Wilms' tumor is considered to be the paradigm of treatment of pediatric solid tumors. However, despite the reported successes, improved survival percentages have been accompanied by delayed sequelae induced by therapy. These include scoliosis, pulmonary fibrosis, reproductive problems, congestive cardiac failure, and gastrointestinal complications (Jaffe et al. 1980). New therapeutic trends have consequently evolved in an effort to reduce or eliminate such complications. These involve in particular modifications in chemotherapy and radiation therapy and constitute a major component of the regimens currently under investigation in group-wide studies (D'Angio et al. 1984; Green 1987).

CONCLUSION

The improved cure rates in Wilms' tumor bear eloquent testimony to the successful application of multidisciplinary treatment. The cornerstone of success is the efficacy of chemotherapy, which has been a fundamental component of the evolving strategies. Current regimens are based on surgicopathologic staging and histologic tumor subtype and are designed to achieve maximum cure with minimal toxicity.

REFERENCES

1. Allen JE, Brecher MJ, Karp MP. 1985. Wilms' tumor—treatment and results: A five-decade experience. *J Surg Oncol* 30:235–239.
2. Asch MJ, Siegel S, White L, et al. 1985. Prognostic factors and outcome in bilateral Wilms' tumor. *Cancer* 56:2524–2529.
3. Baum ES, Gaynon P, Greenberg L. 1981. Phase II trial of cisplatin in refractory childhood cancer: Children's Cancer Study Group report. *Cancer Treat Rep* 85:815–822.
4. Bishop HC, Tefft M, Evans AE, et al. 1977. Survival in bilateral Wilms' tumor: Review of 30 National Wilms' Tumor Study cases. *J Pediatr Surg* 12:631–638.
5. Beckwith JB. 1983. Wilms' tumor and other renal tumors of childhood: A selective review from the National Wilms' Tumor Study Pathology Center. *Hum Pathol* 14:481–492.
6. Blatt J, Russo P, Taylor S. 1986. Extrarenal rhabdoid sarcoma. *Med Pediatr Oncol* 14:221–226.
7. Bleyer WA, Krivit W, Chard RL. 1979. Phase II study of VM-26 in acute leukemia, neuroblastoma and other refractory childhood malignancies: A report from the Children's Cancer Study Group. *Cancer Treat Rep* 63:977–981.
8. Bolande RP. 1983. Congenital mesoblastic nephroma of infancy. *Perspect Pediatr Pathol* 1:227–250.
9. Bonnin J, Rubinstein LJ, Palmer NF. 1984. The association of embryonal tumor originating in the kidney and in the brain. *Cancer* 54:2137–2146.

10. Bove KE, McAdams AJ. 1976. The nephroblastomatosis complex and its relationship to Wilms' tumor: A clinicopathologic treatise, in Rosenberg H, Bolande R (eds): *Perspectives in Pediatric Pathology*, vol 3. Chicago: Year Book Medical Publishers, pp 185–222.

11. Bracken RB, Sutow WW, Jaffe N, et al. 1982. Preoperative chemotherapy for Wilms' tumor. *Urology* 19:55–60.

12. Breslow N, Churchill G, Beckwith JB. 1985. Prognosis for Wilms' tumor patients with nonmetastatic disease at diagnosis: Results of the Second National Wilms' Tumor Study. *J Clin Oncol* 3:521–531.

13. Breslow NE, Churchill G, Nesmith B. 1986. Clinicopathologic features and prognosis for Wilms' tumor patients with metastases at diagnosis. *Cancer* 58:2501–2511.

14. Broecker BH, Perlmutter AD. 1986. Management of unresectable Wilms' tumor. *Urology* 24:170–174.

15. Camitta B, Kun L, Glicklich M, et al. 1982. Doxorubicin vincristine therapy for Wilms' tumor: A pilot study. *Cancer Treat Rep* 66:1791-1794.

16. Cassidy JR, Tefft M, Filler RM, et al. 1973. Considerations in the radiation therapy of Wilms' tumor. *Cancer* 32:598–608.

17. Chard RL, Krivit W, Bleyer WA. 1979. Phase II study of VP-16-213 in childhood malignant disease: A Children's Cancer Study Group report. *Cancer Treat Rep* 63:1755–1759.

18. Coggins PR, Ravden RG, Eisman SM. 1959. Clinical pharmacology and preliminary evaluation of Cytoxan (cyclophosphamide). *Cancer Chemother Rep* 3:9–11.

19. D'Angio GJ. 1962. Clinical and biological studies of actinomycin D and roentgen irradiation. *Am J Roentgenol* 87:106–109.

20. D'Angio GJ, Beckwith JB, Breslow NE, et al. 1980. Wilms' tumor: An update. *Cancer* 45:1791–1798.

21. D'Angio GJ, Evans AE, Breslow N, et al. 1984. Results of the Third National Wilms' Tumor Study (NWTS-3): A preliminary report (abstract). *Proc Am Assoc Cancer Res* 25:183.

22. D'Angio GJ, Evans AE, Breslow NE. 1976. The treatment of Wilms' tumor: Results of the National Wilms' Tumor Study. *Cancer* 38:633–646.

23. D'Angio GJ, Evans AE, Breslow N, et al. 1981. The treatment of Wilms' tumor: Results of the Second National Wilms' Tumor Study. *Cancer* 47:2304–2311.

24. D'Angio GJ, Farber S, Maddock CL. 1959. Potentiation of x-ray effects of actinomycin-D. *Radiology* 73:175–177.

25. De Campo JF. 1986. Ultrasound of Wilms' tumor. *Pediatr Radiol* 16:21–24.

26. Dennicol NT, Koff WJ. 1984. Bilateral Wilms' tumor: Successful nonsurgical treatment. *J Brazilian Urol* 10:34–36.

27. Douglass EC, Look AT, Webber B, et al. 1986. Hyperdiploidy and chromosomal rearrangements define the anaplastic variant of Wilms' tumor. *J Clin Oncol* 4:975–981.

28. Douglass EC, Wilimas JA, Doty G, et al. 1987. Cis-platinum/VP-16 (DDP/VP) initial therapy in high risk (HR) Wilms' tumor (WT) (abstract). *Proc Am Assoc Cancer Res* 28:221.

29. Ducos R, Warrier R, Arensman R, et al. 1987. Needle biopsy and preoperative chemotherapy for massive unilateral and bilateral Wilms' tumor. *Pediatr Surg Int* 2:42–45.

30. Dungar DE, Malpas JS, Graham-Pole JR, et al. 1981. The use of four drug combination chemotherapy (DAVE) in the treatment of advanced Wilms' tumor. *Cancer Chemother Pharmacol* 5:211–215.

31. Fairley KF, Barrie JD, Johnson W. 1972. Sterility and testicular atrophy related to cyclophosphamide therapy. *Lancet* 1:568–569.

32. Farber S. 1966. Chemotherapy in the treatment of leukemia and Wilms' tumor. *JAMA* 198:826–836.

33. Farber S, D'Angio GJ, Evans A. 1960. Clinical studies of actinomycin D with special reference to Wilms' tumor in children. *Ann NY Acad Sci* 89:421–424.

34. Farewell VT, D'Angio GJ, Breslow N. 1981. Retrospective validation of a new staging system for Wilms' tumor. *Cancer Clin Trials* 4:167–171.

35. Fernbach DJ, Martyn DT. 1966. Role of dactinomycin in the improved survival of children with Wilms' tumor. *JAMA* 195:1005–1009.

36. Filler RM, Tefft M, Vawter GF, et al. 1969. Hepatic lobectomy in childhood: Effects of x-ray and chemotherapy. *J Pediatr Surg* 4:31–41.

37. Finkelstein JZ, Hittle RE, Hammond GD. 1969. Evaluation of a high dose cyclophosphamide regimen in childhood tumors. *Cancer* 23:1239–1242.

38. Fossati-Bellani F, Gasparini M, Bonadonna G. 1975. Adriamycin in Wilms' tumor previously treated with chemotherapy. *Eur J Cancer* 11:593–595.
39. Gillidoga AC, Corazon M, Tan TC, et al. 1976. The cardiotoxicity of doxorubicin and daunomycin in children. *Cancer* 37:1070–1078.
40. Green DM. 1987. The treatment of advanced or recurrent malignant genitourinary tumors in children. *Cancer* 60:602–611.
41. Greenwood RD, Rosenthal A, Cassidy R, et al. 1974. Constrictive pericarditis in childhood due to mediastinal irradiation. *Circulation* 50:1033–1039.
42. Guarda LA, Ayala AG, Jaffe N, et al. 1984. Chemotherapy induced histologic changes in Wilms' tumors. *Pediatr Pathol* 2:197–206.
43. Heideman RL, Haase GM, Foley CL, et al. 1985. Nephroblastomatosis and Wilms' tumor. *Cancer* 55:1446–1451.
44. Hou LT, Holman RL. 1961. Bilateral nephroblastomatosis in a premature infant. *J Pathol Bacteriol* 82:249–255.
45. Huff DS. 1973. Nodular renal blastema, nephroblastomatosis and Wilms' tumor: A report of two cases. *Am J Pathol* 70:23a–24b.
46. Jaffe N. 1977. Metastasis in malignant childhood tumor: The role of "adjuvant" therapy and the utility of multidisciplinary treatment. *Semin Oncol* 4:117–126.
47. Jaffe N, Link M, Cohen D, et al. 1981. High-dose methotrexate in osteogenic sarcoma. *NCI Monogr* 56:201–206.
48. Jaffe N, McNeese M, Mayfield JK, et al. 1980. Childhood urologic cancer therapy-related sequelae and their impact on management. *Cancer* 45:1815–1822.
49. Jaffe N, Murray J, Traggis D, et al. 1977. Multiple disciplinary treatment for childhood sarcoma. *Am J Surg* 133:405–413.
50. Jayalakshmamma B, Pinkel D. 1976. Urinary bladder toxicity following pelvic irradiation and simultaneous cyclophosphamide therapy. *Cancer* 38:701–707.
51. Jones B, Breslow NE, Takashima J. 1984. Toxic deaths in the Second National Wilms' Tumor Study. *J Clin Oncol* 2:1028–1032.
52. Kamalakor P, Freeman AI, Higby DJ. 1977. Clinical response and toxicity with cis-dichlorodiammine-platinum (II) in children. *Cancer Treat Rep* 61:835–839.
53. Kay R, Tank E. 1986. The current management of bilateral Wilms' tumor. *J Urol* 135:983–985.
54. Kidd JM. 1970. Exclusion of certain renal neoplasms from the category of Wilms' tumor. *Am J Pathol* 58:16a.
55. Kim TN, Zaalor GS, Baum ES, et al. 1985. Recurrence of Wilms' tumor after apparent cure. *J Pediatr* 107:44–49.
56. Kogan SJ, Marans H, Sontoreneau M, et al. 1986. Successful treatment of renal vein and vena caval extension of nephroblastoma by preoperative chemotherapy. *J Urol* 136:312–317.
57. Kumar APM, Wrenn EL Jr, Flemming ID. 1975. Preoperative therapy for unresectable malignant tumors in children. *J Pediatr Surg* 10:657–669.
58. Laster WR Jr, Mayo JG, Simpson-Herren L, et al. 1969. Success and failure in the treatment of solid tumor: II. Kinetic parameters and "cell cure" of moderately advanced carcinoma 755. *Cancer Chemother Rep* 53:169–188.
59. Lemerle J, Voute PA, Tournade MF, et al. 1983. Effectiveness of preoperative chemotherapy in Wilms' tumor: Results of an International Society of Pediatric Oncology (SIOP) clinical trial. *J Clin Oncol* 1:604–609.
60. Lemerle J, Voute PA, Tournade MF, et al. 1976. Preoperative versus post-operative radiotherapy, single versus multiple course actinomycin-D in the treatment of Wilms' tumor. *Cancer* 38:647–654.
61. Loh W, Ortega JA, Wolff J, et al. 1987. Cis-platinum/VP-16 for the retrieval of Wilms' tumor relapsing on chemotherapy (abstract). *Proc Am Soc Clin Oncol* 6:222.
62. Machin GA. 1980a. Persistent renal blastema (nephroblastomatosis) as a frequent precursor of Wilms' tumor: A pathological and clinical review. Part 1. Nephroblastomatosis in content of embryology and genetics. *Am J Pediatr Hematol Oncol* 2:165–171.
63. Machin GA. 1980b. Persistent renal blastema (nephroblastomatosis) as a frequent precursor of Wilms'

tumor: A pathological and clinical review. Pt 2. Significance of nephroblastomatosis in the genesis of Wilms' tumor. *Am J Pediatr Hematol Oncol* 2:253–261.

64. Malcolm AW, Jaffe N, Folkman MJ, et al. 1980. Bilateral Wilms' tumor. *Int J Radiat Oncol Biol Phys* 6:167–174.

65. Marsden HB, Lawler W, Kumar PM. 1978. Bone metastasizing renal tumor of childhood: Morphological and clinical features and differences from Wilms' tumor. *Cancer* 42:1922–1928.

66. Medical Research Council Working Party on Embryonal Tumor in Childhood. 1978. Management of nephroblastoma in childhood. *Arch Dis Child* 53:112–119.

67. Mills BA, Roberts RW. 1979. Cyclophosphamide-induced cardiomyopathy. *Cancer* 43:2223–2226.

68. Omar R, Davidian MM, Marcus JR, et al. 1986. Significance of the "maturation" of metastasis from Wilms' tumor after therapy. *J Surg Oncol* 33:239–242.

69. Ortega JA, Higgins GR, Williams KO, et al. 1980. Vincristine, dactinomycin and cyclophosphamide (VAC) chemotherapy for recurrent metastatic Wilms' tumor in previously treated children. *J Pediatr* 96:502–504.

70. Pinkel D, Camitta B, Kun L, et al. 1982. Doxorubicin cardiomyopathy in children with left-sided Wilms' tumor. *Med Pediatr Oncol* 10:483–488.

71. Pratt CB, Hayes A, Green AA. 1981. Pharmacokinetic evaluation of cisplatin in children with malignant solid tumors: A phase II study. *Cancer Treat Rep* 65:1021–1026.

72. Reiman TA, Siegel MJ, Shackelford GD. 1986. Wilms' tumor in children: Abdominal CT and US evaluation. *Radiology* 160:501–505.

73. Schabel FM Jr. 1975. Concepts for systemic treatment of micrometastases. *Cancer* 35:15–24.

74. Shimizu H, Jaffe N, Eftekhari F. 1987. Massive Wilms' tumor: Sonographic demonstration of therapeutic response without alteration in size. *Pediatr Radiol* 17:493–494.

75. Skipper HE, Schabel FM Jr, Wilcox WS. 1965. Experimental evaluation of potential anticancer agents: XIV. Further study of certain basic concepts underlying chemotherapy of leukemia. *Cancer Chemother Rep* 45:5–28.

76. Steinfeld AD, Crowley CA, O'Shea PA, et al. 1984. Recurrent and metastatic mesoblastic nephroma in infancy. *J Clin Oncol* 2:956–960.

77. Sullivan MP. 1968. Vincristine (NSC-67574) therapy for Wilms' tumor. *Cancer Chemother Rep* 52:481–484.

78. Sullivan MP, Sutow WW, Cangir A. 1967. Vincristine sulfate in management of Wilms' tumor. *JAMA* 202:381–386.

79. Sutow WW. 1967. Cyclophosphamide (NSC-2671) in Wilms' tumor and rhabdomyosarcoma. *Cancer Chemother Rep* 51:407–409.

80. Sutow WW. 1979. Wilms' tumor: Retrospect and prospect, in: *Care of the Child with Cancer.* New York, American Cancer Society, pp 62–70.

81. Sutow WW, Thurman WG, Windmiller J. 1963. Vincristine (leucoristine) sulfate in the treatment of children with metastatic Wilms' tumor. *Pediatrics* 32:880–887.

82. Tan CTC, Dargeon HW, Burchenal JH. 1959. Effect of actinomycin D in cancer in childhood. *Pediatrics* 24:544–561.

83. Taylor SR, Nunez C. 1984. Fine needle aspiration biopsy in a pediatric population: Report of 64 consecutive cases. *Cancer* 54:1449–1453.

84. Telander RL, Gilchrist GS, Burgert EO, et al. 1980. Bilateral massive nephroblastomatosis in infancy. *J Pediatr Surg* 15:163–166.

85. Tournade MF, Lemerle J, Sarazin E, et al. 1986. Tumors of the kidney, in Voute PA, Barrett A, Bloom HJG, et al. (eds): *Cancer in Children,* 2nd ed. Berlin, Springer Verlag, pp 252–264.

86. Tucker MA, Meadows AT, Bocce JD, et al. 1984. Secondary leukemia (SC) after alkylating agents (AA) for childhood cancer (abstract). *Proc Am Soc Clin Oncol* 3:85.

87. van Leeuwen EH, Postma A, Oosterhuis JW. 1987. An analysis of histology and DNA-ploidy in primary Wilms' tumors and their metastases and a study of the morphological effects of therapy. *Virchows Arch [A]* 410:487–494.

88. Voute PA, Tournade MF, Delemarre JFM, et al. 1987. Preoperative chemotherapy (CT) as first treatment in children with Wilms' tumor: Results of the SIOP Nephroblastoma Trials and Studies (abstract). *Proc Am Soc Clin Oncol* 6:223.

89. Wagget J, Koop CE. 1970. Wilms' tumor: Preoperative radiotherapy and chemotherapy in the management of massive tumors. *Cancer* 26:338–340.
90. Wagner CW, Parresh RA. 1981. Use of preoperative chemotherapy and radiation therapy in patients with Wilms' tumor. *Am Surg* 47:190–194.
91. Wang JJ, Cortex E, Sinks LF. 1971. Therapeutic effect and toxicity of adriamycin in patients with neoplastic disease. *Cancer* 23:237–243.
92. Wolff JA, D'Angio GJ, Hartman J, et al. 1974. Long-term evaluation of a single versus multiple courses of actinomycin-D therapy of Wilms' tumor. *N Engl J Med* 290:84–86.
93. Wolff JA, Krivit W, Newton WA, et al. 1968. Single versus multiple dose dactinomycin therapy of Wilms' tumor: Controlled cooperative study conducted by the Children's Cancer Study Group A. *N Engl J Med* 279:290–294.

PART II

Genital Tumors

Cancer of the Prostate: Clinically Significant Advances

Andrew C. von Eschenbach, M.D.

Alberto G. Ayala, M.D.

Since the introduction of endocrine therapy in 1941, little progress of clinical significance has occurred in the management of advanced prostate cancer. There has been no major improvement in the survival rate of patients with metastatic disease despite a variety of endocrine manipulations and numerous trials of chemotherapeutic agents. Our concern over lack of progress is magnified when we realize that the absolute and relative incidences of prostate cancer are increasing, owing to an increase in the population at risk and a concomitant increase in the frequency of occurrence of prostate cancer. Statisticians estimate that by the year 2,000 over 125,000 cases of prostatic cancer will be diagnosed each year. At present, prostate cancer accounts for 10% of cancer deaths among men and is the third leading cause of cancer death. If we are to improve on these survival statistics, we must acquire a more comprehensive understanding of the biology of prostate cancer and define strategies for early detection and selection of therapy as well as develop more effective treatment. Recent research is beginning to lead to clinical progress: increased knowledge about the histologic variants of prostate cancer and the impact of histologic differentiation on selection of therapy.

HISTOPATHOLOGY

Prostatic Carcinoma and Variants: Pathologic Findings of Clinical Significance

During the last decade we have learned significantly more about the clinicopathologic correlations of prostatic carcinoma. Particularly valuable has been the development of a grading system that can predict not only survival but also metastases to regional lymph nodes (Gleason 1977). In addition, the research of McNeal (1965), McNeal and Bostwick (1986), and McNeal et al. (1986) has contributed significantly to our understanding of the histogenesis of prostatic carcinoma.

Acinar prostatic carcinoma is the most common form of the disease, composing approximately 96% to 98% of all the prostatic carcinomas. Today, however, a group of less well-known prostatic tumors are slowly emerging as distinct clinical entities. Identifying these tumors pathologically is crucial to the prognosis and to the therapy selected. In the following discussion, we describe the differential pathologic findings of ductal (endometrioid) adeno-carcinoma, transitional cell carcinoma, and small cell carcinoma of the prostate.

Ductal (Endometrioid) Adenocarcinoma

Although a few cases of ductal carcinoma were reported in the early literature (Belter and Dodson 1970; Dube et al. 1972), Dube and associates in 1973 published the first large series of cases of this neoplasm. Only two relatively large series have been added, one by Bostwick et al. (1985) and one by Epstein and Woodruff (1986). At The University of Texas M. D. Anderson Cancer Center we have collected 35 cases, 24 of which were from patients seen and treated at UT M. D. Anderson Cancer Center and the remainder seen in consultation (Ro et al. 1988).

Like acinar carcinoma, ductal prostatic carcinoma arises in the seventh decade of life. Clinically, it manifests itself by urinary obstruction, hematuria, or both. Seventeen of the 24 patients seen at UT M. D. Anderson Cancer Center presented with one or both of these symptoms. Physical examination revealed an abnormal prostate in 3 patients, and in 2 bone pain was a presenting symptom. Bone metastases are usually osteoblastic but may be lytic or mixed. Metastases may be accompanied by elevated serum levels of acid phosphatase. Eight of 19 patients with metastases in our series also had elevated serum levels of acid phosphatase, although in 3 of these the level was not determined until after hormonal therapy had begun.

Dube and associates (1973) classified their cases into tumors arising from primary and secondary ducts and found that the two differed in histologic and biologic characteristics. We, too, have divided ductal carcinomas into two histologic groups, group A and group B. Group A tumors are comparable to the primary-duct carcinomas of Dube et al. They consist of an exuberant papillary growth with stalks lined by single or stratified layers of tall columnar epithelium involving stroma (Fig 21–1A and B). The cells show basally located nuclei, prominent nucleoli, and abundant mitoses. Cytoplasm is usually abundant. Large ducts are involved also by the same type of proliferation. In contrast, group B adenocarcinomas are located chiefly in smaller prostatic ducts. The ducts are several times enlarged and filled with glandulopapillary structures containing cells similar to those of type A. Neither pattern,

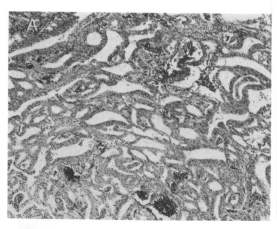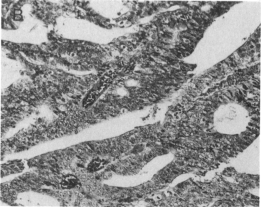

FIG 21–1.
Ductal (endometrioid) adenocarcinoma of the prostate. **A,** this tumor displays a pattern reminiscent of endometrial carcinoma, as manifested by an intricate array of glandular structures (×60). **B,** tumor cells lined by a pleomorphic epithelium with prominent nucleoli and numerous mitoses (×150).

however, is pure, since each may contain a minor component of the other. The exuberant papillary pattern seen in group A may be explained by the fact that once the tumor has reached the urethra there is no longer any prostatic stroma to hold the growth down. Interestingly, 52.9% of these lesions were accompanied by a concomitant low-grade acinar prostatic adenocarcinoma (MDAH grade 1, Gleason's combined score up to 4) (Ro et al. submitted for publication), which was about equally distributed between patterns A and B. The microacinar carcinoma was focal in the majority of our cases, but in two it was multifocal.

Prostatic ductal adenocarcinoma resembles adenocarcinoma of the endometrium in histologic pattern. Melicow and Patcher (1967), and later Melicow and Tannenbaum (1971), described a carcinoma arising in the utricle that had an endometrioid pattern. Since the utricle, also called uterus masculinus, is the male homologue of the uterus, they believed that the neoplasm was an endometrial carcinoma of the prostatic utricle and was endocrine responsive, similar to endometrial carcinomas. If this theory were valid, then castration or estrogen therapy would be inappropriate for these cases. Since then, confusion and debate have raged in the literature over whether a ductal carcinoma is different from an endometrioid carcinoma of utricular origin, or whether all carcinomas with an endometrioid pattern are ductal in origin. The work of Ro et al. (1988), demonstrating both prostatic acid phosphatase and prostate-specific antigen present in carcinomas with endometrioid features, further confirms a prostatic ductal origin rather than a utricular origin.

Transitional Cell Carcinoma of the Prostate

Transitional cell carcinoma arising from the prostatic ducts and extending down into the acinar units was identified many years ago by several investigators (Melicow and Hollowell 1952; Ende et al. 1963; Johnson et al. 1972). Pathologically, this tumor resembles a transitional cell carcinoma of the bladder of high-grade malignancy; the clue for diagnosis is the finding of tumor arising in the ducts and extending into the acinar units (Johnson et al. 1972). The tumor may be localized to the ducts, but it may also transgress the basement membranes and invade the prostatic stroma.

From the clinical point of view, transitional cell carcinoma of the prostate can be a manifestation of three different processes: a primary tumor of the prostatic ducts, a ductal prostatic involvement of transitional cell carcinoma in situ of the bladder, or a synchronous or asynchronous ductal manifestation of bladder carcinoma (Johnson et al. 1972). Primary transitional cell prostatic tumors develop in a patient's sixth or seventh decade. Bladder transitional cell carcinoma and transitional cell carcinoma in situ arise over the same age range as the primary process (Johnson et al. 1972).

There are no specific symptoms for primary transitional cell prostatic carcinoma, and it may be silent. Obstruction, hematuria, or both may be observed, or a mass may be recognized on digital examination. When transitional cell carcinoma of the prostate occurs as a secondary manifestation of bladder carcinoma, the prostate may show some irregularities or may be totally normal, evidencing no clinical or physical finding at all. It behooves the urologist to obtain a biopsy of the prostate to confirm or rule out prostatic disease. For the pathologist, it is very important to distinguish in situ carcinoma from invasive carcinoma, because the prognosis and management are different. Originally Johnson et al. (1972) suggested that transitional cell carcinoma in situ (T_{is}) could be managed conservatively with a transurethral resection alone, but when the prostatic stroma was invaded, radical therapy using radiotherapy, radical prostatectomy, or both was necessary. Many years of experience, however, have demonstrated that prostatic T_{is} cannot be managed conservatively because the disease recurs. Furthermore, invasive prostatic transitional cell carcinoma cannot be controlled with radical surgery or radiotherapy alone because it is prone to metastasize rapidly. Radical surgery is the management of choice for both processes, but aggressive chemotherapy must also be instituted if stromal invasion has occurred. Recent experience at UT M. D. Anderson Cancer Center has shown that metastasis can be eradicated with combination chemotherapy (Dexeus et al. 1987).

Small Cell Carcinoma of the Prostate

Small cell carcinoma of the prostate is an extremely rare, yet very important, type of high-grade prostatic neoplasm. It is composed of small undifferentiated cells similar to the cells of oat cell carcinoma. Reports of this tumor in the prostate began to appear in the 1970s with examples of a Cushing's syndrome (Vuitch and Mendelsohn 1982) and adrenocortico-tropic hormone (ACTH)-producing tumors (Wenk et al. 1977). The experience at UT M. D. Anderson Cancer Center has been with 20 patients seen in a period of over 20 years (Ro et al. 1987; Tetu et al. 1987). Patients ranged in age from 30 to 89 years (median, 67 years); the majority was older than 50. Presenting symptoms were related to obstruction and included dysuria, nocturia, and urgency.

The neoplasm may comprise small cell carcinoma only or small cell carcinoma coexisting with a microacinar adenocarcinoma (Figs 21–2 and 21–3). Among the 20 patients in our series, 9 presented with a microacinar carcinoma 7 months to 8 years (median, 18 months) before they developed the small cell carcinoma. The initial microacinar adenocarcinomas in these 9 patients were stage A in 5, C in 1, and D in 3. In the 11 patients who first had small cell carcinoma, 6 tumors were pure small cell carcinoma and 5 had a microacinar carcinoma component. Ten of these tumors were stage D and one stage B.

The grades of microacinar carcinoma in the nine patients whose initial biopsy did not show small cell carcinoma, according to the MDAH grading system, were grade 1 in four, grade 2 in one, grade 3 in three, and grade 4 in one (Tetu et al. 1987). In 6 of these 9 patients, the ratio of small cell carcinoma to microacinar carcinoma at the time the small cell carcinoma was recognized ranged from 30:70 to 90:10. The other three patients had no residual adenocarcinoma. Distant metastases were frequently present. The pelvic lymph nodes were the most common site followed by the liver, lungs, and bone.

Treatment was recorded for 19 of the 20 patients and was not uniform. Twelve were

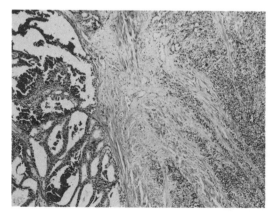

FIG 21–2.
Small cell carcinoma of the prostate. A low-power view showing diffuse sheets of small cells on the *right side* and glandular carcinoma on the *left* (×60).

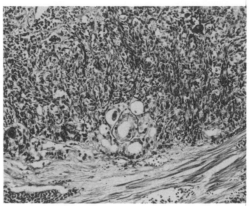

FIG 21–3.
Small cell carcinoma of the prostate. A cluster of microacinar carcinoma is surrounded by small cells of intermediate size (×150).

treated with transurethral resection, hormonal manipulation, and adjuvant radiation or chemotherapy (in 6) or radiation and chemotherapy (in 6). Hormonal manipulation included administration of exogenous estrogen, orchiectomy, or both. The tumors of the other 7 patients were not resected, but one or more of the following modalities were instituted: chemotherapy, radiation therapy, or hormonal therapy.

Eleven of the 20 patients died of their disease. Their median overall survival duration was 10 months, and 9 were alive with disease from 3 to 60 months after initial diagnosis. However, 3 of those surviving had extremely advanced disease.

Summary

These rare variants of prostatic carcinoma are distinct clinicopathologic entities. Identifying them accurately is the responsibility of the pathologist; treating them effectively is a challenge for the urologist.

Acinar Carcinoma

The most frequent malignant transformation that occurs in the prostate is acinar adenocarcinoma. From inception, this tumor can assume a variety of clinical expressions ranging from the indolent tumor that never presents a threat to the patient to the rapidly progressive malignancy that results in early metastasis and ends in death from disease. An intermediate type grows slowly over a long period of time. Its slow local growth is evidenced first by a palpable mass in the prostate; later in its course, tumor cell clones metastasize to lymph nodes and then to bones and viscera.

This heterogeneity in clinical expression reflects both a variation among tumor cells and differences in host factors. The existence of such variable behavior presents a great challenge to urologists, who must determine which of several possible treatments is best for an individual patient. An intelligent choice among no therapy, transurethral resection, radical prostatectomy, irradiation, hormonal therapy, or chemotherapy requires not only a precise determination of the extent of tumor burden but also an understanding of the cancer's natural history.

Historically, the method for selecting a treatment plan has been to group tumors homogeneously by stage, employing a system such as that proposed by Whitmore (1956).

However, as Whitmore (1984) subsequently pointed out, because tumors do not progress clearly from one stage to the next and because, within a given stage, response to therapy varies widely, stage is a static and imprecise prognosticator.

Several variations have been introduced to define homogeneous groups more precisely (Fig 21–4), but no consensus is currently available. For example, with regard to advanced disease, extracapsular extension of the primary tumor is divided into stage C_1 and C_2, depending on the tumor size and whether it appears fixed to the pelvic sidewall. Metastatic disease, too, is divided into categories: stage D_0 indicates only an elevation of serum prostatic acid phosphatase without apparent clinical or radiographic metastasis; stage D_1 is defined as the presence of pelvic lymph node metastasis below the common iliac artery, confirmed either clinically or pathologically; and stage D_2 indicates either lymph node metastasis beyond the pelvis or osseous or visceral disease.

Despite these subcategories, staging systems remain inadequate for predicting outcome of therapy. It is apparent that, in addition to the extent of tumor burden at the time of evaluation, the malignant potential of the tumor is an important factor that affects the rate of tumor progression and, perhaps, response to therapy. Thus, ability to differentiate a tumor by determining its histologic grade has affected the ability to select appropriate therapy. Using both clinical stage and histologic grade of the tumor in selecting therapy and assessing prognosis has had a major impact on treatment for patients with prostatic cancer.

STAGING OF PROSTATE CANCER

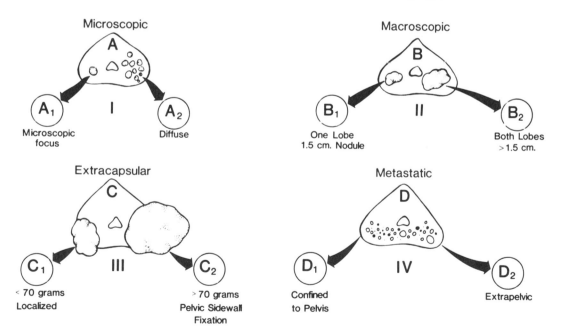

FIG 21–4.
Staging systems for prostate cancer. Tumor burden is broadly categorized as microscopic intracapsular, macroscopic intracapsular, extracapsular extension, and metastatic disease. (From von Eschenbach AC. 1981. *Cancer of the Prostate. Current Problems in Cancer*, vol 5, no. 12. Chicago, Year Book Medical Publishers, p 27. Used by permission.)

SELECTION OF THERAPY

Tumor Assessment: The Basis for Therapy Choice

It now appears to be appropriate to consider the selection of therapy to be a process based on tumor burden as evidenced by stage and malignant potential as reflected by tumor grade. Therefore the clinician can look at this process in terms of a decision matrix (Fig 21–5). Using this model, we can identify clearly low-stage, low-grade tumors for which local modalities of therapy can be considered curative. Similarly, only systemic therapy is capable of controlling high-stage, high-grade tumors. The major challenge for the future is to define methods that can detect tumors when they are still in a state amenable to total extirpation by surgery or irradiation. Recent advances in the technology of ultrasonography have made available high-resolution transducers of 7.0-MHz or higher frequency that are adapted to transrectal probes for transverse and longitudinal examinations of the internal architecture of the prostate.

Preliminary reports by Lee (1987) suggest that this method can discover early prostate cancer by detecting small hypoechoic foci in the prostate indicative of tumor deposits not identifiable by digital rectal examination. In his experience with 1,343 examinations, transrectal ultrasound had an overall detected prevalence rate for cancer of 2.1% and a positive

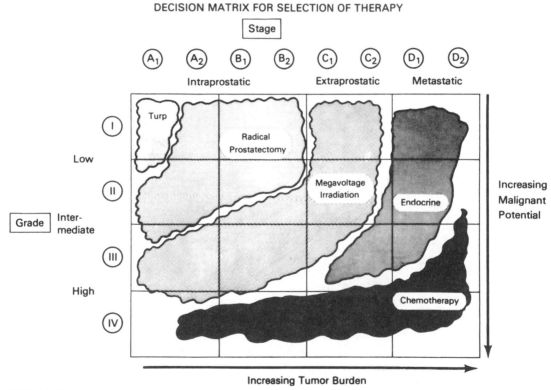

FIG 21–5.
Decision matrix for therapy selection. Increasing tumor grade is correlated with increasing malignant potential, and increasing tumor stage is correlated with increasing tumor burden. *TURP* = transurethral resection of the prostate. (From Johnson DE, Swanson DA, von Eschenbach AC. 1984. Tumors of the genitourinary tract, in Smith DR (ed): *Urology,* ed 11. Los Altos, Calif, Lange Medical Publications, p 349. Used by permission.)

predictive value of 31% compared to rates for digital rectal examination of 1.0% and 27%, respectively. Experience with a larger group of patients is necessary to determine, first, the number of false positive and false negative examinations, and second, whether ultrasonography has any value for screening and detecting early prostate cancer. A multicenter national cooperative trial is currently underway to examine the role of ultrasound as a screening method for detecting early-stage prostate cancer. Ultrasound has also been employed as an objective method of determining the extent of tumor and the presence of extracapsular extension, and serial examinations of prostate tumor size have been used to measure therapy response. Although many questions regarding the accuracy of prostate ultrasound are unanswered, this imaging technique holds great promise for objective assessment of the primary tumor.

Another advance significant to the assessment of tumor burden is the introduction of prostate-specific antigen (PSA) as a serum marker for prostate cancer. This glycoprotein, like prostatic acid phosphatase (PAP), is a tissue-specific antigen for prostate epithelial cells. It is, therefore, not a marker of prostate cancer, but when present in elevated amounts in the serum of patients with prostate cancer, it serves as a relative index of tumor burden. Monitoring serum levels of both PSA and PAP can determine tumor regression in response to therapy. Likewise, elevations of these marker values may serve as the first indicator of relapse following therapy. Evaluating 82 patients with progressing disease, Lange et al. (1986) reported that PSA, PAP, or both were elevated in 95%; they believe these two markers can be used to monitor patients for evidence of progression after initially successful therapy.

Therapeutic Options

Despite extensive efforts to determine precisely the most appropriate form of therapy, the clinician still must deal with a great deal of uncertainty. The reason is the apparent overlap in efficacy between treatment strategies. It is in these transition zones that so much confusion and controversy exist regarding selection of therapy. With regard to systemic therapy for advanced disease, for example, controversial areas include the selection and timing of endocrine therapy and the role of chemotherapy. A great deal of pessimism has been engendered by the failure of therapy to achieve cure or "long-term cancer-free survival." There are, however, some recent developments of clinical significance that can perhaps provide some optimism for the future.

Endocrine Therapy

Hormonal therapy has been available for the past 45 years. Tumors respond in 80% to 90% of patients, and at times the response can be very dramatic; however, complete responses are rare and the duration of response is limited. Eventually tumor progresses or relapses— in most patients after a mean of 24 months—and the median survival duration for patients with metastatic disease is 36 months despite therapy. The frustration of failing to achieve cures was further compounded when the Veterans Administration Cooperative Urological Research Group (VACURG) reported no difference in survival duration when various forms of endocrine therapy were compared to placebo (VACURG 1967; Byar 1973). These facts led to a very pessimistic view of the role of endocrine therapy for metastatic prostate cancer. It was considered to be only palliative, and as a result many clinicians have chosen to allow patients to go untreated until disease becomes symptomatic. A number of recently emphasized caveats can dispel this unfortunate pessimistic conclusion. Early endocrine therapy does prevent disease progression and can lengthen the survivals of patients with advanced disease.

When the VACURG study determined the probability of patients with stage III tumors progressing to stage IV, they discovered that 60% of those treated initially with placebo had progressed by 8 years as compared with approximately 15% of those patients treated initially with estrogen (Byar 1973). This suggests that endocrine therapy provides more than symptomatic palliation and is able to influence the disease process.

In the VACURG studies, Hurst and Byar (1973) reported that patients treated with placebo who subsequently progressed were then usually treated with hormonal therapy. However, they were analyzed for survival as placebo patients. Among 223 patients with stage IV (metastatic) disease originally assigned to placebo, 133 (60%) were taken off study after a median of 9 months and, presumably, then received hormonal treatment. In addition to early progression of disease, the survival durations of patients were adversely affected when they were treated initially with placebo.

In an analysis of cause of death by initial treatment (Byar 1977), the death rate from prostatic cancer for the 223 patients with stage IV disease in study 1 who were treated initially with placebo was 47%, as compared with 38% for 216 patients treated with orchiectomy and estrogen. For patients with either stage III or stage IV disease, combined survival curves after 7 years demonstrated a poorer survival rate for placebo-treated patients than for those treated initially with endocrine therapy. It is therefore reasonable to conclude that endocrine therapy instituted at the time metastatic disease is diagnosed does lengthen patient survival and reduce the death rate from prostatic cancer, although death from competing causes continues to occur at a high frequency in this age group. From the VACURG data, Jordan et al. (1977) conclude that estrogen therapy would be indicated initially if cardiovascular complications could be avoided.

Recently, Labrie et al. (1986) have suggested that total androgen ablation instituted at the time of diagnosis could significantly improve survival rates over those of historical controls. Labrie initially reported that the combination of a luteinizing hormone-releasing hormone (LH-RH) agonist and an antiandrogen could effectively deprive tumor cells of stimulation by androgens of both testicular and adrenal origin. He reported a positive objective response in 125 of 131 patients and a probability of survival of 89% at 2 years. More recently, prospective randomized trials evaluating this strategy but using standard methods of suppressing or eliminating testicular androgen have failed to demonstrate any significant advantage for total androgen ablation. However, the introduction of LH-RH agonists has provided clinicians with an alternative method of therapy that is effective in consistently reducing circulating testosterone to castrate levels without the side effects associated with estrogens or the need for irreversible surgical castration.

Regardless of what strategy of androgen deprivation is employed, responses are not permanent, and eventually, in most patients, tumor progresses. Although there is no evidence that further androgen ablation lengthens survival, clinicians have long known that surgical or chemical adrenalectomy or hypophysectomy can significantly palliate pain. Recently, Trachtenberg and Pont (1984) and others have recognized that the oral antifungal agent, ketoconazole, blocks the cytochrome P-450-mediated synthesis of androgen and is an effective method of suppressing both adrenal and testicular androgens. For patients with symptomatic progressing disease after standard endocrine therapy, oral ketoconazole in a dose of 200 mg every 8 hours can provide temporary subjective improvement and is a safe and effective new addition to our treatment armamentarium.

Chemotherapy

Regardless of the efficacy of androgen ablation, it would seem that improving the survival of patients with advanced prostatic cancer is dependent on developing a therapeutic strategy other than hormonal therapy. As a result, much emphasis has been placed on the search for effective chemotherapeutic agents. The cooperative trials of the National Prostate Cancer Project (Gibbons 1981) served to focus the efforts of many investigators on the evaluation of single chemical agents as treatment of hormone-refractory prostate cancer. Although their results demonstrated the ability of some chemotherapeutic agents either to induce objective regression or at least to stabilize progressive disease, no single agent emerged as superior.

More recent efforts have been directed at combining effective single agents to produce a greater response with a minimum of toxicity. At UT M. D. Anderson Cancer Center, Logothetis et al. (1983) have achieved a 48% objective response rate with the combination of doxorubicin (Adriamycin), mitomycin C, and 5-fluorouracil (DMF). Of significance in this study is the recognition that response rate and duration of survival varied with the metastatic site and tumor burden. When patients were stratified according to extent of osseous metastasis and visceral metastasis, the problem of heterogeneity in prostatic cancer again became apparent. Metastatic sites varied in their response to chemotherapeutic agents: 8 out of 9 lung metastases regressed significantly more than comparable osseous metastases. In the latter, however, although the magnitude of response was less, the duration of response was greater. As a result, the longest survivals occurred among patients with osseous metastases limited to the axial skeleton.

These differences in magnitude and duration of response have provided a basis on which to stratify patients in future trials to define more effective chemotherapy regimens.

CONCLUSION

Despite much progress in cancer therapy, the treatment of patients with advanced prostatic cancer is frustrated by our failure to detect the disease at an early stage when total tumor ablation is possible and our failure to develop effective systemic therapy that can completely and permanently eradicate disease. Future developments of clinical significance should stem from our understanding of the biology of prostate cancer rather than from clinical empiricism. Our efforts will focus on earlier detection, initiating therapy when the tumor burden is smallest, and developing effective combinations of chemoendocrine therapy.

REFERENCES

1. Belter LF, Dodson AI Jr. 1970. Papillomatosis and papillary adenocarcinoma of the prostate: A case report. *J Urol* 104:880–883.
2. Bostwick DG, Kindrachuk RW, Rouse RV. 1985. Prostatic adenocarcinoma with endometrioid features: Clinical, pathologic, and ultrastructural findings. *Am J Surg Pathol* 9:595–609.
3. Byar DP. 1973. The Veterans Administration Cooperative Urological Research Group's studies of cancer of the prostate. *Cancer* 32:1126–1130.
4. Byar DP. 1977. VACURG studies on prostatic cancer and its treatment, in Tannenbaum M (ed): *Urologic Pathology: The Prostate.* Philadelphia, Lea & Febiger, pp 241–267.
5. Dexeus FH, Logothetis CJ, Samuels ML, et al. 1987. Complete responses in metastatic transitional cell carcinoma of the prostate with cis-platin regimens. *J Urol* 137:122–125.
6. Dube VE, Farrow GM, Greene LF. 1973. Prostatic adenocarcinoma of ductal origin. *Cancer* 32:402–409.
7. Dube VE, Joyce GT, Kennedy E. 1972. Papillary primary duct adenocarcinoma of the prostate. *J Urol* 107:825–826.
8. Ende N, Woods LP, Shelley HS. 1963. Carcinoma originating in ducts surrounding the prostatic urethra. *Am J Clin Pathol* 40:183–189.

9. Epstein JI, Woodruff JM. 1986. Adenocarcinoma of the prostate with endometrioid features: A light microscopic and immunohistochemical study of ten cases. *Cancer* 57:111–119.

10. Gibbons RP, Investigators, National Prostatic Cancer Project Cooperative Clinical Trials. 1981. Co-operative trial of single and combined agent protocols. *Urology* 7 (suppl):48–52.

11. Gleason DF. 1977. Histologic grading and clinical staging of prostatic carcinoma, in Tannenbaum M (ed): *Urologic Pathology: The Prostate*. Philadelphia, Lea & Febiger, pp 171–197.

12. Hurst KS, Byar DP. 1973. An analysis of the effects of changes from the assigned treatment in a clinical trial of treatment for prostate cancer. *J Chron Dis* 26:314–324.

13. Johnson DE, Hogan JM, Ayala AG. 1972. Transitional cell carcinoma of the prostate. *Cancer* 29:287–293.

14. Jordan WP Jr, Blackard CE, Byar DP. 1977. Reconsideration of orchiectomy in the treatment of advanced prostate carcinoma. *South Med J* 70:1411–1413.

15. Labrie F, Dupont A, Giguere M, et al. 1986. Advantages of the combination therapy in previously untreated and treated patients with advanced prostate cancer. *J Steroid Biochem* 25:877–883.

16. Lange PH, Ercole CJ, Vessella RL. 1986. Tumor markers in follow up of initial therapy of prostate cancer, in Lange PH (ed): *Tumor Markers in Prostate Cancer: Symposium Proceedings*. Excerpta Medica, pp 16–23.

17. Lee F. 1987. Transrectal ultrasound in the diagnosis, staging, guided needle biopsy, and screening for prostate cancer, in McLeary RD, Lee F (eds): *The Use of Transrectal Ultrasound in the Diagnosis and Management of Prostate Cancer*. New York, Alan R. Liss, pp 73–109.

18. Logothetis CJ, Samuels ML, von Eschenbach AC, et al. 1983. Doxorubicin, mitomycin-C, and 5-fluorourocil (DMF) in the treatment of metastatic hormonally refractory adenocarcinoma of the prostate with a note on the staging of prostate cancer. *J Clin Oncol* 6:368–379.

19. McNeal JE. 1965. Morphogenesis of prostatic cancer. *Cancer* 18:1659–1666.

20. McNeal JE, Bostwick DG. 1986. Intraductal dysplasia: A premalignant lesion of the prostate. *Hum Pathol* 17:64–71.

21. McNeal JE, Reese HH, Redwine EA, et al. 1986. Cribriform adenocarcinoma of the prostate. *Cancer* 58:1714–1719.

22. Melicow MM, Hollowell JW. 1952. Intraurothelial cancer. Carcinoma in situ, Bowen's disease of the urinary system: Discussion of thirty cases. *J Urol* 68:763–772.

23. Melicow MM, Patcher MR. 1967. Carcinoma of prostatic utricle (uterus masculinus). *Cancer* 20:1715–1722.

24. Melicow MM, Tannenbaum M. 1971. Endometrial carcinoma of uterus masculinus (prostatic utricle): Report of six cases. *J Urol* 106:892–902.

25. Ro JY, Ayala AG, Wishnow KI, et al. 1988. Prostatic duct adenocarcinoma with endometrioid features: Immunohistochemical and electron microscopic study. *Semin Diagn Pathol* 5:301–310.

26. Ro JY, Tetu B, Ayala AG, et al. 1987. Small cell carcinoma of the prostate. II: Immunohistochemical and electron microscopic study of 18 cases. *Cancer* 59:977–982.

27. Tetu B, Ro JY, Ayala AG, et al. 1987. Small cell carcinoma of the prostate: A clinicopathologic study of 20 cases. Pt I. *Cancer* 59:1803–1809.

28. Trachtenberg J, Pont A. 1984. Ketoconazole therapy for advanced prostate cancer. *Lancet* 2:433–435.

29. Veterans Administration Co-Operative Urological Research Group (VACURG). 1967. The treatment and survival of patients with cancer of the prostate. *Surg Gynecol Obstet* 124:1011–1017.

30. Vuitch MF, Mendelsohn G. 1981. Relationship of ectopic ACTH production to tumor differentiation: A morphologic and immunohistochemical study of prostatic carcinoma with Cushing's syndrome. *Cancer* 47:296–299.

31. Wenk RE, Bhagavan BS, Levy R, et al. 1977. Ectopic ACTH, prostatic oat cell carcinoma and marked hypernatremia. *Cancer* 40:773–778.

32. Whitmore WF Jr. 1956. Hormone therapy in prostatic cancer. *Am J Med* 21:697–713.

33. Whitmore WF Jr. 1984. Natural history and staging of prostate cancer. *Urol Clin North Am* 11:205–220.

Chapter 22

Histologic Grade, Clinical Stage, and Response to Diethylstilbestrol Therapy for Prostate Carcinoma

Donald F. Gleason, M.D., Ph.D.

It has proved difficult to evaluate the results of treatment of prostate cancer because of its very variable and often prolonged clinical course, ranging from rapidly progressive fatal cancer to documented tumors that never do progress. Just to compare two treatments, many patients must be followed for many years to average out this variability.

The variability is reduced by defining standardized clinical stages—A, B, C, D (or I, II, III, IV, in the Veterans Administration [VA] studies)—which have predictable average clinical behavior and help prescribe appropriate treatment. There is general agreement that small, well-differentiated stage A tumors rarely progress and therefore do not need any immediate, potentially harmful treatment. Radical prostatectomy is not logical treatment for advanced metastatic cancer (stage D). However, between those two extremes lies a substantial area of varied and occasionally shifting opinion.

The histologic structure (grade) of prostate cancer also separates patients into groups with predictable tumor behavior, but that possibility is not widely applied. About 2% of stage A tumors do progress to death, and the histologic grade can predict the probability of that progression.

Unfortunately for the clinicians who would like more precise predictions of tumor behavior, normal biologic variation will always prevail around the average predicted behavior. We can only provide strong probabilities, as is true in many of the difficult areas of medical practice.

The possibility that tumors of different microscopic structure might respond differently to treatment has not been explored systematically. Unfortunately, there do not appear to be (cannot be?) any completely controlled trials of x-ray or chemotherapy. The author has no special experience with radiation therapy or chemotherapy, but the Veterans Administration Cooperative Urological Research Group (VACURG) studies of cancer of the prostate provided extensive data on diethylstilbestrol (DES) therapy. This chapter examines the relationships between the histologic grade and clinical stage and the response to DES therapy.

HISTOLOGIC GRADING—THE VETERANS ADMINISTRATION ("GLEASON") GRADING SYSTEM

For more than 45 years there have been many reports of strong correlations between the histologic structure and the biologic behavior of prostate cancers: well-differentiated tumors progress slowly or not at all; poorly differentiated tumors progress more rapidly. Unfortunately, the necessarily subjective nature of histologic grading makes it difficult to adopt previously published systems, and almost every author proposed a new and different grading system.

The VACURG studies were prospective, controlled, and randomized comparisons of the conventional systemic treatment alternatives of that time (1960–1975): DES, orchiectomy, orchiectomy plus DES—and placebo. Radical prostatectomy was performed in the appropriate patients. The results of the VACURG studies are generally known (VACURG 1967; Byar 1972, 1973; Blackard et al. 1978).

The VACURG studies produced yet another grading system (Gleason et al. 1974; Gleason 1977), which was standardized with a simple drawing that enabled many other pathologists to adopt it, confirm its value, and evaluate its reproducibility (Corriere et al. 1970; Kramer et al. 1980; Paulson et al. 1980; Thomas et al. 1980; Bain et al. 1982). The VA ("Gleason") grading system considered only the degree of glandular dedifferentiation and the relationship of the tumor to the prostate stroma. Cytologic details were not included; they were strongly correlated with the histologic grades and appeared to "tell the same story" without increasing the range or strength of the histologic-biologic correlations.

The system identified five histologic grades. An effort was made to assign only one grade to each tumor, but more than one grade was clearly present in about half of the cases. A primary grade (predominant by area) and a secondary grade (lesser area) were recorded simply as two digits, e.g., 2-3 or 5-4. For uniformity in analysis, single-grade tumors were also identified with two digits, e.g., 2-2 or 4-4.

The separate primary and secondary grades yielded strong and very similar correlations with the subsequently observed death rates, and a very interesting phenomenon was noted: the cancer death rates for patients with two different grades of tumor were intermediate between the cancer death rates for patients with the pure forms of those two grades (Fig 22–1). Thus, in contradistinction to the time-honored aphorism, prostate cancer is not "as bad as its worst part" but behaves more in proportion to its average grade. Therefore, the primary and secondary grades were added together, obtaining the scaling effect of "averaging" but omitting division by two. This avoided fractional grades and created a new histologic score (see Fig 22–1), which could range from 2 to 10 (grade 1 + 1 = score 2; grade 5 + 5 = score 10).

The histologic score was the most powerful single parameter correlating with the biologic malignancy of prostate cancer encountered in the VACURG studies. As in Figure 22–1, it correlated very strongly with the subsequently observed total and cancer-specific death rates. There were no cancer deaths with score 2 tumors (pure grade 1), and there was a steady progression of cancer death rates to over 30% cancer deaths per year with histologic score 10 (pure grade 5 tumor).

The histologic score correlated strongly with the percent of patients with metastases in various organs identified at autopsy, years later. It correlated also with initial pretreatment observations such as the presence or absence of hydronephrosis, metastases, and elevated level of serum acid phosphatase. In general, the histologic score correlated to some degree with almost any parameter logically related to the biologic malignancy of prostatic cancer (Gleason 1977).

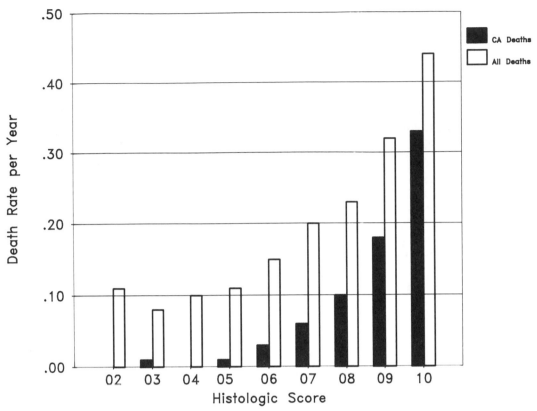

FIG 22–1.
Death rates by histologic scores (primary + secondary grades). Note that the death rates for odd-numbered scores (two different grades) fall between the death rates for even-numbered scores (mostly pure single-grade tumors). *DES* = diethylstilbestrol.

CLINICAL STAGING

Many other observations, of course, correlate well with the subsequent course of cancer of the prostate. Most of these have the quality of "mileposts" along the course of the progression of the cancer: tumor size, extension of tumor through the capsule, lymph node metastases, elevated serum acid phosphatase, distant metastases, etc. The histologic score correlates with the *rate* at which the tumors progress while the "mileposts" indicate *how far* the tumors have progressed.

Various combinations of these "mileposts" identify the clinical stage of the tumor. The clinical stages are very powerful predictors of survival and thus limit the choice of treatments to a substantial degree. The VACURG studies used the simple clinical stages of that time:

Stage I   No palpable tumor, no metastases.
Stage II   Palpable, localized tumor, no metastases.
Stage III   Palpably extended tumor, no metastases.
Stage IV   Metastases present and/or high acid phosphatase level.

This simple staging system produced the expected strong correlations with subsequent mortality. There was also definite correlation between the clinical stages and the histologic scores, with more low-score tumors in stages I and II and more high-score tumors in stages III and IV. However, both clinical stage and histologic score had strong independent predictive powers for mortality. The cancer mortality for patients who had stage III tumors with a high histologic score was worse than that for patients who had stage IV tumors with a lower score. The VACURG also developed a simple but powerful category score, which combines the clinical stage and histologic score into a single number (Gleason 1977). It was confirmed (Sogani et al. 1985) but has not been widely used. It predicts survival at least as effectively as the subdivided clinical stages.

RELATIONSHIP OF CLINICAL STAGE AND HISTOLOGIC SCORE TO DIETHYLSTILBESTROL THERAPY

The VACURG data confirmed the favorable response to DES therapy (reduction of cancer-specific death rates by roughly half). The favorable effect decreased mildly for (VA) stage III compared with stages I and II, and again for stage IV compared with stage III (Fig 22–2). This minor shift is probably entirely accounted for by the higher average histologic scores found in the higher stages.

There appeared to be a systematic relationship between histologic scores and the favorable response to DES therapy (Fig 22–3). There was no detectable response in the best-differentiated tumors (score 2, 3, 4, 5) and an increasingly favorable response in the intermediate

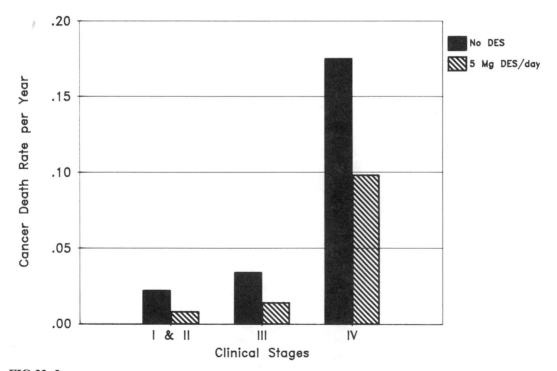

FIG 22–2.
Cancer-specific death rates by clinical stages. Note that the marked reduction of cancer death rates with diethylstilbestrol (*DES*) therapy decreases slightly in the higher stages.

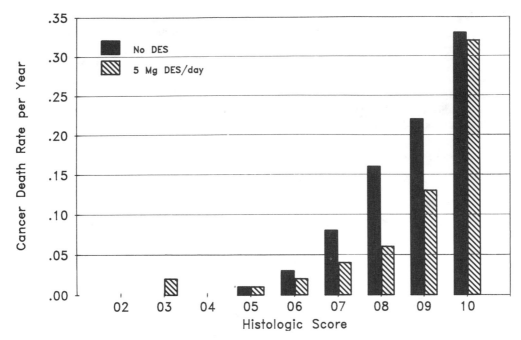

FIG 22–3.
Cancer (*CA*)-specific death rates by histologic scores, comparing death rates with and without diethylstilbestrol (*DES*) therapy.

tumors (scores 6, 7, 8). The favorable response decreased in score 9 tumors, and score 10 tumors responded minimally, if at all.

This apparently systematic association is probably a nonspecific phenomenon, unrelated to any unique attributes of the specific histologic structures. That is, the low-score, well-differentiated tumors have such low rates of progression and cancer death that a favorable effect simply cannot be observed. The intermediate–histologic-score tumors (6, 7, 8) associated with higher cancer death rates apparently retain certain normal metabolic mechanisms and can respond to the DES treatment. The poorly differentiated (scores 9 and 10) tumors appear to lose the metabolic mechanisms that promote the response to DES.

DO PROSTATE CANCERS BECOME MORE MALIGNANT WITH TIME?

It is currently popular to interpret the correlation of higher grade tumor with more extensive tumor (clinical stage) as proof of a *linear progression of malignancy with time*. This is a hypothesis that prostatic cancers progress through the clinical stages to death because of increasing histologic and biologic malignancy: "This tumor is poorly differentiated and widely disseminated because it was present for a long time and steadily became more malignant."

However, all the observed data can be explained just as well by a hypothesis of *biologic determinism*, postulating a constant degree of histologic grade and biologic malignancy from the beginning of the tumor, followed by steady growth and progression at a rate that is specific for that grade of tumor: "This tumor is poorly differentiated and widely disseminated because it was very malignant from the beginning and progressed very rapidly."

Surprisingly, there are apparently no published data relating tumor grades at autopsy to tumor grades during life. However, the consistency of correlation between histologic and biologic malignancy during life, noted by many authors, suggests that it is not common for tumors of low histologic grade to become more highly malignant.

Histologic grade and clinical stage *are* definitely but incompletely correlated. That is, almost the entire range of histologic grades may be found in any of the clinical stages, although the highest-grade tumors are rare in the lower stages and the lowest-grade tumors are very rare in the highest clinical stages.

Apparent explosive increases in malignancy do occur, but they are rare exceptions. Only a mild and inconsistent upward drift in average histologic score could be detected in the limited number of repeat biopsies in the VACURG study. The increases usually consisted of the higher grade overgrowing the lower grade in two-grade tumors. Most commonly the histologic score remained the same. In a few cases, the score actually decreased, but these were probably "sampling errors" in small biopsies.

There is no trend to higher-grade tumors with advancing age at diagnosis. Highly malignant tumors do occur in some younger men and appear to have been present for a short time.

There is autopsy evidence that low-grade tumors remain low-grade for long periods of time. Careful studies reveal a surprising incidence of prostate cancers beginning about age 40 years, increasing steadily with age, and reaching levels as high as 80% of men in their tenth decade. Most of these tumors are small, low-grade, had caused no difficulty, and clearly had been present for many years. For example, if the rough incidence of these tumors is 10% at age 55, 20% at age 65, and 30% at age 75, then two thirds of the tumors in the 75-year-old men must have been present for more than 10 years and one third must have been present for more than 20 years! They provide the troublesome tumors found unexpectedly in tissue resected during life (stage A and some stage B).

The autopsy data and the long survivals for patients with the low-grade tumors diagnosed during life could not prevail if increasing biologic/histologic malignancy were inexorable and frequent.

CONCLUSIONS

The clinician must react most directly, of course, to the clinical stage of the tumor, but the histologic grade (or score) of the tumor is also a powerful predictive variable and should be incorporated into the treatment decisions, along with the patient's age and general state of health.

Diethylstilbestrol therapy definitely improves survival of patients with prostatic cancer but is probably effective only for tumors with VA histologic scores greater than 5. A constant histologic and biologic malignancy is quite consistent with the natural history of prostatic cancer, and it is not necessary to postulate a progressive increase in malignancy with time.

REFERENCES

1. Bain G, Koch M, Hanson J. 1982. Feasibility of grading carcinomas. *Arch Pathol Lab Med* 106:265–267.
2. Blackard C, Doe R, Mellinger G, et al. 1978. Incidence of cardiovascular disease in patients receiving diethylstilbestrol for carcinoma of the prostate. *Cancer* 26:249–256.
3. Byar D. 1972. Treatment of prostatic cancer: Studies by the Veterans Administration Cooperative Urological Research Group. *Bull NY Acad Med* 48:751–766.

4. Byar D. 1973. The Veterans Administration Cooperative Urological Research Group's studies of cancer of the prostate. *Cancer* 32:1126–1130.

5. Corriere J, Cornog J, Murphy J. 1970. Prognosis in patients with carcinoma of the prostate. *Cancer* 25:911–918.

6. Gleason D. 1977. Histologic grading and clinical staging of carcinoma of the prostate, in Tannenbaum M (ed): *Urologic Pathology: The Prostate.* Philadelphia, Lea & Febiger, pp 171–197.

7. Gleason D, Mellinger G, Veterans Administration Cooperative Urological Research Group. 1974. Prediction of prognosis for prostatic carcinoma by combined histological grading and clinical staging. *J Urol* 111:58–64.

8. Kramer S, Spahr J, Brendler C, et al. 1980. Experience with Gleason's histopathologic grading in prostatic cancer. *J Urol* 124:223–225.

9. Paulson D, Piserchia P, Gardner W. 1980. Predictors of lymphatic spread in prostatic adenocarcinoma. *J Urol* 123:697–699.

10. Sogani P, Israel A, Lieberman P, et al. 1985. Gleason grading of prostatic carcinoma: A predictor of survival. *Urology* 25:223–227.

11. Thomas R, Lewis R, Sarma D, et al. 1980. Aid to accurate staging: Histopathologic grading in prostatic cancer. *J Urol* 128:726–728.

12. The Veterans Administration Cooperative Urological Research Group. 1967. Carcinoma of the prostate: Treatment comparisons. *J Urol* 98:516–522.

Chapter 23

Leuprolide vs. Diethylstilbestrol for Metastatic Prostate Cancer: A Multicenter Study

Marc B. Garnick, M.D.

Linda J. Swanson, Ph.D.

Devorah T. Max, M.D.

for the Leuprolide Study Group

For the past 40 years since Huggins and Hodges observed that surgical castration or diethylstilbestrol (DES) could bring relief of symptoms from metastatic prostate cancer, these have been the two standard therapies for the initial treatment of that disease (Huggins and Hodges 1941; Huggins et al. 1941). However, during that time the search for less toxic and more acceptable forms of therapy has continued.

The potent analogues of gonadotropin-releasing hormone (GnRH) offer an important alternative to DES or orchiectomy. These analogues have substitutions in the sixth and tenth amino acid positions (Fig 23–1). Chronic administration of these analogues, to both animals and man, results in an initial stimulation, followed by inhibition, of the release of follicle-stimulating hormone (FSH) and luteinizing hormone (LH) (Belchetz et al. 1978; Linde et al. 1981). The suppression of LH and FSH leads to a decrease in circulating testosterone levels, critical in the treatment of prostate adenocarcinoma (Borgmann et al. 1982; Ahmed et al. 1983; Allen et al. 1983; Fauré et al. 1983; Koutsilieris and Tolis 1983; Walker et al. 1983; Waxman et al. 1983; Garnick and Glode 1984).

METHODS

The efficacy and safety of the superactive analogue of GnRH, leuprolide, were compared to those of DES in patients with previously untreated stage D_2 prostate cancer. The study was conducted in 20 centers in the United States, Canada, and Mexico beginning in October 1981.

On entry into the study, patients were randomly assigned to receive leuprolide, 1 mg

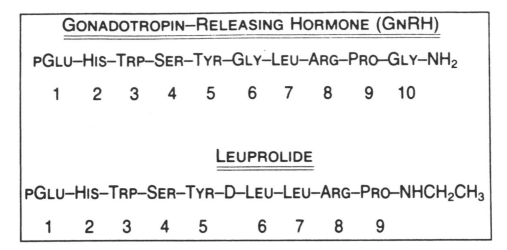

FIG 23–1.
Amino acid sequence of native gonadotropin-releasing hormone and leuprolide. (From Garnick MB, Glode LM. 1984. Leuprolide versus diethylstilbestrol for metastatic prostate cancer. *N Engl J Med* 311:1281–1286. Used by permission.)

subcutaneously daily, or DES, 3 mg orally per day. Ninety-eight patients were randomized to the leuprolide arm as initial treatment, and 101 were randomized to the DES arm. Patients could cross over to the other treatment when disease progressed or when side effects were intolerable. When disease progressed or if side effects were intolerable on the second treatment, patients were discontinued from the study and were monitored from that time on to determine survival. Patients were examined every 6 weeks during the study and were evaluated for objective response every 3 months. Objective response was determined using the criteria of the National Prostatic Cancer Project (Schmidt et al. 1980) (Table 23–1).

Entrance Criteria

Patients were enrolled in the study who met the following entrance criteria: carcinoma of the prostate with bone metastases, lymph node metastases above the aortic bifurcation, or metastases to other soft tissues (stage D_2); two measurable or evaluable manifestations of prostate cancer (e.g., metastases, nodules in the prostate, or elevated serum acid phosphatase level); performance status no higher than 2 according to the Eastern Cooperative Oncology Group scale (ambulatory for more than 50% of waking hours, unless incapacitated by bone pain); no previous systemic therapy or radiotherapy, except for local radiotherapy of non-indicator lesions; complete recovery from the effects of major surgery; and informed consent given voluntarily.

Exclusion Criteria

Patients were excluded from the study if they had had an orchiectomy. In addition, they were excluded if they had a history of other cancer or of life-threatening renal, hepatic, or cardiovascular disease or if their life expectancy was less than 3 months because of cancer.

There were no significant differences in patient characteristics with respect to age, performance status, acid phosphatase levels, tumor burden, or cardiovascular history between the two initial treatment groups at study entry (Table 23–2).

TABLE 23–1.
National Prostatic Cancer Project for Evaluation of Clinical Responses to Treatment of Prostate Cancer*

Response	Tumor Masses	Elevated Acid Phosphatase	Osteoblastic Lesions	Osteolytic Lesions	Hepatomegaly/Abnormal LFTs†	Weight, Symptoms, Performance Status
Complete response (all, if present)	Complete disappearance No new lesions	Normalized	Disappeared	Recalcified	Normalized/normalized	No deterioration
Partial response (all, if present)	>50% reduction of at least 1 mass	Normalized	No progression	Recalcification of some	30% decrease/30% decrease	No deterioration
Objectively stable—no change (all, if present)	No increase in size by >25% No new lesions	Decreased in value	Stabilized	Not worse	No increase by >30%/not worse	No deterioration
Progression (any of following)	Increase in size by >25% New lesions	Increase in acid and/or alkaline phosphatase with other evidence of progression				Deterioration

*From Garnick MB, Glode LM, 1984. Leuprolide versus diethylstilbestrol for metastatic prostate cancer. *N Engl J Med* 311:1281–1286. Used by permission.
†LFTs = liver-function tests.

TABLE 23–2.
Characteristics of Evaluable Patients With Metastatic
Prostate Cancer Treated With Leuprolide or
Diethylstilbestrol (DES)*

Variable	Leuprolide Group (n = 98)	DES Group (n = 101)
Age—mean (range)	69 (46–87)	71 (43–96)
Performance status 0-1— no. of patients (%)	76 (82)	76 (80)
Prostatic acid phosphatase (ng/ml)—mean ± SD	22 ± 34	31 ± 72
Initial serum testosterone (ng/dl)—mean ± SD	410 ± 214	409 ± 210
High tumor burden—no. of patients (%)[†]	72 (77)	75 (79)
Cardiovascular history—no. of patients (%)[‡]	68 (73)	67 (71)

*From Garnick MB, Glode LM. 1984. Leuprolide versus diethylstilbestrol for metastatic prostate cancer. *N Engl J Med* 311:1281–1286. Used by permission.
[†]High tumor burden is defined as one of the following: three or more bone lesions, liver lesions (with or without bone lesions), or lung and bone lesions.
[‡]Includes patients with any cardiovascular abnormalities noted on the electrocardiogram, in the physical examination, or in the medical history and patients receiving concomitant cardiovascular medication.

RESULTS AND DISCUSSION

Serum testosterone (T) and dihydrotestosterone (DHT) levels during the study are shown in Figures 23–2 and 23–3. After an initial increase (not shown), T and DHT levels fell to castration levels (less than 50 ng/dl) by weeks 3 and 4 and remained there throughout the study. The mean T and DHT levels remained at castration levels for both groups during the period of drug administration.

The best objective responses determined at or beyond week 12 for evaluable patients, 92 initially treated with leuprolide and 94 with DES, are shown in Table 23–3. Eighty-six percent of the patients in the leuprolide group (complete response [CR], partial response [PR], and stable disease [NC]: 1% + 37% + 48%) and 85% of the patients initially treated with DES (CR + PR + NC: 2% + 44% + 39%) had a favorable response (no progression) to treatment. Two percent of the evaluable patients initially treated with DES and 11% of those initially treated with leuprolide showed progressive disease at or before week 12. Among evaluable patients, 3% of those receiving leuprolide and 13% of those receiving DES were considered to have failed at the week-12 point because of intolerable side effects. They had either crossed over to the alternative therapy or discontinued therapy.

With the initiation of GnRH analogue administration, including leuprolide, testosterone production is stimulated, with peak levels occurring about 3 days later (Warner et al. 1983). Temporary increases in bone pain and obstructive symptoms, possibly related to tumor stimulation, have been reported concomitant with the initial increase in testosterone (Borgmann et al. 1982; Warner et al. 1983; Garnick and Glode 1984). The evaluation of early changes in acid phosphatase level and bone pain during the first 12 weeks of therapy is shown in Table 23–4.

Patients were examined at weeks 1, 2, and 4 to determine whether or not there was a

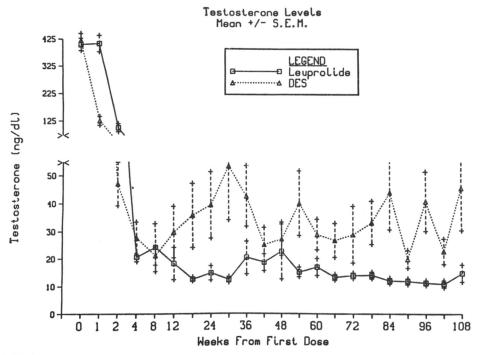

FIG 23–2.

Mean (± SEM) serum testosterone levels over 108 weeks of study. The number of patients studied (N) decreased from 89 to 27 in the leuprolide group and from 82 to 24 in the diethylstilbestrol (*DES*) group as patients discontinued study. At any point N was never less than 12. (From Swanson LJ, Garnick MB. 1987. Leuprolide versus diethylstilbestrol for metastatic prostate cancer, in Klijn JGM, Paridaens R, Foekens JA (eds): *Hormonal Manipulation of Cancer: Peptides, Growth Factors and New (Anti) Steroidal Agents.* Monograph Series of the European Organization for Research on Treatment of Cancer, vol 18. New York, Raven Press, pp 301–308. Used with permission.)

TABLE 23–3.

Best Objective Response to Treatment*†

Response	Leuprolide (n = 92)		DES (n = 94)	
	No.	%	No.	%
CR	1	1	2	2
PR	34	37	41	44
NC	44	48	37	39
No progression	79	86	80	85
PD	10	11	2	2
SE	3	3	12	13

*From Garnick MB, Glode LM. 1984. Leuprolide versus diethylstilbestrol for metastatic prostate cancer. *N Engl J Med* 311:1281–1286. Used by permission.
†DES = diethylstilbestrol; CR = complete response; PR = partial response; NC = no change; PD = progressive disease; SE = patients discontinued secondary to side effects.

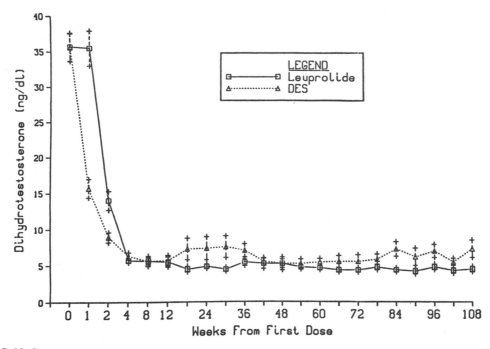

FIG 23–3.
Mean (± SEM) serum dihydrotestosterone levels over 108 weeks of study. The number of patients studied (N) varies as described in the legend to Figure 23–2. *DES* = diethylstilbestrol. (From Swanson LJ, Garnick MB. 1987. Leuprolide versus diethylstilbestrol for metastatic prostate cancer, in Klijn JGM, Paridaens R, Foekens JA (eds): *Hormonal Manipulation of Cancer: Peptides, Growth Factors and New (Anti) Steroidal Agents.* Monograph Series of the European Organization for Research on Treatment of Cancer, vol 18. New York, Raven Press, pp 301–308. Used with permission.)

temporary worsening of symptoms such as bone pain or an increase in the acid phosphatase level. Although bone pain had increased at week 1 in 7 patients receiving leuprolide and 1 receiving DES, this difference was not statistically significant and had disappeared by week 2. Patients in both groups showed an increase in the acid phosphatase level at week 1, which continued to be observed at weeks 2 and 4 in only the leuprolide group. Differences between the two groups only at weeks 2 and 4 were statistically significant ($P < .05$). The fact that acid phosphatase levels continued to be elevated at weeks 2 and 4 in patients receiving leuprolide suggests that these patients responded more slowly to treatment than patients treated with DES, presumably because of the initial increases in testosterone. By week 12, however, no significant differences between the two groups remained.

The majority of patients in both groups showed either a decrease or no change in acid phosphatase levels between weeks 1 and 12. There were no significant differences between the groups by week 12.

The evaluations of the overall subjective response to treatment, performance status, and bone pain at week 12 are shown in Table 23–5.

Patients in both groups showed improvement in overall subjective response to treatment (53%, leuprolide; 61%, DES), in performance status (41%, leuprolide; 36%, DES), and in bone pain (73%, leuprolide; 69%, DES). There were no differences between the two groups in the number of patients who improved, remained stable, or worsened for these three variables.

TABLE 23–4.
Early Assessment of Acid Phosphatase and
Bone Pain*[†]

Week	Leuprolide (No.)		DES (No.)	
	AP	BP	AP	BP
1	26	7	21	1
2	27[‡]	6	12[‡]	6
4	19[‡]	8	4[‡]	5
12	11	3	5	7

*From Garnick MB, Glode LM. 1984. Leuprolide versus diethylstilbestrol for metastatic prostate cancer. *N Engl J Med* 311:1281–1286. Used by permission.
[†]AP = acid phosphatase; BP = bone pain
[‡]$P<.05$.

TABLE 23–5.
Subjective Response to Treatment at Week 12*

	Leuprolide						DES[†]					
	Improved		Same		Worse		Improved		Same		Worse	
Criterion	No.	%	No.	%	No.	%	No.	%	No.	%	No.	%
Overall subjective response	48	53	35	39	7	8	51	61	21	33	5	6
Performance status	37	41	37	41	16	18	30	36	40	48	13	16
Bone pain severity (if present)	32	73	9	20	3	7	33	69	9	19	6	13

*Adapted from Garnick MB, Swanson LJ, Max DT. In press. A randomized prospective evaluation of leuprolide versus diethylstilbestrol in the treatment of stage D_2 prostate cancer: Results of a multicenter study, in Coffey DS, Resnick M, Dorr A, et al. (eds): *The Management of Prostate Cancer*. New York, Plenum Publishing Corp. Used with permission.
[†]DES = diethylstilbestrol.

The time to treatment failure of patients with evaluable stage D_2 disease is shown in Figure 23–4. There were no differences between the two groups.

Figure 23–5 exhibits the distributions of time from start of study to death for evaluable patients receiving leuprolide and DES. No differences were observed between the two groups. It is important to note that when survival is examined, one is not comparing the survival rates of patients treated only with DES to those of patients treated only with leuprolide. Rather, one is comparing the survival of patients treated with leuprolide as first treatment followed by DES, any other treatment, or no treatment, to the survival of patients treated with DES as primary therapy, followed by leuprolide, another treatment, or no treatment. The two curves, then, include cohorts of patients who crossed over to the alternative treatment. The two cohorts do not make similar contributions to the two survival curves, and a bias in favor of the DES group may be present.

The importance of the long-term complications of DES therapy in elderly men with prostate cancer is becoming increasingly clear. Although reducing the DES to 1 mg/day may reduce toxicity, this dose may not be as effective as the standard therapy of 3 mg/day in reducing testosterone to castrate level (Robinson and Thomas 1971). In the present study, patients receiving DES, 3 mg/day, showed significantly more gynecomastia, peripheral edema, and nausea than did those receiving leuprolide (Table 23–6). A greater number of patients in the DES group also had thrombosis, pulmonary emboli, and myocardial infarction, although these differences were not significant.

Fifteen patients (3 on leuprolide and 12 on DES) discontinued their initial therapy before week 12 owing to adverse reactions. Eight of 12 receiving DES discontinued because of

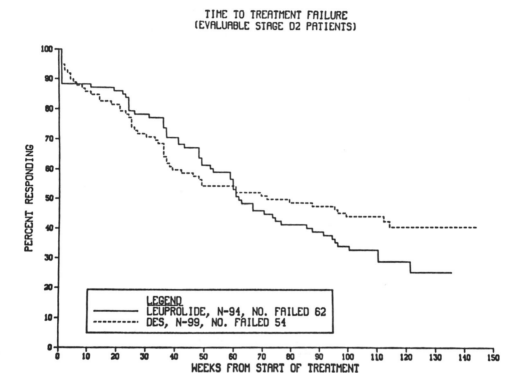

FIG 23–4.
Time to failure of the initial treatment for evaluable stage D_2 patients treated with leuprolide or diethylstilbestrol (*DES*). (From Swanson LJ, Garnick MB. 1987. Leuprolide versus diethylstilbestrol for metastatic prostate cancer, in Klijn JGM, Paridaens R, Foekens JA (eds): *Hormonal Manipulation of Cancer: Peptides, Growth Factors and New (Anti) Steroidal Agents.* Monograph Series of the European Organization for Research on Treatment of Cancer, vol 18. New York, Raven Press, pp 301–308. Used with permission.)

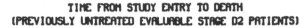

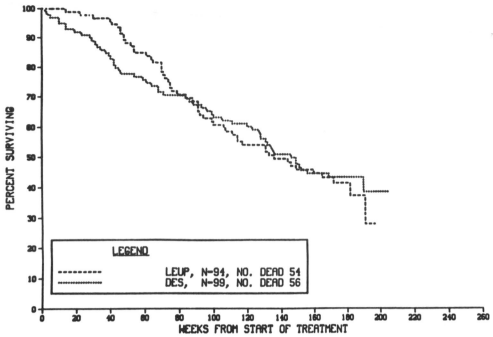

FIG 23–5.

Time from study entry to death of evaluable stage D_2 patients initially treated with leuprolide or diethylstilbestrol *(DES).* (From Swanson LJ, Garnick MB. 1987. Leuprolide versus diethylstilbestrol for metastatic prostate cancer, in Klijn JGM, Paridaens R, Foekens JA (eds): *Hormonal Manipulation of Cancer: Peptides, Growth Factors and New (Anti) Steroidal Agents.* Monograph Series of the European Organization for Research on Treatment of Cancer, vol 18. New York, Raven Press, pp 301–308. Used with permission.)

TABLE 23–6.
Adverse Side Effects in Patients Receiving Leuprolide or DES*[†]

Side Effect	Leuprolide Group (n = 98)	DES Group (n = 101)	P Value
Hot flashes	51	11	<.00001
Gynecomastia/breast tenderness	3	49	<.00001
Nausea/vomiting	5	17	<.02
Edema	2	16	<.0008
Thrombosis/phlebitis/pulmonary emboli	1	7	.065
Myocardial infarction, angina, or congestive failure	3	5	NS

*From Garnick MB, Glode LM. 1984. Leuprolide versus diethylstilbestrol for metastatic prostate cancer. *N Engl J Med* 311:1281–1286. Used by permission.
[†]DES = diethylstilbestrol; NS = not significant.

cardiovascular side effects, while none of the 3 receiving leuprolide discontinued for those reasons.

In conclusion, leuprolide is a safe and effective treatment for metastatic prostate cancer. It is an important alternative treatment for prostate cancer for patients who do not want to undergo orchiectomy or who cannot tolerate DES because of the risk of cardiovascular complications.

REFERENCES

1. Ahmed SR, Brooman PJC, Shalet SM, et al. 1983. Treatment of advanced prostatic cancer with LHRH analogue ICI 118630: Clinical response and hormonal mechanisms. *Lancet* 2:415–419.
2. Allen JM, O'Shea JP, Mashiter K, et al. 1983. Advanced carcinoma of the prostate: Treatment with a gonadotropin releasing agonist. *Br Med J* 286:1607–1609.
3. Belchetz PE, Plant TM, Nakai Y, et al. 1978. Hyophysial responses to continuous and intermittent delivery of hypothalamic gonadotropin-releasing hormone. *Science* 202:631–633.
4. Borgmann V, Hardt W, Schmidt-Gollwitzer M, et al. 1982. Sustained suppression of testosterone production by the luteinising-hormone releasing-hormone agonist buserelin in patients with advanced prostate carcinoma: A new therapeutic approach? *Lancet* 1:1097–1099.
5. Fauré N, Lemay A, Laroche B, et al. 1983. Preliminary results on the clinical efficacy and safety of androgen inhibition by the LHRH agonist alone or combined with an antiandrogen in the treatment of prostatic carcinoma. *Prostate* 4:601–624.
6. Garnick MB, Glode LM, for the Leuprolide Study Group. 1984. Leuprolide versus diethylstilbestrol for metastatic prostate cancer. *N Engl J Med* 311:1281–1286.
7. Garnick MB, Swanson LJ, Max DT. In press. A randomized prospective evaluation of leuprolide versus diethylstilbestrol in the treatment of stage D_2 prostate cancer: Results of a multicenter study, in Coffey DS, Resnick M, Dorr A, et al. (eds): *The Management of Prostate Cancer.* New York, Plenum Publishing Corporation.
8. Huggins C, Hodges CV. 1941. Studies on prostatic cancer. I. The effect of castration, of estrogen and of androgen injection on serum phosphatases in metastatic carcinoma of the prostate. *Cancer Res* 1:293–297.
9. Huggins C, Stevens RE Jr, Hodges CV. 1941. Studies on prostatic cancer. II. The effects of castration on advanced carcinoma of the prostate gland. *Arch Surg* 43:209–223.
10. Koutsilieris M, Tolis G. 1983. Gonadotropin-releasing hormone agonist analogues in the treatment of advanced prostatic carcinoma. *Prostate* 4:569–577.
11. Linde R, Doelle GC, Alexander N, et al. 1981. Reversible inhibition of testicular steroidogenesis and spermatogenesis by a potent gonadotropin-releasing hormone agonist in normal men: An approach toward the development of a male contraceptive. *N Engl J Med* 305:663–667.
12. Robinson MRG, Thomas BS. 1971. Effect of hormonal therapy on plasma testosterone levels in prostatic carcinoma. *Br Med J* 4:391–394.
13. Schmidt JD, Scott WW, Gibbons R, et al. 1980. Chemotherapy programs of the National Prostatic Cancer Project. *Cancer* 45:1937–1946.
14. Swanson LJ, Garnick MB. 1987. Leuprolide versus diethylstilbestrol for metastatic prostate cancer, in Klijn JGM, Paridaens R, Foekens JA (eds): *Hormonal Manipulation of Cancer: Peptides, Growth Factors and New (Anti) Steroidal Agents.* Monograph Series of the European Organization for Research on Treatment of Cancer, vol 18. New York, Raven Press, pp 301–308.
15. Walker KJ, Nicholson RI, Turkes AO, et al. 1983. Therapeutic potential of the LHRH agonist, ICI 118630, in the treatment of advanced prostatic cancer. *Lancet* 2:413–415.
16. Warner B, Worgul TJ, Drago J, et al. 1983. Effect of very high dose D-leucine[6]-gonadotropin-releasing hormone proethylamide on the hypothalamic-pituitary testicular axis in patients with prostatic cancer. *J Clin Invest* 71:1842–1853.
17. Waxman JH, Wass JAH, Hendry WF, et al. 1983. Treatment with gonadotrophin releasing hormone analogue in advanced prostatic cancer. *Br Med J* 286:1309–1312.

Chapter 24

Buserelin (HOE-766) as Treatment of Advanced Prostatic Carcinoma

Buserelin Protocol 301 Study Group*

The recognition by Huggins in 1941 that prostate cancer cells were androgen dependent (Huggins et al. 1941) inaugurated a continuing search for the ideal method of androgen ablation. Orchiectomy, estrogen administration, or both have been the principal strategies of therapy but are not without their drawbacks. Surgical castration is psychologically traumatic and at times associated with significant operative morbidity. Estrogens in therapeutic dosages have been associated with exacerbation of cardiovascular disease, the occurrence of thrombophlebitis, and gynecomastia.

In 1971 Schally synthetically produced gonadotropin-releasing hormone (GnRH), a decapeptide found in the hypothalamus, which controls release of luteinizing hormone (LH) from the pituitary (Schally et al. 1971). A number of analogues of naturally occurring GnRH were soon synthesized, and it was recognized that chronic administration of very potent analogues would result in initial overstimulation and then depletion of LH receptors in the pituitary. This depletion results in a decline of LH release that is paralleled by a decline in the production of testosterone by the testes. The administration of luteinizing hormone-releasing hormone (LH-RH) analogues therefore became recognized as an effective therapeutic strategy for producing a medical castration.

Buserelin (Suprefact) was produced by scientists at Hoechst AG (West Germany) by substituting at the sixth site in the peptide chain of natural GnRH the amino acid glycine with D-serine-O-tert-butyl ether and by replacing the terminal glycinamide with ethylamide, resulting in a nonapeptide. This new compound called buserelin has a serum half-life similar to that of natural GnRH but, after binding to the receptor, is resistant to degradation by arylamidase, resulting in a prolonged and more intense receptor blockade that is, however, completely reversible on cessation of the drug.

Repeated stimulation with buserelin at a high dosage invokes an initial surge of LH release owing to saturation of the pituitary receptors, which results in a transient rise of the serum level of testosterone. As buserelin administration is continued, LH production falls very rapidly, causing a profound decline in the serum testosterone level similar to that achieved by surgical castration. This castrate level of testosterone is maintained for as long as sufficient drug is administered, either by daily subcutaneous injections or by nasal insuf-

*A. C. von Eschenbach, N. L. Block, S. J. Childs, N. Fauré, V. P. Hollander, D. T. Mininberg, J. E. Pontes, R. T. Huben, C. A. Presant, M. C. Schwarz, M. S. Soloway, B. Stein, R. S. Swerdloff, S. S. Klioze, J. W. Kosola, T. P. Spiro.

flation three times daily, thus providing a very effective method of therapy for advanced prostate cancer.

In the early 1980s, pilot clinical trials using buserelin to treat prostate cancer were inaugurated by investigators in Canada and Germany. Early reports and references cited therein (Fauré et al. 1985; Tolis and Koutsilieris 1985; Waxman et al. 1985; Wenderoth and Jacobi 1985) confirmed that the objective regression and subjective improvement that accompanied the administration of buserelin were comparable to those achieved by standard endocrine therapy. Moreover, the medication was easily administered and free of any serious side effects.

Because of its effectiveness and encouraging potential advantages, a cooperative trial of buserelin was conducted among 12 institutions (Table 24–1) in North America to (1) confirm its clinical usefulness as a method of achieving testosterone suppression, (2) evaluate its safety, and (3) determine its efficacy in achieving objective tumor regression and symptomatic improvement in patients with advanced prostatic cancer.

MATERIALS AND METHODS

This nonrandomized, noncomparative study of patients with locally advanced (stage C) or metastatic (stage D) disease was begun in November 1982. Some patients who were treated with estrogen or underwent orchiectomy were admitted for comparison; however, because accrual was small, historical controls have been substituted in the analysis.

A total of 249 patients were enrolled, 211 of whom received buserelin and 38 standard

TABLE 24–1.
Institutions Participating in Buserelin Trial

Institution	Investigator	No. of Patients
University of Miami School of Medicine Miami, Fla.	N. Block	70
Brookwood Medical Center Birmingham, Ala.	S. Childs	14
Hospital St. Francois d'Assise Quebec City, Quebec	N. Fauré	21
Mount Sinai Medical Center New York, N.Y.	V. Hollander	13
Cornell Medical Center New York, N.Y.	D. Mininberg	23
Roswell Park Memorial Institute Buffalo, N.Y.	E. Pontes/R. Huben	5
St. Vincent Medical Center Los Angeles, Calif.	C. Presant	16
Hematology and Oncology Associates of Virginia Richmond, Va.	M. Schwarz	12
University of Tennessee Center for Health Sciences Memphis, Tenn.	M. Soloway	24
Temple University Medical Center Philadelphia, Pa.	B. Stein	4
Harbor-UCLA Medical Center Torrance, Calif.	R. Swerdloff	25
The University of Texas M.D. Anderson Cancer Center Houston, Tex.	A. von Eschenbach	22
Total	12 investigators	249

endocrine therapy, 3 with diethylstilbestrol (DES) and 35 with orchiectomy. Five enrolled patients have been excluded from all analyses because of absent data. Of the 244 remaining, 17 had stage C, 29 stage D_1, and 198 stage D_2 disease. Data for all 244 patients were sufficient to evaluate for safety; however, 23 patients (22 buserelin-treated and 1 after orchiectomy) have been excluded from the efficacy-of-treatment analysis because of protocol violations.

Buserelin was first administered to the 211 patients as a subcutaneous injection of 500 μg every 8 hours for 7 days. Following this induction, 151 patients were maintained on subcutaneous injections of 200 μg once daily, and 56 patients received an intranasal spray of 400 μg three times a day. From the 211 patients assigned to buserelin, sufficient data were available to evaluate the safety of the drug in 207 and the efficacy of therapy in 185.

Because the 38 patients in this study who received DES or underwent orchiectomy were too few to serve as meaningful controls, the protocol data were compared with data from historical controls. Data were obtained for 166 patients who underwent primary endocrine therapy for stage D_2 prostate cancer in the National Prostatic Cancer Project (NPCP) protocols numbers 500 and 1,300 (Murphy et al. 1983, 1986). These data were analyzed and compared to data from 147 fully evaluable patients with stage D_2 disease who received buserelin. Analysis of prognostic variables demonstrated that the groups were comparable. The only statistically significant difference was that the buserelin-treated patients entered the study with histories of a higher frequency of pain and a greater weight loss. The patients enrolled in the NPCP trials either underwent orchiectomy or received DES, 1 mg orally three times a day. The majority of patients received estrogen only and are designated as the DES group. To include the few treated by orchiectomy in the analysis, those treated by either DES or orchiectomy (Orch) are combined as DES/Orch. It should be remembered, however, that this classification designates not the combination of therapies but use of one or the other.

To evaluate the impact of initial therapy and the long-term effectiveness of treatment, the efficacy of buserelin therapy was analyzed in terms of early (up to 12 weeks) progression-free survival, long-term progression-free survival (2 years), and life survival. Other factors analyzed were the effect of buserelin therapy on testosterone suppression, signs and symptoms of prostate cancer including performance status, and selected laboratory values (Table 24–2). The results of this study have been reported previously in detail (von Eschenbach 1987) and are summarized here.

RESULTS

Suppression of Testosterone

Buserelin is effective at achieving prolonged suppression of serum testosterone (T) to castrate levels. After rising briefly during the first week, mean serum testosterone levels began to fall rapidly, and by week 3 were below 100 ng/dl. Thereafter, serum T levels were sustained at these castrate levels for the 24 months of observation; mean serum testosterone levels fluctuated in the range of 30 to 40 ng/dl (Table 24–3).

The values of serum testosterone for patients who received buserelin are comparable to those of patients who received DES or underwent orchiectomy (Fig 24–1). Buserelin was ineffective in achieving medical castration in only 8 of 185 patients. Although there is no statistically significant difference in mean testosterone levels between the intranasal (IN) and subcutaneous (SC) routes of buserelin administration, the values were higher for the IN group than for the SC group. Some fluctuation of serum testosterone values did occur. After the serum testosterone level of patients with stage D_2 disease was first suppressed, it rose again to above 100 ng/dl at least once in 8 of 30 patients (26.7%) who received buserelin intranasally;

TABLE 24–2.
Schedule of Observations, Buserelin Trial*†

Evaluation	Before Treatment	wk 1	wk 2	wk 3	wk 4 / mo 1	wk 8 / mo 2	wk 12 / mo 3	mo 4	mo 5	mo 6	mo 7	mo 8	mo 9	mo 10	mo 11	mo 12	After 1 yr (every 3 mo)
Medical history	+																
Physical examination	+		+		+	+	+	+	+	+	+	+	+	+	+	+	+
Laboratory tests‡																	
Hematology	+				+		+			+			+			+	+
Blood chemistry	+				+		+			+			+			+	+
Acid/alkaline phosphatase	+				+	+	+			+			+			+	+
Urinalysis (general)	+				+		+			+			+			+	+
Endocrinology‡																	
Testosterone‡	+	+	+	+	+	+	+	+	+	+	+	+	+	+	+	+	+
DHT, E2, T4, PRL	+					+				+			+			+	+
LH-RH test or LH and FSH	+				+		+			+			+			+	+
Synacthen test or F test†	+						+			+						+	+
HOE-766 antibody titration	+															+	Every 12 mo
Clinical evaluation																	
Ultrasound test of prostate	(+)					(+)	(+)			(+)			(+)			(+)	(+)
CT of prostate and pelvis	+									+						+	Every 6 mo
Flowmetry	+					+	+			+			+			+	+
Chest x-ray	+						+			+						+	Every 6 mo
Bone scan	+						+			+						+	+
Bone x-ray (if indicated)	(+)						(+)			(+)						(I)	(+)
ECG	+									+						+	Every 6 mo
IVP or radionuclide urogram	(+)						(+)			(+)						(+)	(+)
Prostate biopsy	+									(+)						+	
Medication administered		+	+	+	+	+	+	+	+	+	+	+	+	+	+	+	+
Side effects recorded		+	+	+	+	+	+	+	+	+	+	+	+	+	+	+	+
Clinical global impression recorded		+	+	+	+	+	+	+	+	+	+	+	+	+	+	+	+

*From Von Eschenbach AC. 1987. Therapeutic applications of buserelin. *Br J Clin Pract* 41:94. Used by permission.
†DHT = dihydrotestosterone; E2 = estradiol; T4 = thyroid function test; PRL = prolactin; LH-RH = luteinizing hormone releasing hormone; LH = luteinizing hormone; FSH = follicle-stimulating hormone; F = cortisol; CT = computed tomography; ECG = electrocardiogram; IVP = intravenous pyelogram; (+) = if indicated or optional.
‡Blood serum samples obtained prior to daily dosing and at follow-up visits.

in comparison, only 21 of 109 similar patients (19.3%) who received buserelin subcutaneously ever exceeded this value. Compliance appeared to be excellent with both forms of administration, but the SC route appeared to be more consistent.

Safety

Buserelin was well tolerated and free of serious side effects. No biochemical or hematologic abnormalities that could be attributed to buserelin therapy were detected.

No drug-related deaths occurred, and almost all side effects attributable to the drug were mild (Table 24–4). The most frequent complaint was vasomotor instability ("hot flashes"), which occurred in over 70% of patients treated with buserelin. Exacerbation of disease

TABLE 24–3.
Mean Serum Testosterone Level Changes in Buserelin Study*

| Time | No. of Patients | Testosterone Levels (ng/dl)[†] | | | |
		Mean	SD	Min.	Max.
				Range	
0	175	416.8	197.7	56	1140
1 wk	175	452.8	330.8	24	2616
2 wk	164	152.1	137.4	16	887
3 wk	161	84.6	93.8	5	729
4 wk	170	69.5	100.5	9	843
2 mo	165	54.5	92.3	2	825
3 mo	160	51.5	75.2	2	544
4 mo	158	37.7	34.9	4	248
5 mo	138	37.0	31.3	2	187
6 mo	137	36.4	37.9	4	285
12 mo	82	34.2	35.4	0	270
15 mo	55	30.8	24.7	10	154
18 mo	47	29.5	28.5	8	157
21 mo	33	30.4	28.9	10	165
24 mo	21	38.9	46.2	7	218

*From von Eschenbach AC. 1987. Therapeutic applications of buserelin. *Br J Clin Pract* 41:95. Used by permission.
[†]SD = standard deviation from the mean; Min. = minimum; Max. = maximum.

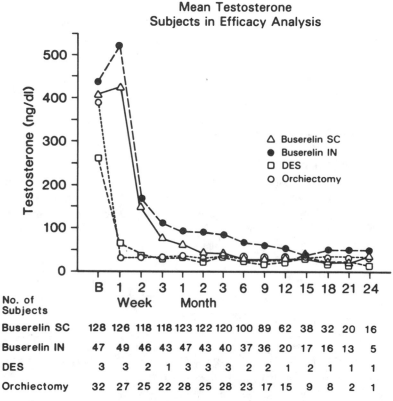

**Mean Testosterone
Subjects in Efficacy Analysis**

△ Buserelin SC
● Buserelin IN
□ DES
○ Orchiectomy

| No. of Subjects | B | 1 | 2 | 3 | 1 | 2 | 3 | 6 | 9 | 12 | 15 | 18 | 21 | 24 |
		Week			Month									
Buserelin SC	128	126	118	118	123	122	120	100	89	62	38	32	20	16
Buserelin IN	47	49	46	43	47	43	40	37	36	20	17	16	13	5
DES	3	3	2	1	3	3	3	2	2	1	2	1	1	1
Orchiectomy	32	27	25	22	28	25	28	23	17	15	9	8	2	1

FIG 24–1.
A comparison over 2 years of the mean serum testosterone values following administration of subcutaneous (*SC*) buserelin, intranasal (*IN*) buserelin, diethylstilbestrol (*DES*), or orchiectomy. (From von Eschenbach AC. 1987. Therapeutic applications of buserelin. *Br J Clin Pract* 41:95. Used by permission.)

TABLE 24–4.
Safety of Buserelin: Side Effects of Treatment*

| | Buserelin Administration | | | |
| | Subcutaneous (n = 151) | | Intranasal (n = 56) | |
Symptom	No.	(%)	No.	(%)
Biochemical abnormality (drug-induced)	0	(0)	0	(0)
Hot flashes	108	(72)	37	(66)
Loss of libido[†]	128	(85)	42	(75)
Impotence[†]	120	(79)	42	(75)
Nasal irritation	—		7	(13)
Headache	—		16	(29)
Flare reactions	2	(1)		
Gynecomastia	4	(2)		
Pruritus	4	(2)		
Gastrointestinal disturbances	5	(2)		

*Adapted from von Eschenbach AC. 1987. Therapeutic applications of buserelin. *Br J Clin Practice* 41:95.
[†]In 50% of patients, loss of libido and impotence were recorded at admission.

symptoms can occur during the first week of therapy owing to the transient rise in serum testosterone level. Most of these "flare" reactions can easily be managed symptomatically; however, severe or catastrophic tumor exacerbations are possible. In this series, two patients (1%) experienced severe clinical flare reactions such as paralysis due to spinal cord compression by tumor. In patients considered to be at risk of a serious flare reaction, androgen production could be temporarily blocked by another agent such as ketoconazole for the first few weeks of therapy.

Efficacy

At the time of data analysis, 101 of 207 patients (49%) who received buserelin were off the study. Sixty patients (29%) were removed because of progressing disease. Twelve patients (6%) died during the study, 3 patients (1%) were removed for serious adverse reactions, and 26 were discontinued for other reasons. Objective tumor response was analyzed according to the NPCP criteria; categories were complete regression (CR), partial regression (PR), stable disease, and progression. The best responses achieved by patients with stage D_2 disease receiving buserelin are compared to the results of stage D_2 patients who received DES or orchiectomy (Orch) in the NPCP protocols in Table 24–5. No significant differences between the buserelin-treated group and the historical controls were evident. Although the CR rates were higher in the historical controls (11% for DES/Orch vs. 3% for buserelin), the overall response rates (CR + PR) are comparable (37% for either DES/Orch vs. 45% for buserelin).

Progression-Free Survival Rates

Stage D_2 buserelin-treated patients in the current trial were compared to historical controls from the NPCP protocols 500 and 1,300 to evaluate early progression-free survival, long-term progression-free survival, and life survival.

Progression-free survival duration was defined as the length of time from study entry to first detection of disease progression or to death. Patients who discontinued therapy before week 12 and had not yet progressed were dropped from the early-progression-free survival

TABLE 24–5.
Response to Treatment by Patients With Stage D_2 Disease*[†]

		Response							
		Complete Regression		Partial Regression		Progression		Stable	
Treatment	No. of Subjects	No.	(%)	No.	(%)	No.	(%)	No.	(%)
Buserelin	142	4	(3)	59	(42)	23	(16)	56	(39)
				[63 (45)][‡]					
DES/Orch[‡]	179	20	(11)	46	(26)	24	(13)	89	(50)
				[66 (37)]					
DES	120	12	(10)	35	(29)	13	(11)	60	(50)
				[47 (39)]					

*Adapted from von Eschenbach AC. 1987. Therapeutic applications of buserelin. *Br J Clin Prac* 41:96.
[†]No statistically significant difference among treatments.
[‡][] = CR + PR; DES = diethylstilbestrol; Orch = orchiectomy.

analysis. Among patients with stage D_2 disease, 5 of 147 treated with buserelin and none of 179 treated with DES/Orch discontinued therapy before the 12-week evaluation. Within the first 12 weeks, 23 (16.2%) of these 142 buserelin-treated patients and 24 (13.4%) of the 179 DES/Orch-treated patients progressed ($P = NS$) and were considered refractory to hormonal treatment.

Those patients who survived progression free beyond 77 days (lower limit for the month 3 assessment) were considered to have received sufficient therapy to be analyzed for long-term progression-free survival; the probability of survival was calculated up to 874 days, which was the longest period of buserelin treatment for any patient. The progression-free survival rates are shown in Table 24–6. No significant difference is apparent in the progression-free rates between patients treated with buserelin and historical controls at any time period after therapy began (Fig 24–2).

Life Survival

Survival data of patients on the buserelin protocol were updated through March 1986 to provide a follow-up sufficiently long to allow life survival rates to be compared adequately with those in the NPCP study. The median survival point for the buserelin-treated patients had not yet been reached. For all subjects who began therapy, there were no significant differences between treatment groups in survival rates at 1 and 2 years (Fig 24–3). An analysis

TABLE 24–6.
Efficacy of Buserelin Vs. Standard Endocrine Therapy (% Surviving)*

		Historical Controls		
Response	Buserelin	DES/Orch[†]	DES	
Early progression-free survival (12 wk)	83.8 ± 3.1	86.6 ± 2.5	89.2 ± 2.8	NS
Long-term progression-free survival (2 yr)	33.9 ± 6.1	42.2 ± 4.0	43.2 ± 4.9	NS
Median duration progression-free survival (days)	488 ± 70	589 ± 68	605 ± 70	NS

*Adapted from von Eschenbach AC. 1987. Therapeutic applications of buserelin. *Br J Clin Pract* 41:96.
[†]DES = diethylstilbestrol; Orch = orchiectomy; NS = not significant.

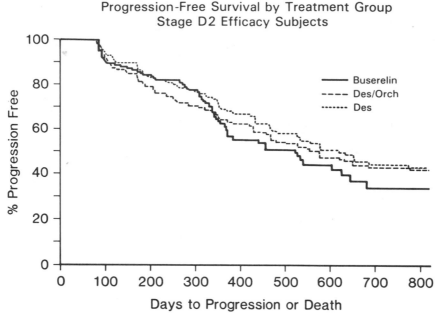

FIG 24–2.

The progression-free survival rates of buserelin-treated patients are comparable to the progression-free survival rates of patients treated with standard endocrine therapy. *DES* = diethylstilbestrol; *Orch* = orchiectomy. (From von Eschenbach AC. 1987. Therapeutic applications of buserelin, *Br J Clin Pract* 41:96. Used by permission.)

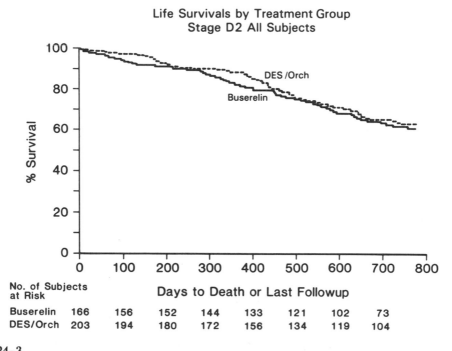

FIG 24–3.

For all patients included in the study, the life survival rates are the same regardless of the form of therapy. *DES* = diethylstilbestrol; *Orch* = orchiectomy. (From von Eschenbach AC. 1987. Therapeutic applications of buserelin. *Br J Clin Pract* 41:97. Used by permission.)

of all subjects in the study shows the 2-year survival rate to be 60.6% for the buserelin-treated patients, 65.0% for those receiving DES, and 63.0% for the DES/Orch group.

If one analyzes only those patients who are in the efficacy portion of the study, the survival results are also comparable. A comparison of results at 1 and 2 years for both groups of patients is shown in Table 24–7 and Figure 24–4. The estimates of survival rate at 2 years were not significantly different between treatment groups. However, at 1 year, patients treated with DES have a statistically significant advantage. This result is most likely because the buserelin-treated group contained a higher proportion of patients who had pain and weight loss at entry into the study and thus were more likely to have a higher early failure rate.

TABLE 24–7.
Comparison of Life Survival Rates: Patients With Stage D_2 Disease*[†]

Survival Time	Survival Rate by Treatment (SD)[‡]			P Value
	Buserelin	DES/Orch	DES	
All patients	n = 166	n = 203	n = 133	
1-yr (410 days)	79.5 ± 3.1	85.0 ± 2.6	88.8 ± 2.8	NS
2-yr (776 days)	60.6 ± 4.0	63.0 ± 3.6	65.0 ± 4.5	NS
Patients evaluable for efficacy	n = 147	n = 179	n = 120	
1-yr (410 days)	80.3 ± 3.3	87.3 ± 2.5	91.3 ± 1.6	DES vs. buserelin .05
2-yr (776 days)	61.9 ± 4.2	65.9 ± 3.8	68.9 ± 4.5	NS

*Adapted from von Eschenbach AC. 1987. Therapeutic applications of buserelin. *Br J Clin Pract* 41:97.
[†]Comparison made by the Kaplan-Meier product limit method.
[‡]SD = standard deviation from the mean; DES = diethylstilbestrol; Orch = orchiectomy; NS = not significant.

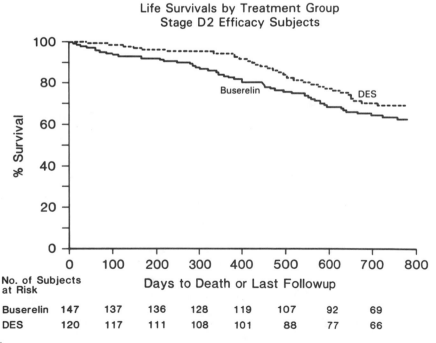

**Life Survivals by Treatment Group
Stage D2 Efficacy Subjects**

No. of Subjects at Risk

Buserelin	147	137	136	128	119	107	92	69
DES	120	117	111	108	101	88	77	66

FIG 24–4.
Among those patients in the efficacy analyses of the study, there is a slight advantage in the life survival rates at 1 year for those patients receiving diethylstilbestrol (*DES*) therapy.

DISCUSSION

These results confirm the experience of others that LH-RH agonists are effective in achieving androgen deprivation of prostatic adenocarcinomas (Eisenberger et al. 1985; Fauré et al. 1985; Tolis and Koutsilieris 1985; Waxman et al. 1985; Wenderoth and Jacobi 1985; Koutsilieris et al. 1986). The magnitude of objective regression of disease for patients receiving buserelin was comparable to that achieved by orchiectomy or the administration of DES. As with standard endocrine therapy, the responses were not permanent, and relapses eventually occurred; the median time to relapse was approximately 20 months in this study.

A comparison with a large series of patients suggests that both progression-free survival rates and overall survival rates are very similar for patients treated with buserelin and standard endocrine manipulation. Buserelin achieved these therapeutic results with minimal toxicity and side effects. The transient rise in serum testosterone level during the first week of therapy may, in a few patients, transiently exacerbate symptoms. Caution should be exercised in treating patients with ominous tumor presentations.

The introduction of LH-RH agonists has at present not significantly improved the survival rates of patients with advanced prostatic cancer. These drugs are, however, a very valuable alternative to standard endocrine therapy because of their safety and ease of administration. At present, the most significant deterrent to their widespread use is their relatively high cost as compared with estrogens and orchiectomy. However, when one considers their ease of administration and freedom from side effects, their cost-benefit ratio becomes much more attractive. Although buserelin has not yet been released by the United States Food and Drug Administration, final approval of pending applications is expected. Trials of a long-acting SC depot lasting 6 to 8 weeks are planned, and once costs are reduced and administration becomes less frequent, the LH-RH agonists should replace estrogen therapy and be a suitable alternative to surgical castration.

REFERENCES

1. Eisenberger MA, Odwyer PJ, Friedman MA. 1985. Gonadotropin hormone-releasing hormone analogues: A new therapeutic approach for prostatic carcinoma. *J Clin Oncol* 4:414–424.
2. Fauré N, Lemay A, Laroche B, et al. 1985. Clinical response and safety of LHRH-agonist treatment in prostatic carcinoma, in Labrie L, Wenderoth UK (eds): *Excerpta Medica. A New Approach to the Treatment of Prostatic Cancer: Buserelin (Suprefact).* New York, Elsevier North-Holland, Inc, pp 17–33.
3. Huggins CB, Stevens RE, Hodges CV. 1941. Studies on prostatic cancer: Effects of castration on advanced carcinoma of the prostate gland. *Arch Surg* 43:209–223.
4. Koutsilieris M, Fauré N, Tolis G, et al. 1986. Objective response and disease outcome in 59 patients with stage D_2 prostatic cancer treated with either buserelin or orchiectomy: Disease aggressivity and its association with response and outcome. *Urology* 27:221–228.
5. Murphy GP, Beckley S, Brady MF, et al. 1983. Treatment of newly diagnosed metastatic prostate cancer patients with chemotherapy agents in combination with hormones versus hormones alone. *Cancer* 51:1264–1272.
6. Murphy GP, Huben RP, Priore R. 1986. Results of another trial of chemotherapy with and without hormones in patients with newly diagnosed metastatic prostate cancer. *Urology* 28:36–40.
7. Schally AV, Arimura A, Baba Y, et al. 1971. Isolation and properties of the FSH and LH-releasing hormone. *Biochem Biophys Res Commun* 43:393–399.
8. Tolis G, Koutsilieris M. 1985. Advanced prostatic carcinoma: A therapeutic challenge, in Labrie L, Wenderoth UK (eds): *Excerpta Medica: A New Approach to the Treatment of Prostatic Cancer: Buserelin (Suprefact).* New York, Elsevier North-Holland, Inc, pp 34–41.

9. von Eschenbach AC. 1987. Buserelin (HOE-766) as treatment of advanced prostatic carcinoma. *Br J Clin Practice* 41:92–99.

10. Waxman JH, Hendry WF, Whitfield HN, et al. 1985. Response and relapse in patients with prostatic cancer treated with buserelin, in Labrie L, Wenderoth UK (eds): *Excerpta Medica: A New Approach to the Treatment of Prostatic Cancer: Buserelin (Suprefact)*. New York, Elsevier North-Holland, Inc, pp 51–58.

11. Wenderoth UK, Jacobi GH. 1985. Three years of experience with the GnRH-analogue buserelin in 100 patients with advanced prostatic cancer, in Labrie L, Wenderoth UK (eds): *Excerpta Medica: A New Approach to the Treatment of Prostatic Cancer: Buserelin (Suprefact)*. New York, Elsevier North-Holland, Inc, pp 42–50.

Chapter 25 _____

Androgen Suppression Using Megestrol Acetate and Minidose Estrogen

Douglas E. Johnson, M.D.

R. Joseph Babaian, M.D.

David A. Swanson, M.D.

Andrew C. von Eschenbach, M.D.

Kenneth I. Wishnow, M.D.

Denise Tenney, R.N.

Preliminary reports by Trachtenberg (1984), Geller (1985), Geller and Albert (1985), Labrie et al. (1985, 1986), and their colleagues have suggested that total androgen ablation (testicular and adrenal) may provide better control and longer survivals for patients with adenocarcinoma metastatic from the prostate than does conventional testicular androgen suppression alone. Investigations by Geller (1985) and Geller and Albert (1985) demonstrated that a combination of minidose estrogen and megestrol acetate significantly blocked both testicular and adrenal androgens. In a small pilot study (Geller et al. 1981) using this regimen, the estrogen appeared to produce minimal, if any, clinically evident biologic side effects. Salt retention and thromboembolism were not noted, and gynecomastia was mild and undisturbing. As a result, we at The University of Texas M. D. Anderson Cancer Center undertook a larger clinical trial to assess more thoroughly the side effects and cardiovascular risks of this combination and to determine whether it produces remission rates better than those achieved with standard therapy for patients who have metastatic prostate cancer.

STUDY POPULATION AND ANALYSIS

Over a 14-month period (May 1984–July 1985), 62 patients with recently diagnosed prostatic carcinoma who had clinical evidence of metastatic disease were treated with an oral combination of megestrol acetate (Megace, 80 mg twice daily) and minidose estrogen (diethylstilbestrol [DES], 0.1 mg, or ethinyl estradiol, 0.05 mg daily) as a means of achieving medical castration. In each instance the diagnosis of prostatic adenocarcinoma had been histologically confirmed at UT M. D. Anderson Cancer Center before treatment began. Fifty-two patients had received no prior therapy, and 10 patients had taken DES for periods ranging from several days to less than 3 months. Disease in all but four patients was assigned a histologic grade, based on the percentage of tumor that was forming glands (Fig 25–1) (Brawn et al. 1982). Patients were stratified according to the extent of their disease into one of three categories: D_0, elevated serum level of prostatic acid phosphatase but no other evidence of metastases—10 patients; D_1, tumor within pelvic lymph nodes, confirmed by staging lymphadenectomy in 24 patients, by lymphangiography combined with needle biopsy in 3, and by computed tomography of the pelvis in 2—29 patients; and D_2, distant nodal, bony, or visceral metastases—23 patients.

Patients ranged in age from 48 to 86 years (median, 66 years). Twenty-three patients (37%) were known to have preexisting cardiovascular disease as evidenced by their having received therapy for hypertension (15), cardiac arrhythmias (4), coronary artery disease (2), aortic aneurysm (1), and cerebral vascular accident (1).

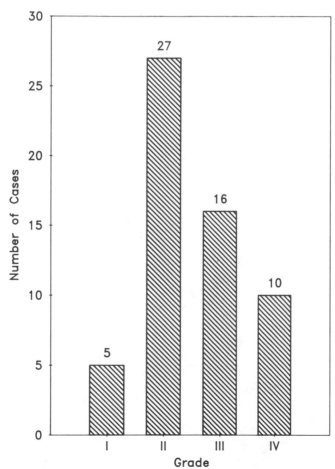

FIG 25–1.
Distribution of primary tumor grades.

Since it was not possible to determine accurately the actual response to therapy of the local tumor and regional nodal metastases, we used the following criteria to assess clinical response: *stable disease*—acid phosphatase level returned to normal, no new lesions appeared, and performance status did not deteriorate; *progressive disease*—acid phosphatase level failed to normalize or, if already normal, it became elevated; measurable lesions increased by 25% or more; or new lesions appeared.

Follow-up consisted of telephone interviews combined with periodic clinic visits, usually at 3- to 4-month intervals, at which time evaluation included a careful physical examination, determination of prostatic acid phosphatase level, serum multiple analyses (SMA), and pertinent radiologic or radionuclide scans to assess metastatic disease. Minimum follow-up time has been 13 months. Serum testosterone levels in 46 patients were measured at periods ranging from 6 to 28 months after therapy began. Serum cortisol levels were determined as dictated by symptoms or clinical findings. Serum levels of aldosterone, estradiol, prolactin, androstenedione, sodium, and potassium were assessed in 10 randomly selected patients 6 months or longer after they started therapy.

RESULTS

Side Effects

Table 25–1 lists the type and frequency of side effects that occurred after therapy began. Penile erections of sufficient turgor for intercourse were maintained in only 2 (6%) of 35 patients known to be potent prior to therapy. Breast enlargement, frequently a major concern to patients, accompanied by tender nipples was recorded in almost three fourths of the patients. One third complained of generalized weakness and loss of energy level. Serum cortisol levels were sufficiently depressed in eight of these latter patients to require cortisone replacement. Peripheral edema became clinically apparent in a fourth of the patients, and weight gain in excess of 10% of pretreatment levels that could not be attributed to fluid retention was observed in another 27%. Although an increased appetite was reported frequently, 12% of patients developed nausea. Interestingly, three patients who were bald noted hair return to a minor degree.

Cardiovascular Complications

Fourteen patients (23%) developed 16 cardiovascular complications. Four patients developed pulmonary emboli, presumably from pelvic veins since they had no history of con-

TABLE 25–1.
Type and Frequency of Side Effects

Side Effects	Population Size*	Frequency	
		No.	%
Impotence	51	49	96
Breast tenderness	54	40	74
Gynecomastia	55	38	69
Lethargy	52	19	37
Peripheral edema	52	15	29
Weight gain ≥10%	52	14	27
Nausea	52	6	12

*Interviews with patients were not sufficiently detailed to provide adequate information in all cases.

current or antecedent phlebitis. Three patients suffered a myocardial infarction; one of these died at 14 months without evidence of active disease. Three patients developed deep-vein thrombosis, and another two suffered with phlebitis. Cerebral vascular accidents occurred in two patients. In addition, one patient developed an unusual vascular occlusive ocular lesion, and another developed severe cardiac arrhythmias.

Hormone Levels

Serum testosterone levels were measured on 93 occasions in 46 patients at periods ranging from 6 to 28 months after therapy was initiated. Although the level was depressed in all instances, levels of 36, 38, 47, 48, 63, 74, 82, 82, 90, and 173 ng/dl were of sufficient concern to physicians for them to increase the estrogen dose slightly, causing the levels to fall to less than 20 ng/dl.

Results of hormone assays performed for 10 randomly selected patients are shown in Table 25-2. The level of androstenedione was consistently depressed, and serum prolactin levels tended to rise slightly. However, results were not consistent for either aldosterone or estradiol: serum aldosterone levels were depressed in 2 patients and elevated in 3; estradiol levels were depressed in 5 and elevated in 2.

Response

Disease failed to regress completely in any patient. Twenty-one patients remain on treatment at periods ranging from 24 to 37 months (median, 26 months). The drug program was discontinued at periods ranging from 6 to 29 months (median, 17 months) in 18 patients (29%), although they had no evidence of progressive disease. Ten of these patients discontinued the drugs because of side effects; 7 were withdrawn from the program because of severe cardiovascular complications; and 1 patient stopped treatment because of the expense. Progressing disease has been documented in 23 patients (37%). Within the first 12 months of therapy, no correlation could be demonstrated between the grade of the primary malignancy and the incidence of progressive disease.

Stage D_0

Four of the 10 patients (40%) were removed from the study without evidence of progressive disease because of side effects (3) or cardiovascular complications (1). Of the remaining

TABLE 25-2.
Hormone Levels in Ten Patients 6 Months or Longer After Beginning Megestrol Acetate and Minidose Estrogen

Aldosterone (ng/dl) (5–30)*	Estradiol (ng/ml) (2–8)	Prolactin (ng/dl) (0–25)	Androstenedione (ng/dl) (70–205)
10	36	18	20
4	8	18	38
27	<5	39	31
4	<5	22	25
37	10	31	22
15	<5	30	20
32	<5	34	–
9	<5	39	<20
35	<5	39	35
11	59	37	<20

*( ) = normal range.

6 patients, 3 have developed progressive disease at 6, 19, and 27 months, and 3 remain free of known metastases with normal acid phosphatase levels at 25 months.

Stage D_1

Nine of 29 patients (31%) have been withdrawn from the study because of side effects (8) or expense of Megace (1) but without progressive disease. Six patients developed progressive disease at periods ranging from 11 to 32 months (median, 24 months). The remaining 14 patients are alive without further metastases after periods ranging from 24 to 36 months (median, 29 months).

Stage D_2

Five of the 23 patients (22%) have been removed from the study because of complications (3) or side effects (2) at 14, 14, 23, 27, and 29 months, respectively, but without progression of their metastases. Fourteen patients developed progressive disease and are off study. The remaining four patients have stable disease after periods ranging from 24 to 37 months (median, 29 months). However, all patients with stage D_2 disease were evaluable after 12 months of therapy; eight (35%) had progressed during this period.

COMMENTS

In 1970 Maltry (1970) presented preliminary data at the 18th Annual Kimbrough Urological Seminar held in San Antonio, Texas, suggesting that megestrol acetate could eradicate previously untreated metastatic carcinoma of the prostate. He showed in serial biopsies of the prostate definite pathologic effects beginning with the formation of cytoplasmic vacuolization and pyknosis of the nuclei, followed by replacement of the malignant cells by hyaline and fibrous tissue. In addition, he reported normalization of elevated prostatic acid phosphatase values, amelioration of pain, and an increased feeling of well-being when patients were treated with 60 to 100 mg megestrol acetate daily. Excited by these findings, we began investigations the following year with the drug, which at that time had not been released commercially in the United States. Although we demonstrated a beneficial clinical response in 92% of previously untreated patients with metastatic prostatic carcinoma, we found that almost half required orchiectomy within 6 months because of progressive disease (Johnson et al. 1975). Consequently, we resumed the use of more conventional therapy (orchiectomy, estrogens, or both).

In our current study, we failed to achieve castrate levels (less than 39.7 ng/dl) in 8 of 46 patients (17%) until we slightly escalated the estrogen dose. This was not surprising, since Klugo et al. (1981) reported that, following bilateral orchiectomy, serum testosterone levels failed to fall to anorchid levels in 11% of their patients, requiring the administration of 1 mg DES to reduce serum testosterone to the anorchid range. The reasons for these findings remain unclear, but they serve to emphasize the necessity for periodic monitoring of serum testosterone levels in all patients receiving hormonal therapy for prostate cancer.

Two major advantages suggested for using combination megestrol acetate and minidose estrogen therapy were the presumed lack of feminizing side effects and the lack of cardiovascular complications. Therefore the gynecomastia and breast tenderness that developed in almost three fourths of our patients were unexpected and most distressing findings. The fact that major cardiovascular complications occurred in 23% of our patients, although also unexpected, should not have been surprising in light of recent reports. Originally, studies reported by the Veterans Administration Cooperative Urological Research Group (1967)

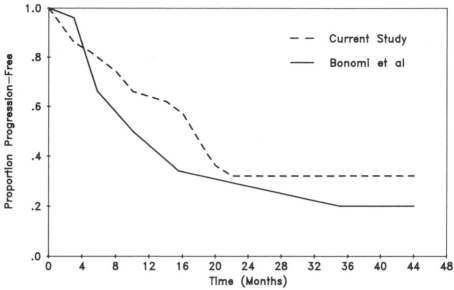

FIG 25–2.
Disease progression (Kaplan-Meier analysis).

showed a higher cardiovascular mortality for patients receiving 5 mg DES than for those treated without estrogen. Although a subsequent study (Bailar and Byar 1970) suggested that a lower dose of DES was not associated with an increased incidence of cardiovascular deaths, Glashan and Robinson (1981) demonstrated in a prospective study that patients receiving 3 mg DES had a significantly higher incidence of cardiovascular complications and deaths than similar patients who underwent orchiectomy. More recently, Henriksson and Edhag (1986) have reported that 25% of patients with prostatic cancer given low-dose estrogen therapy suffered major cardiovascular events during the first year, while the patients treated with orchiectomy had none. We did not exclude patients with preexisting cardiovascular disease from our treatment program, but we could find no evidence suggesting that these were the patients who developed the higher incidence of cardiovascular complications. Twenty-three patients in our study (37%) had received treatment for preexisting cardiovascular disease before starting therapy, and only 4 of them developed a major cardiovascular event during therapy.

Some investigators may argue that we have monitored too few patients in each substage sufficiently long to reach a definite conclusion about remission rates, but our experience with patients presenting with stage D_2 disease suggests that this therapy produces no better results than standard therapy. Koutsilieris and colleagues (1986), in a comparative study evaluating 59 patients recently diagnosed with stage D_2 prostate cancer and treated either with a leuteinizing hormone-releasing hormone agonist (buserelin) or with orchiectomy, reported relapse rates within 1 year of 27% and 22%, respectively. In our study we found that 35% of our patients receiving megestrol acetate and minidose estrogen had progressed within 12 months.

Recently, Bonomi and associates (1985) studied 25 patients with symptomatic stage D_2 prostatic cancer treated with megestrol acetate as initial hormonal therapy. They concluded that the response rate and median survival duration appeared comparable to those achieved with estrogen therapy or orchiectomy. When one compares our results using combination megestrol acetate and low-dose estrogens to theirs with megestrol acetate alone, few differences in time to progression are noted (Fig 25–2).

In light of the high incidence of feminizing side effects (69%–74%), a higher than expected rate of cardiovascular complications (23%), an unexpected need for cortisone replacement (13%), and failure to obtain better results over standard therapy for patients with stage D_2 disease, we have concluded that this regimen offers no advantage over standard therapy.

REFERENCES

1. Bailar JC III, Byar DP. 1970. Estrogen treatment for cancer of the prostate: Early results with 3 doses of diethylstilbestrol and placebo. *Cancer* 26:257–261.
2. Bonomi P, Pessis D, Bunting N, et al. 1985. Megestrol acetate used as primary hormonal therapy in stage D prostatic cancer. *Semin Oncol* 12:36–39.
3. Brawn PN, Ayala AG, von Eschenbach AC, et al. 1982. Histologic grading study of prostate adenocarcinoma: The development of a new system and comparison with other methods. A preliminary study. *Cancer* 49:525–532.
4. Geller J. 1985. Rationale for blockade of adrenal as well as testicular androgens in the treatment of advanced prostate cancer. *Semin Oncol* 12:28–35.
5. Geller J, Albert JD. 1985. Adrenal androgen blockade in relapsed prostate cancer. *Eur J Cancer Clin Oncol* 21:1127–1131.
6. Geller J, Albert J, Yen SS, et al. 1981. Medical castration with megestrol acetate and minidose of diethylstilbestrol. *Urology* 17(suppl):27–33.
7. Glashan RW, Robinson MR. 1981. Cardiovascular complications in the treatment of prostatic carcinoma. *Br J Urol* 53:624–627.
8. Henriksson P, Edhag O. 1986. Orchidectomy versus oestrogen for prostatic cancer: Cardiovascular effects. *Br Med J* 293:413–415.
9. Johnson DE, Kaesler KE, Ayala AG. 1975. Megestrol acetate for treatment of advanced carcinoma of the prostate. *J Surg Oncol* 7:9–15.
10. Klugo RC, Farah RN, Cerny JC. 1981. Bilateral orchiectomy for carcinoma of prostate: Response of serum testosterone and clinical response to subsequent estrogen therapy. *Urology* 17:49–50.
11. Koutsilieris M, Fauré N, Tolis G, et al. 1986. Objective response and disease outcome in 59 patients with stage D_2 prostatic cancer treated with either buserelin or orchiectomy. *Urology* 27:221–228.
12. Labrie F, Dupont A, Belanger A, et al. 1986. Combined blockade with a pure antiandrogen (flutamide) should be used without interruption in all patients with previously untreated or treated advanced prostate cancer, in Baulieu EE, Iacobelli S, McGuire WL (eds): *Endocrinology and Malignancy: Basic and Clinical Issues. Proceedings of the First International Congress on Cancer and Hormones.* London, Parthenon Publishing, pp 348–359.
13. Labrie F, Dupont A, Belanger A, et al. 1985. Combination therapy with flutamide and castration (LHRH agonist or orchiectomy) in advanced prostate cancer: A marked improvement in response and survival. *J Steroid Biochem* 23:833–841.
14. Maltry E. 1970. Use of megestrol acetate (a new progestational agent) in the treatment of carcinoma of the prostate in *Proceedings of the Kimbrough Urological Seminar, 18th Annual Meeting, 1970.* Norwich, Eaton Laboratories, pp 135–137.
15. Trachtenberg J. 1984. Ketoconazole therapy in advanced prostatic cancer. *J Urol* 132:61–63.
16. Veterans Administration Cooperation Urological Research Group. 1967. Carcinoma of the prostate: Treatment comparisons. *J Urol* 98:516–522.

Chapter 26

Ketoconazole Therapy for Hormonally Refractive Prostate Cancer

R. Joseph Babaian, M.D.

Douglas E. Johnson, M.D.

Denise M. Tenney, R.N.

HISTORICAL PERSPECTIVE

At the time of initial presentation, approximately 40% of the patients with prostate cancer already have metastatic disease (Whitmore 1973). The relationship between hormone dependency and growth in this neoplasm was first posited in 1941 by Huggins and Hodges. Although hormonal therapy is not curative and has only palliative intent, it induces either a regression or stabilization of neoplastic cell proliferation in approximately 75% of patients with systemic disease. The mechanism of action that results in the treatment response is a decrease in the circulating androgen concentration, which leads to a reduction in the intracellular concentration of dihydrotestosterone and, subsequently, to a diminution of protein synthesis by the neoplastic prostate cells.

Historically, the mainstay of treatment for metastatic disease has been to reduce the serum level of androgen, approximately 95% of which is produced by the testicles and 5% by the adrenals. Therapeutically, this reduction has been accomplished by one of two classical procedures, bilateral orchiectomy or administration of diethylstilbestrol (DES). The choice of treatment has most often been determined by physician preference, since neither modality has demonstrated any cancer-inhibitory advantage over the other.

Within the last several years, considerable effort has been expended searching for alternative hormonal regimens (Trachtenberg and Pont 1984; Geller and Albert 1985; Labrie et al. 1985; Johnson et al. 1988). This endeavor has been pursued for several reasons: first, a cure for prostatic cancer has not yet been found and the mean duration of conventional hormonal therapy response (2 years) is relatively short; second, the potential psychological trauma associated with orchiectomy is occasionally unacceptable; third, side effects are associated with oral estrogen therapy, namely thromboembolism, myocardial ischemia, gynecomastia, and fluid retention; and fourth, current chemotherapeutic regimens are ineffective in eliciting objective durable responses.

Ketoconazole

The use of ketoconazole as a potential inhibitor of both testicular and adrenal androgen synthesis was reported initially by Pont et al. (1982a, b). These investigators observed the development of gynecomastia in patients receiving ketoconazole for systemic fungal infections, which prompted them to study the effects of the drug on both testicular androgen production and adrenal steroid synthesis. These findings led to the proposal of ketoconazole as a treatment for metastatic prostate cancer. Subsequently, Trachtenberg et al. (1983) have advocated ketoconazole as a primary alternative treatment for metastatic prostate cancer.

Pharmocokinetics

Ketoconazole   (*cis*-1-acetyl-4[4-[[2-(2,4-dichlorophenyl)-2-(1H-imidazol-1-ylmethyl)-1,3-dioxolan-4-yl] methoxyl]phenyl]) piperazine is an imidazole derivative with antifungal properties. It has been reported to be effective in some cases of infection caused by *Coccidioides immitis, Candida* species, *Blastomyces dermatitidis, Histoplasma capsulatum,* and *Cryptococcus neoformans* (Resirepo 1980). Its mechanism of action is the inhibition of 14-demethylation, which prevents the conversion of lenosterol to ergosterol (Van den Bossche et al. 1980; Willemsens et al. 1980). Ketoconazole has also been shown to inhibit the conversion of lenosterol to cholesterol in mammalian cells (Van den Bossche et al. 1980; Willemsens et al. 1980). These actions are the result of the inhibition of a wide variety of cytochrome P-450-dependent enzymes (Rajfer et al. 1986). The testis appears to be more sensitive than the adrenal to the steroidogenesis blockade of ketoconazole. It has been postulated that the site of this blockade is 17,20-desmolase and 17α-hydroxylase, which catalyze the conversion of C-21 steroidal precursors to C-19 sex steroids (Rajfer et al. 1986).

THE UNIVERSITY OF TEXAS M. D. ANDERSON EXPERIENCE

Patients and Methods

Between March 1986 and April 1987, 38 patients with hormone-refractory metastatic prostate cancer were treated with ketoconazole at The University of Texas M. D. Anderson Cancer Center. Thirty-one of these patients were ultimately considered evaluable and seven were not. One died of a myocardial infarction before his reassessment, 3 had subjective disease progression within 8 weeks of starting ketoconazole therapy, 1 was lost to follow-up, and 2 developed side effects (1 nausea and vomiting and 1 pruritus) that required early cessation of therapy. In every patient, ketoconazole produced a castrate level of serum testosterone: less than 20 ng/dl in 14 patients and from 20 to 39 ng/ml (median, 21 ng/ml) in the remaining 17. The patients ranged in age from 55 to 84 years (median, 69 years). Prior hormonal therapy had consisted of bilateral orchiectomy alone in 12 patients, combination orchiectomy and diethylstilbestrol in 9 patients, diethylstilbestrol only in 4 patients, combination megestrol acetate and low-dose estrogen in 1 patient, and only a luteinizing hormone-releasing hormone (LH-RH) agonist in 5 patients.

Metastatic disease was present in the axial skeleton of 19 patients, in the axial skeleton and long bones of 5 patients, in osseous sites and lymph nodes (supraclavicular, 1; retroperitoneum 2) in 3 patients, in bone and viscera (lung, 2) in 2 patients, and in lymph nodes only (inguinal, 1; retroperitoneal, 1) in 2 patients. The serum prostatic acid phosphatase (PAP) level, as determined by the Roy test, was normal for 12 patients and elevated for 19. The median PAP value at presentation was 1.2 milliunits (mU)/ml (range 0.2–21.8 mU/ml). The median serum alkaline phosphatase level was 164 mU/ml (range, 60–>350 mU/ml) at the time ketoconazole therapy was initiated.

The dose of oral ketoconazole was 400 mg every 8 hours for 14 patients and 200 mg every 8 hours for 17 patients. Those patients who were taking the 200-mg dose were also maintained on hormonal therapy (DES or LH-RH) if they had not had an orchiectomy. Most patients taking the higher dose were given trimethobenzamide hydrochloride, 200 mg, for nausea 45 to 90 minutes before they took the ketoconazole. To decrease gastric toxicity, some patients began by taking the lower dose for 1 week and then changed to the higher 400-mg dose.

Clinical response was monitored by frequent telephone conversations as well as regularly scheduled clinic visits. The patients were evaluated by monthly follow-up liver function tests and PAP analysis. Bone scans were obtained prior to beginning therapy, at 3 months, and whenever progressive disease was clinically suspected. The median time of follow-up has been 3 months (range, 3–13 months).

Results

Four patients (13%) have had a partial response that has been maintained for a median of 11 months. Pain has completely resolved in 2 of these 4 patients. Bone scans have shown significant improvement in 3 patients who presented with abnormal scans (Fig 26–1); in the

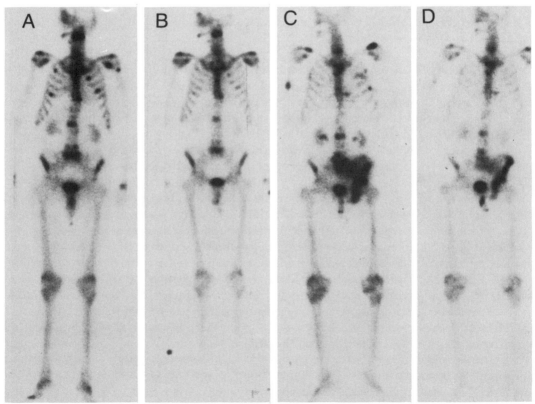

FIG 26–1.
Pretreatment bone scans of two patients (**A** and **C**) compared with scans of the same patients made during ketoconazole therapy (**B** and **D**).

fourth patient the size of a biopsy-proved involved inguinal lymph node decreased 75%. Disease stabilization lasting from 3 to 12 months was observed in 12 patients. Disease progressed in 15 patients, and they are no longer receiving ketoconazole. The median time to progression in this group was 3 months (range, 6 weeks to 5 months).

Pain is a symptom frequently associated with the failure of conventional hormonal therapy. Twenty-three patients (74%) presented with this symptom. Pain decreased in 16 patients (70%)—usually within a week—and completely disappeared in 5 (22%) for a median of 9 months (range, 3–13 months). In the 11 whose pain responded partially, improvement lasted for a median duration of 3.5 months (range, 1–12 months), after which pain intensified in 6 patients.

The serum PAP level was elevated in 19 patients when ketoconazole therapy was initiated. Levels returned to normal in 5 of these patients and remained so for a median period of 6 months (range, 5–6 months). Disease progressed objectively in 1 of these patients at 9 months, accompanied by an abnormally elevated PAP level.

In general, ketoconazole was fairly well tolerated: only 2 patients were withdrawn from the study because of drug intolerance (nausea and vomiting, one; pruritus, one). Twenty-two patients had no early adverse effects, but 7 experienced nausea (mild, 4; moderate, 1; and severe, 2). Thirteen patients developed late toxicity, which consisted of mild nausea in 8, mild fatigue in 5, pruritus, rash, or both in 3, and a mildly elevated alkaline phosphatase level in 1. No late drug sequelae developed in 18 patients.

THERAPEUTIC CONSIDERATIONS FOR HORMONE-REFRACTORY PATIENTS

Physicians are frequently confronted with patients who have failed conventional hormonal therapy. These patients can generally be divided into a small group of asymptomatic patients and a larger group with symptomatic and progressive bone disease. Are there any treatment modalities currently available that can either improve the quality of their lives or increase their median expected survival of 7 months?

Chemotherapy, with its known toxicities, has produced no meaningful prolongation of survival and provides little palliation except for some patients with severe symptoms. The initial reports of Labrie et al. (1986), Geller et al. (1985), and others suggesting higher response rates and longer survivals for patients with metastatic prostate cancer treated by total androgen ablation have prompted a number of clinical trials to evaluate the effects of complete androgen deprivation in patients who have failed conventional hormonal therapy.

Whether or not adrenal androgens significantly stimulate prostate cancer growth in vivo has not yet been firmly established. Even less certain is whether adrenal androgen can be converted to dihydrotestosterone in significant amounts. Although the studies of Harper et al. (1974) and Geller et al. (1984) suggest that adrenal androgens are converted into dihydrotestosterone in the prostate, no human data are available to ascertain whether the amount of dihydrotestosterone produced is biologically important for tumor growth. Animal data reported by Bartsch et al. (1983) suggest that it may be.

Labrie et al (1986) reported using an LH-RH agonist (leuprolide) and an antiandrogen (flutamide) to treat 204 patients who had progressed after treatment by orchiectomy, estrogen, or LH-RH agonists alone. They reported an objective response rate of 14% (28 patients) and a disease-stabilization rate of 33% (67 patients) during a mean follow-up of 690 days. Allen and associates (1983) reported two cases of a favorable response to the combination of LH-RH agonist and ketoconazole in previously hormone-refractory patients.

Reports of other investigators including Smith et al. (1973), Bhanalaph et al. (1974), Drago et al. (1984), and Murry and Pitt (1985) have demonstrated approximately a 33% response (partial objective regression and objective stability) and a survival of approximately 1 year for patients relapsing after orchiectomy when adrenal androgen blockade was employed. More recently, Williams et al. (1986) reported a 30% objective and a 50% subjective clinical response rate for ketoconazole therapy in 20 patients with hormone-refractory disease. However, the durations of response are not reported by the authors. These investigators also noted no significant difference in results between patients receiving 400 mg ketoconazole and those receiving the 200-mg dose.

CONCLUSION

Ketoconazole, which blocks adrenal androgen production, can elicit an objective response in a small number of patients. Disease stabilization occurs in a significant proportion of patients, but whether this represents treatment effect or the natural history of the disease in these patients is not known. Ketoconazole can produce subjective improvement in pain, usually within a relatively short period of time. Since ketoconazole is fairly well tolerated, we advocate that, before considering chemotherapy with its known morbidity and questionable efficacy, the physician institute a trial of ketoconazole therapy, using 200 mg every 8 hours, for patients who are effectively maintained at castrate androgen levels.

REFERENCES

1. Allen JM, Kerle DJ, Ware H, et al. 1983. Combined treatment with ketoconazole and luteinising hormone-releasing hormone analogue: A novel approach to resistant progressive prostatic cancer. *Br Med J* 287:1766.
2. Bartsch W, Knobbe G, Voight KD. 1983. Regulation and compartmentalization of androgens in rat prostate and muscle. *J Steroid Biochem* 19:929–937.
3. Bhanalaph T, Vorkarakis MJ, Murphy GP. 1974. Current status of bilateral adrenalectomy for advanced prostatic carcinoma. *Ann Surg* 179:17–23.
4. Drago JR, Santen RJ, Lipton A. 1984. Clinical effect of aminoglutethimide, medical adrenalectomy, in treatment of 43 patients with advanced prostatic carcinoma. *Cancer* 53:1447–1450.
5. Geller J, Albert JD. 1985. Adrenal androgen blockade in relapsed prostate cancer. *Eur J Cancer Clin Oncol* 21:1127–1131.
6. Geller J, Albert JD, Nachtsheim DA, et al. 1984. Comparison of prostatic cancer tissue dihydrotestosterone levels at the time of relapse following orchiectomy or estrogen therapy. *J Urol* 132:693–696.
7. Harper ME, Pile A, Peeling WB. 1974. Steroids of adrenal origin metabolized by human prostatic tissue both in vivo and in vitro. *J Endocrinol* 60:117–125.
8. Huggins C, Hodges CV. 1941. Studies on prostatic cancer: The effect of castration, of estrogen, and of androgen injection on serum phosphatases in metastatic carcinoma of the prostate. *Cancer Res* 1:293–297.
9. Johnson DE, Babaian RJ, von Eschenbach AC, et al. 1988. Ketoconazole therapy for hormonally refractive metastatic prostate cancer. *Urology* 31:132–134.
10. Labrie F, Dupont A, Belanger A, et al. 1986. Combined blockade with a pure antiandrogen (flutamide) should be used without interruption in all patients with previously untreated or treated advanced prostate cancer, in Baulieu EE, Iacobelli S, McGuire WL (eds): *Endocrinology and Malignancy: Basic and Clinical Issues. Proceedings of the First International Congress on Cancer and Hormones.* London, Parthenon Publishing.

11. Labrie F, Dupont A, Belanger A, et al. 1985. Combination therapy with flutamide and castration (LHRH agonist or orchiectomy) in advanced prostate cancer: A marked improvement in response and survival. *J. Steroid Biochem* 23:833–841.

12. Murry R, Pitt P. 1985. Treatment of advanced prostatic cancer, resistant to conventional therapy, with aminoglutethimide. *Eur J Cancer Clin Oncol* 21:453–458.

13. Pont A, Williams PL, Azhar S, et al. 1982a. Ketoconazole blocks testosterone synthesis. *Arch Intern Med* 142:2137–2140.

14. Pont A, Williams PL, Loose DS, et al. 1982b. Ketoconazole blocks adrenal steroid synthesis. *Ann Intern Med* 97:370–372.

15. Rajfer J, Sikka SC, Rivera F, et al. 1986. Mechanism of inhibition of human testicular steroidogenesis by oral ketoconazole. *J Clin Endocrinol Metab* 63:1192–1198.

16. Resirepo A, Sievens DA, Utz JP. 1980. First International Symposium on Ketoconazole. *Rev Infect Dis* 2:519–699.

17. Smith RB, Walsh PC, Goodwin WE. 1973. Cyproterone acetate in the treatment of advanced carcinoma of the prostate. *J Urol* 110:106–108.

18. Trachtenberg J, Pont A. 1984. Ketoconazole therapy for advanced prostate cancer. *Lancet* 2:433–435.

19. Trachtenberg J, Halpern N, Pont A. 1983. Ketoconazole: A novel and rapid treatment for advanced prostate cancer. *J Urol* 130:152–153.

20. Van den Bossche H, Willemsens G, Cools W, et al. 1980. In vitro and in vivo effects of the antimycotic drug ketoconazole on sterol synthesis. *Antimicrob Agents Chemother* 17:922–928.

21. Whitmore WF Jr. 1973. The natural history of prostate cancer. *Cancer* 32:1104–1112.

22. Willemsens G, Cools W, Van den Bossche H. 1980. Effect of miconazole and ketoconazole on sterol synthesis in a subcellular fraction of yeast and mammalian cells, in Van den Bossche H (ed): *The Host-Invader Interplay.* New York, Elsevier North-Holland, pp 691–694.

23. Williams G, Kerle DJ, Ware HA, et al. 1986. Objective responses to ketoconazole therapy in patients with relapsed progressive prostatic cancer. *Br J Urol* 58:45–51.

Radical Prostatectomy and Adjuvant Treatment for High-Stage ($T_3N_0M_0$; $T_{0-3}N_{1-2}M_0$) Cancer of the Prostate

Horst Zincke, M.D.

Treatment for localized, that is stage B (T_1, T_2), adenocarcinoma of the prostate by using interstitial and/or external-beam radiation or radical prostatectomy has provided similarly good results as measured by survival rate and by local and systemic control (Cupps et al. 1980; Guerriero et al. 1980; Benson et al. 1984; Whitmore 1984). One can assume that at least a comparable and probably a larger group of patients presents with stage C (T_3) or D_1 (T_{0-3} $N_{1-2}M_0$ [tumor, node, metastasis]) disease. However, because the use of radical prostatectomy has traditionally been limited to patients with stage B disease, only a small group of the entire population of patients with cancer of the prostate has benefitted from radical prostatectomy.

The treatment of stages C and D_1 disease has been controversial (Zincke et al. 1986; Zincke in press) because of the belief that radical prostatectomy benefits only the patient with truly localized cancer of the prostate—that is, clinically and surgically intracapsular disease—even though, at the time of surgery, extracapsular disease is found in up to 50% of those clinically staged B_2. Thus, despite the dogmatic contention that patients with more than stage B disease should not undergo radical prostatectomy, this actually has happened to a large number of patients. Further compounding the treatment problem is the fact that many urologists have performed perineal prostatectomies only, without concomitant pelvic lymphadenectomy. Thus, even after surgery, information about the status of pelvic lymph nodes has not been available, and staging has been inaccurate. Often only monotreatment has been recommended, so that many of these patients who had a perineal prostatectomy and were found to have local surgical stage C disease did not receive adjuvant treatment, either locally or systemically. Hence, the opportunity for adjuvant treatment was lost.

Urologists have been opposed to treating patients with large lesions surgically because of the fear of residual cancer, the frequent presence of involved pelvic lymph nodes, and, occasionally, their technical inability to master the operation. This lack of confidence among surgeons, because they have experienced poor results in dealing with extracapsular disease, has made way for other treatment modalities (hormonal manipulation or radiotherapy) to be used for patients with high-stage disease. However, the large tumor bulk encountered in stages C and D_1 disease is often associated with undifferentiated cancer, and the problems of local and systemic control have become apparent in recent years. Published radiation results document unsatisfactory local and systemic control in these patients (Bagshaw 1985; Bagshaw et al. 1985), and we have also been concerned with the associated morbidity, particularly local. Radiation has recently provided palliation of extracapsular disease, including stage D_1 (Bagshaw 1985; Bagshaw et al. 1985), but at a late stage, morbidity may necessitate palliative exenterative procedures for severe local symptoms (Zincke in press).

It is our contention that the goals of therapy for patients with clinical stage C and surgical stage D_1 disease should include both prolonged survival and control of local progression, resulting in a decrease of local complications and possibly in an improved quality of life. In our experience, this can be achieved with combinations of two or more therapeutic modalities: surgery, hormonal manipulation, and radiation (Zincke et al. 1986; Zincke in press). In this chapter, I present our extended experience in managing clinical and pathologic stage C and pathologic stage D_1 disease by bilateral pelvic lymphadenectomy and radical retropubic prostatectomy. I emphasize the beneficial effect of adjuvant treatment in the form of orchiectomy, radiotherapy, or both, and identify pathologic predictors of this locally advanced disease.

RADICAL PROSTATECTOMY FOR PATHOLOGIC STAGE C ($pT_3N_0M_0$) ADENOCARCINOMA OF THE PROSTATE

Recently we completed an analysis of 384 patients who were found to have pathologic stage C disease after bilateral pelvic lymphadenectomy and radical retropubic prostatectomy (Zincke in press). Among these patients, disease in 70 (18%) had been clinically staged C. The mean age of the 384 patients was 64 years, and the mean follow-up was 4.5 years (range, ≥1–18 years). Thirty patients (8%) died of prostatic cancer. The observed 5- and 10-year survival rates (Kaplan-Meier) were 87% and 67%, respectively, similar to the expected survival rates of an age-matched control group (83% and 64%, respectively) (Fig 27–1). Although any comparison with other studies, in particular those in which external-beam radiation was used, is fraught with problems, we have tried to compare our series with that of Bagshaw and associates (1985), a series of 384 patients, which attained 5- and 10-year overall survival rates of 60% and 36%, respectively (see Fig 27–1). In our series, the disease-specific survival rate at 10 years was a favorable 81% ± 8%, whereas in a series of Bagshaw and associates of 310 patients, it was 40% (Fig 27–2) (Bagshaw et al. 1985). Overall, progression occurred in 96 of our patients (25%). The overall projected nonprogression rates of our patients at 5 and 10 years were 71% and 52%, respectively; 15% and 29% of all patients were projected to have local recurrence at 5 and 10 years, respectively (Fig 27–3). Grade (Fig 27–4), seminal vesicle involvement, and tumor bulk (not shown) were also significantly associated with local and systemic progression.

We found that, similar to results in a previous study (Zincke et al. 1986), the presence of residual cancer (usually treated by adjuvant therapy) was not significantly related to systemic or local progression (Fig 27–5). Local progression occurred in 15% (41) of 280 patients who did not receive adjuvant treatment, but in only 2% (1) of the 62 who underwent adjuvant orchiectomy or radiation treatment ($P = .016$). Radiation alone (25 patients) reduced local recurrence to 0%. Remarkably, local recurrence (60% of which occurred in ≤2 years) did not occur beyond 8 years, but systemic progression occurred as late as 12 years after surgery. Systemic progression was markedly decreased by concomitant bilateral orchiectomy (4/37 patients) as compared with no adjuvant treatment (43/280) ($P = .38$, adjusted for grade).

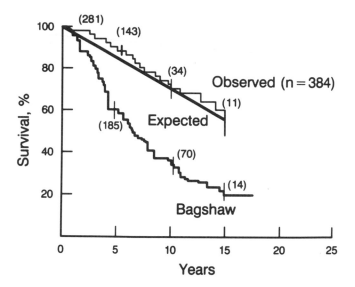

FIG 27–1.

Kaplan-Meier survival curve for 384 patients with pathologic stage C (pT₃) prostate cancer treated with bilateral pelvic lymphadenectomy and radical retropubic prostatectomy with or without adjuvant treatment compared with expected survival curve of an age- and sex-matched control group from North Central United States. This curve is compared to the curve for 384 patients treated by external-beam radiation (Bagshaw 1985). (Numbers within parentheses represent patients under observation at that time.)

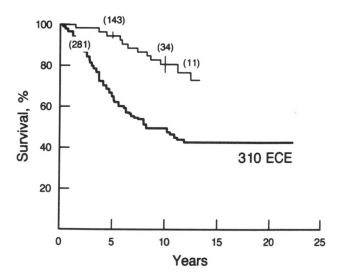

FIG 27–2.

Upper curve represents disease-specific (prostate cancer) survival rate of 384 patients with pathologic stage C (pT₃) prostate cancer treated with bilateral pelvic lymphadenectomy and radical retropubic prostatectomy with or without adjuvant treatment. Lower curve represents 310 patients who received external-beam radiation for stage C disease (Bagshaw 1985). ECE = extracapsular extension. (Numbers within parentheses represent patients under observation at that time.)

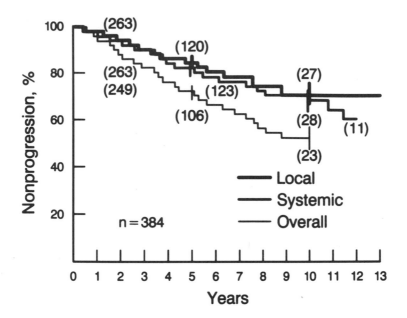

FIG 27–3.
Local, systemic, and overall nonprogression curves (Kaplan-Meier) for 384 patients with stage C (pT₃) prostate cancer treated with bilateral pelvic lymphadenectomy and radical retropubic prostatectomy with or without adjuvant treatment. (Numbers within parentheses represent patients under observation at that time.)

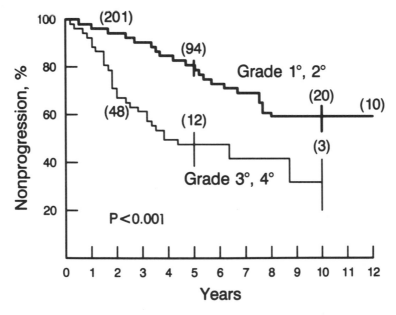

FIG 27–4.
Overall nonprogression curve (Kaplan-Meier) according to tumor grade for 384 patients with pathologic stage C (pT₃) prostate cancer who underwent bilateral pelvic lymphadenectomy and radical retropubic prostatectomy with or without adjuvant treatment. (Numbers within parentheses represent patients under observation at that time.)

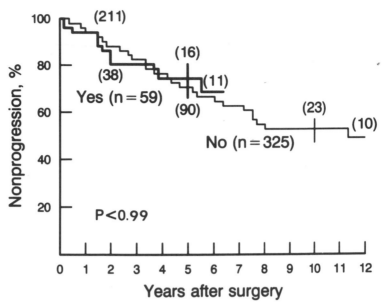

FIG 27–5.
Kaplan-Meier curves of nonprogression according to presence of residual cancer for 384 patients with pathologic stage C (pT_3) prostate cancer treated with bilateral pelvic lymphadenectomy and radical retropubic prostatectomy with or without adjuvant treatment. (Numbers within parentheses represent patients under observation at that time.)

RADICAL PROSTATECTOMY FOR CLINICAL STAGE C ($T_3N_XM_0$) ADENOCARCINOMA OF THE PROSTATE

Previously we reported (Zincke et al. 1986) on 101 patients (mean age, 64 years) who had limited but unequivocal clinical stage C cancer of the prostate who underwent bilateral pelvic lymphadenectomy and radical retropubic prostatectomy. There was no evidence for metastasis on radionuclide bone scans and roentgenograms. Follow-up ranged from 0.5 to 17 years (mean, 4.9 years). Of these 101 patients, 50 had had surgery at least 5 years earlier and 10 at least 10 years before this analysis. Follow-up was complete and included examinations quarterly in the first year, biannually in the second year, and annually thereafter, if there was no evidence for disease progression. Disease was judged to be progressing if there was biopsy-proved local recurrence or if radionuclide bone scans or roentgenograms became positive. An abnormal prostatic acid phosphatase serum level was not judged to be an indicator of metastatic disease without concomitant evidence on roentgenograms, bone or computed tomographic scans, or digital rectal examination. Analysis was performed according to grade and bulk of the local tumor, presence of residual disease, number of positive lymph nodes, and adjuvant treatment.

Fifty-two of the 101 patients had positive pelvic lymph nodes, one third of whom did not receive any adjuvant treatment. The most frequently administered adjuvant treatment was orchiectomy, with or without additional treatment (30 and 12 patients with pathologic stages D_1 and C disease, respectively). Survival analysis by the Kaplan-Meier method indicated that the observed survival data of the 101 patients were similar to the expected survival data of an age- and sex-matched control group of the general population of the North Central United Stages (Fig 27–6). The fact that the nonprogression curve continues to decline over a 10-year period lends credence to the impression that cure cannot be obtained in this difficult population of patients with locally advanced disease.

Residual cancer was identified in 16 patients and did not affect survival or progression; these patients usually received adjuvant radiation, orchiectomy, or both. None of the patients who had received either orchiectomy or radiation had evidence of local recurrence at any time during their follow-up (Table 27–1), but among the 47 patients who received no adjuvant treatment, 13 (28%) had a local recurrence. Three of 6 patients who had been treated with diethylstilbestrol (DES) also had a local recurrence. However, among the 16 patients who had local recurrence, 13 did not have any adjuvant treatment and 3 had received DES; none of them had residual cancer (Table 27–2). As in our larger series of surgical stage C lesions (pT$_3$), local recurrence was definitely related to tumor grade but not to number of positive lymph nodes or residual cancer.

The results in the subgroup of 52 patients who had positive lymph nodes were similar to the results observed in previous (Zincke and Utz 1983; Zincke in press) and present analyses

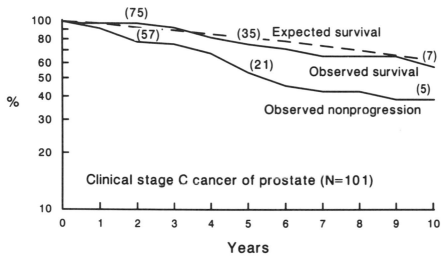

FIG 27–6.
Survival of 101 patients with clinical stage C adenocarcinoma of prostate. Curves of expected survival, overall survival, and observed nonprogression are shown. Expected survival is based on 1970 United States life tables for North Central United States. Arithmetic scale was used for abscissa and logarithmic scale was used for ordinate. (From Zincke H, Utz DC, Taylor WF. 1986. Bilateral pelvic lymphadenectomy and radical prostatectomy for clinical stage C prostatic cancer: Role of adjuvant treatment for residual cancer and in disease progression. *J Urol* 135:1199–1205. Used by permission.)

TABLE 27–1.
Local Recurrence After Radical Surgery for Clinical Stage C Adenocarcinoma of the Prostate (n = 101) According to Adjuvant Treatment

Treatment	No. of Patients	Local Recurrence	
		No.	%
No adjuvant treatment	47	13	28
Diethylstilbestrol (DES)	6	3	50
Adjuvant radiation and/or orchiectomy (with or without DES)	48	0	

TABLE 27–2.
Patients With Local Recurrences After Radical Surgery for
Clinical Stage C Adenocarcinoma of Prostate and No Residual
Cancer (n = 16)

Pathologic Stage	Adjuvant Treatment	Time to Local Recurrence (mo)	Survival (mo)
C+	No	26	97
C+	No	67	95
C	DES[§]	16	47*
C	No	12	61
C	No	25	49
C	No	81	99
C	No	30	42
C	No	52	104
D_1	DES	58	202
D_1[†]	No	56	88
D_1[†]	No	13	46
D_1[†]	No	9	36*
D_1	No	4	66[‡]
D_1[†]	DES	18	51[‡]
D_1[†]	No	10	76
D_1	No	7	48*

*Died of cancer.
[†]Seminal vesicle positive.
[‡]Died of unrelated cause.
[§]DES = diethylstilbestrol.

of patients with D_1 disease. Specifically, of the 30 patients who had immediate adjuvant orchiectomy, 91% were projected to be disease free at 5 years compared with 11% of 22 who had not received adjuvant treatment and were disease free at 5 years ($P<.0001$) (Fig 27–7,A). Although orchiectomy did not result in a significantly prolonged survival, the 5-year survival rate was a favorable 91% compared with 58% when orchiectomy was not used ($P=.09$) (Fig 27–7,B).

TREATMENT OF STAGE D_1 ($pT_{0-3}N_{1-2}M_0$) ADENOCARCINOMA OF THE PROSTATE

Treatment recommendations for stage D_1 of the disease have been limited and have included observation, hormonal treatment, or radiotherapy. Unfortunately, categorical and anecdotal statements have prevailed in the discussion of the treatment of this disease, and no series has been published that used the approach we prefer at the Mayo Clinic—a combination of radical prostatectomy and immediate adjuvant orchiectomy. Single treatment only (surgery or conservative [hormonal and/or radiation]) has resulted in a greater than 50% progression rate at 5 years. The largest conservative series apart from ours (Zincke et al. 1987) is that of Bagshaw (1985), who projected 5- and 10-year survival rates of 50% and 20%, respectively, for 61 patients undergoing external-beam radiation.

Our experience compares favorably with these results (Fig 27–8). Since our first favorable report on 39 patients in 1978 (Zincke 1978), radical prostatectomy has been prospectively performed for patients with D_1 disease and, since 1981, has been combined more or less regularly with immediate bilateral orchiectomy (Zincke et al. 1981). This approach has resulted in favorable tumor-free survival rates compared to those from conservative treatment approaches (Zincke et al. 1987). Furthermore, the local complication rate in our prostatectomy

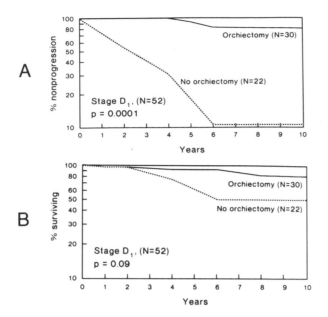

FIG 27-7.
Relationship between adjuvant orchiectomy and rates of nonprogression (**A**) and survival (**B**) in 52 patients with pathologic stage D_1 prostate cancer. (From Zincke H, Utz DC, Taylor WF. 1986. Bilateral pelvic lymphadenectomy and radical prostatectomy for clinical stage C prostatic cancer: Role of adjuvant treatment for residual cancer and in disease progression. *J Urol* 135:1199–1205. Used by permission.)

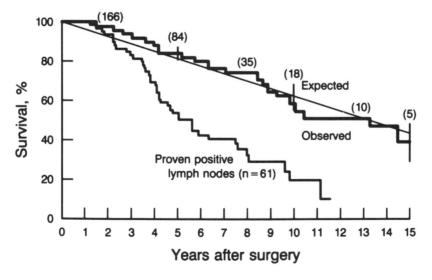

FIG 27-8.
Kaplan-Meier survival curves of 231 patients with stage D_1 prostate cancer who had undergone bilateral pelvic lymphadenectomy and radical retropubic prostatectomy with or without adjuvant treatment compared to expected survival. Comparison is to a group of 61 patients with stage D_1 prostate cancer treated with external-beam radiation (Bagshaw 1985). (Numbers within parentheses represent patients under observation at that time.)

series was significantly below that of conservative treatment approaches ($P = .02$) (Zincke et al. 1987). The morbidity and mortality with radical surgery for this advanced local stage have been low (Patterson and Zincke 1984).

We have analyzed records of 231 patients who were monitored for a minimum of 1 and up to 19.6 years (mean, 4.6 years). Their age range was from 40 to 77 years (mean, 63.9 years). That this represents a patient group with a very unfavorable prognosis is evident by the observations that almost half of the patients had undifferentiated cancer (grades 3 and 4) and 48% had more than 10 cm³ of tumor bulk (Table 27–3). Admittedly, multiple nodes ($\geqslant 3$) were involved in only 28% of the patients. Residual cancer was found in 68 (29%), and seminal vesicle involvement was a frequent finding (64%). Seventy-five of the patients (33%) presented with clinical stage C disease, and 40% originally had clinical stage B_2 disease. An abnormally elevated prostatic acid phosphatase level was found in 41 patients (19%). Adjuvant treatment was administered to 170 (74%); the most frequently administered treatment was orchiectomy, with or without some additional form of treatment (oral hormones or radiation) in 131 patients. Adjuvant treatment was related to number of positive nodes. The mean number of involved nodes in those without adjuvant treatment was 1.87, but in those undergoing orchiectomy or DES treatment, it was 2.48 or 2.65 nodes, respectively (Table 27–4).

TABLE 27–3.
Characteristics of 231 Patients With Pathologic Stage D_1 (pT_{0-3} N_{1-2} M_0) Prostate Cancer

Characteristic	Patients No.	%
Grade		
2	117	51
3,4	114	49
Tumor bulk		
<10 cm³	101	44
≥10 cm³	130	56
Seminal vesicles positive		
Yes	147	64
No	84	36
Number of positive nodes		
1	107	46
2	59	26
≥3	65	28
Residual cancer		
Yes	68	29
No	163	71
Clinical stage		
A	5	2
B_1	43	19
B_2	93	40
C	90	39
Acid phosphatase +/or tartrate-inhibited fraction		
Elevated	41	19
Normal	177	81
Unknown	13	
Adjuvant treatment		
Yes	170	74
No	61	26

TABLE 27–4.
Number of Positive Nodes as Related to Adjuvant Treatment (n = 231)

Adjuvant Treatment	No. of Patients	No. Positive Nodes				
		Mean	Range	1(%)	2(%)	≥3(%)
None	61	1.87	1–8	56	25	19
Orchiectomy (+)	131	2.48	1–9	41	27	33
Diethylstilbestrol (≤3 mg)	31	2.65	1–16	55	16	29
Radiation only	8	1.89	1–4	37	50	13

Whereas overall survival (see Fig 27–8) (5-, 10-, and 15-year survival rates of 84%, 62%, and 39%, respectively) compared favorably to that reported after conservative treatment (Bagshaw 1985) for this disease (overall deaths 40, 17%), the overall death rate from prostatic cancer was only 9% (Fig 27–9) (91% and 74% survivors at 5 and 10 years, respectively). Overall progression occurred in 66 patients (29%). Specifically, local recurrence (none ≥6 years) was detected in only 25 patients or 11% of the entire series (Fig 27–10). Immediate adjuvant orchiectomy (n = 131) significantly ($P = .0004$) reduced progression compared with no treatment (n = 61) or DES (n = 31) or irradiation (n = 8) (Fig 27–11). Five- and 10-year nonprogression rates for the orchiectomy group were 79% and 75%, respectively, as compared with 47% at 5 years for the 61 patients without adjuvant treatment. No patient in the orchiectomy group had progressing disease after 5 years, and only 15 (11%) of that group progressed at all. These favorable nonprogression rates after adjuvant orchiectomy result also in excellent cause-specific–death survival figures; only 6 (<5%) have died of disease, and the projected 10-year survival rate is 81% ± 16% (Fig 27–12).

As in our previous studies (Zincke and Utz 1983; Zincke in press), when patients received no adjuvant treatment, we found no correlation, apart from number of positive nodes (Fig 27–13), between rates of progression and cause-specific survival and the usual pathologic variables, including tumor grade according to Mayo or Gleason, tumor bulk measured in

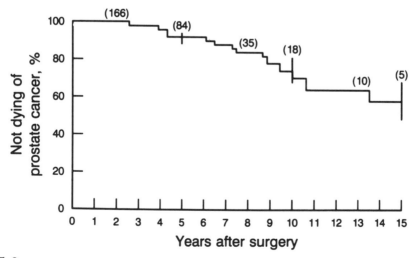

FIG 27–9.
Kaplan-Meier cause-specific (prostate cancer) survival curves for 231 patients with stage D₁ prostate cancer who had undergone a radical prostatectomy with or without adjuvant treatment. (Numbers within parentheses represent patients under observation at that time.)

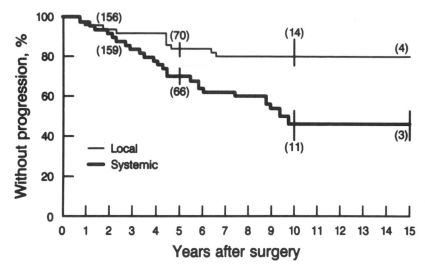

FIG 27–10.
Kaplan-Meier curves of nonprogression according to systemic and local progression for 231 patients with stage D_1 prostate cancer who had undergone bilateral pelvic lymphadenectomy and radical retropubic prostatectomy with or without adjuvant treatment. (Numbers within parentheses represent patients under observation at that time.)

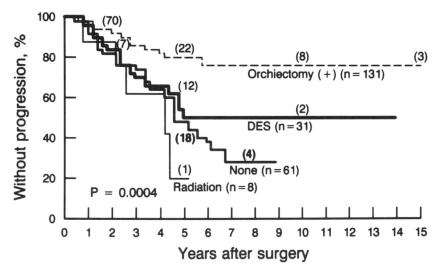

FIG 27–11.
Kaplan-Meier curves of nonprogression comparing immediate orchiectomy (n=31) with diethylstilbestrol (DES) treatment (n=31) or irradiation (n=8) for 231 patients with stage D_1 prostate cancer who had undergone bilateral pelvic lymphadenectomy and radical retropubic prostatectomy. (Numbers within parentheses represent patients under observation at that time.)

cubic centimeters, seminal vesicle involvement, prostatic acid phosphatase value (Utz et al. 1987; Zincke in press), or residual cancer.

In search of a pathologic variable that could be predictive of disease outcome, we used, in addition to traditional techniques, flow cytometry and analysis of tumor nuclear DNA content for a group of 91 patients who were monitored for at least 5 years (Winkler et al.

1988). Thirty-eight of this group (42%) showed a diploid DNA pattern, 41 (45%) had a tetraploid DNA pattern, and 12 (13%) had a DNA aneuploid pattern. At 5 years, the *actual* nonprogression rate for those patients with diploid tumors was 92%, and at 10 years it was 84% (Fig 27–14). Patients with a tetraploid or aneuploid DNA histogram had 5- and 10-year nonprogression rates of less than 50% or 10%, respectively, significantly lower ($P<.0001$) than those of patients who had a diploid pattern. Similar differences ($P<.001$) were found for cause-specific survival (Fig 27–15). None of the patients with a diploid pattern died of cancer, but 44% of the patients with an abnormal histogram on flow cytometry were projected to be dead of disease at 10 years.

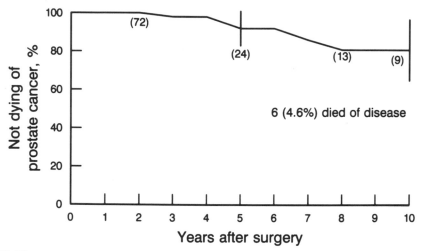

FIG 27–12.
Kaplan Meier curve of cause-specific (prostate cancer)–death survival rates of 130 patients who underwent immediate adjuvant orchiectomy. (Numbers within parentheses represent patients under observation at that time.)

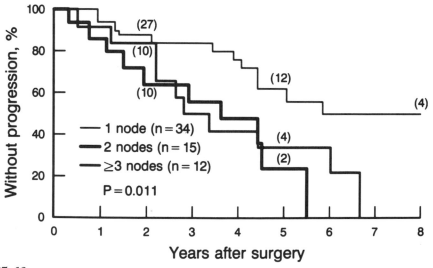

FIG 27–13.
Kaplan-Meier curves of nonprogression according to number of positive nodes for 61 patients with stage D_1 prostate cancer who had undergone bilateral pelvic lymphadenectomy and radical retropubic prostatectomy without immediate adjuvant treatment. (Numbers within parentheses represent patients under observation at that time.)

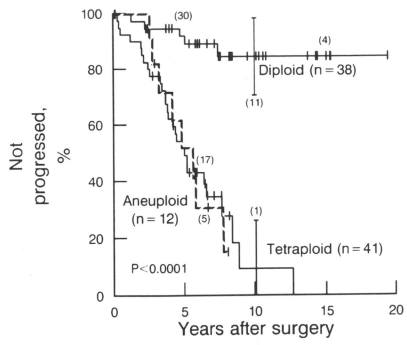

FIG 27–14.
Kaplan-Meier curves of nonprogression according to ploidy pattern for 91 patients with stage D_1 prostate cancer (follow-up ≤5 years) who had undergone bilateral pelvic lymphadenectomy and radical retropubic prostatectomy with or without adjuvant treatment. (Numbers within parentheses represent patients under observation at that time.)

CONCLUSION

Careful review of the literature, our own experience, and a recent consensus conference support the general impression that radiotherapy—when disease has been surgically staged— and radical prostatectomy provide roughly similar progression and survival results at intervals up to 10 years for patients with localized (≤pT_2) cancer of the prostate.

Satisfactory results have not been achieved when treatment is for locally advanced prostate cancer—pathologic (pT_3) and limited clinical (cT_3) stage C disease and pathologic stage D_1 disease ($pT_{0-3}N_{1-2}M_0$). Each of these stages is usually associated with a high percentage of undifferentiated cancers and an unfavorable ploidy pattern as well as large tumor bulk. Also, at least 90% of the patients with pathologic D_1 disease have locally extracapsular disease (Zincke et al. 1987). Conservative treatment (monotherapy) using hormonal manipulation or radiation has accomplished only moderate to poor local and systemic control, particularly when the cancer is stage D_1 (Bagshaw 1985; Bagshaw et al. 1985). The past, present, and projected future results from conservative monotreatment of cancers in these stages are unacceptable to a large and growing group of treating physicians.

Combination treatment as proposed and practiced at the Mayo Clinic has provided excellent results as far as local and systemic progression and survival are concerned and seems also to improve quality of life. The morbidity associated with the combined treatment is minimal (Patterson and Zincke 1984), and local complication rates are significantly lower than those encountered with conservative treatments (Zincke et al. 1987).

In 1983, we reported significantly reduced progression rates for patients with stage D_1

disease whose treatment was radical prostatectomy and immediate orchiectomy; we have now observed excellent cause-specific–death survival rates as well (Zincke and Utz 1983; Zincke et al. 1987; Zincke in press). Whereas for stage C disease, grade, ploidy pattern, seminal vesicle involvement, and tumor bulk are important variables affecting disease outcome, only number of involved nodes (uncorrected for abnormal ploidy pattern), ploidy pattern itself, and adjuvant hormonal treatment (orchiectomy) have predictive value for stage D_1 disease. At this time, the influence on cancer death of orchiectomy and ploidy pattern combined awaits further study. The finding that, once nodal disease is present, ploidy pattern is a highly significant predictor of disease outcome is a recent observation (Winkler et al. 1988) that reveals a significant relationship between DNA pattern and the rates of progression and cause-specific death. It also explains some of the controversial results presented in the literature.

Data presented from our institution justify the continuing use of combination treatments for locally advanced prostate cancer (stages C and D_1). To tailor adjuvant treatment modalities to specific disease forms (i.e., DNA ploidy, local stage), prospective studies combining radical prostatectomy with different forms of adjuvant treatment should be undertaken. Stratification factors should include not only the usual pathologic variables (tumor grade, seminal vesicle involvement, tumor bulk, number of positive nodes, residual cancer, and levels of prostate-specific antigen and prostatic acid phosphatase) but also DNA ploidy patterns. As far as treatment of D_1 disease is concerned, prospective studies should concentrate on the patient with a nondiploid tumor, because it is this pathologic variable that seems to respond poorly even to our proposed combination treatment of radical prostatectomy and orchiectomy.

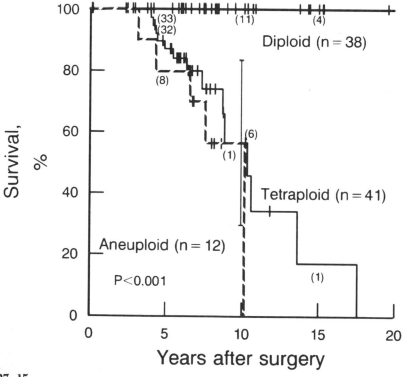

FIG 27–15.
Kaplan-Meier curves according to ploidy pattern for cause-specific (prostate cancer) survival of 91 patients with stage D_1 prostate cancer (follow-up ≤5 years) who had undergone bilateral pelvic lymphadenectomy and radical retropubic prostatectomy. (Numbers within parentheses represent patients under observation at that time.)

REFERENCES

1. Bagshaw MA. 1985. Potential for radiotherapy alone in prostatic cancer. *Cancer* 55(suppl 9):2079–2085.
2. Bagshaw MA, Ray GR, Cox RS. 1985. Radiotherapy of prostatic carcinoma: Long- or short-term efficacy (Stanford University experience). *Urology* 25(suppl 2):17–23.
3. Benson RC Jr, Tomera KM, Zincke H, et al. 1984. Bilateral pelvic lymphadenectomy and radical retropubic prostatectomy for adenocarcinoma confined to the prostate. *J Urol* 131:1103–1106.
4. Cupps RE, Utz DC, Fleming TR, et al. 1980. Definitive radiation therapy for prostatic carcinoma: Mayo Clinic experience. *J Urol* 124:855–859.
5. Guerriero WG, Carlton CE Jr, Hudgins PT. 1980. Combined interstitial and external radiotherapy in the definitive management of carcinoma of the prostate. *Cancer* 45(suppl 7):1922–1923.
6. Patterson DE, Zincke H. 1984. Perioperative complications of pelvic lymphadenectomy and radical retropubic prostatectomy for stages C and D1 prostate cancer. *Urology* 23:243–246.
7. Utz WJ, Zincke H, Utz DC. 1987. Significance of preoperatively elevated acid phosphatase in patients undergoing radical prostatectomy for stage D1 disease (abstract). Annual meeting of the North Central Section, American Urological Association, Detroit, Mich, p 123.
8. Whitmore WF Jr. 1984. Interstitial I-125 implantation in the management of localized prostatic cancer. *Prog Clin Biol Res* 153:513–527.
9. Winkler H, Rainwater L, Myers RP, et al. 1988. Stage D1 prostatic adenocarcinoma: Significance of nuclear DNA ploidy patterns studied by flow cytometry. *Mayo Clin Proc* 63:103–112.
10. Zincke H. In press. Bilateral pelvic lymphadenectomy and radical retropubic prostatectomy for stage C or D1 adenocarcinoma of the prostate: Possible beneficial effect of adjuvant treatment. *NCI Monograph*.
11. Zincke H. 1978. Updated experience on management of cancer of the prostate at the Mayo Clinic, in Rost A, Fiedler U (eds): *Proceedings of the International Symposium on the Treatment of Carcinoma of the Prostate*. West Berlin, University Press, pp 57–67.
12. Zincke H, Utz DC. 1983. Radical surgery for stage D1 prostate cancer. *Semin Urol* 1:253–260.
13. Zincke H, Fleming TR, Furlow WL, et al. 1981. Radical retropubic prostatectomy and pelvic lymphadenectomy for high-stage cancer of the prostate. *Cancer* 47:1901–1910.
14. Zincke H, Utz DC, Taylor WF. 1986. Bilateral pelvic lymphadenectomy and radical prostatectomy for clinical stage C prostatic cancer: Role of adjuvant treatment for residual cancer and in disease progression. *J Urol* 135:1199–1205.
15. Zincke H, Utz DC, Thulé PM, et al. 1987. Treatment options for patients with stage D_1 ($T_{0-3}N_{1-2}M_0$) adenocarcinoma of the prostate. *Urology* 30:307–315.

Chapter 28

Cytotoxic Chemotherapy for Advanced Cancer of the Prostate: Memorial Sloan-Kettering Cancer Center Experience*

Howard I. Scher, M.D.

Tracy Smart-Curley, R.N.

D. David Dershaw, M.D.

Robin C. Watson, M.D.

Jerome Nisselbaum, Ph.D.

Morton Schwartz, Ph.D.

Alan Yagoda, M.D.

Chemotherapy has a limited role in prostatic cancer. In a recent review, only 8% of 1,683 patients treated with chemotherapy achieved a complete or partial remission (Eisenberger et al. 1987). Further, no randomized clinical trial has demonstrated a survival benefit using chemotherapy alone. The evaluation of new agents in disease-oriented phase-II trials requires a clear end point of response to assess antitumor activity. The difficulties encountered in prostatic cancer relate primarily to the clinical manifestations of the disease (Yagoda 1983).

In contrast to the situation with untreated patients, in whom retroperitoneal lymphade-nopathy or a local prostatic mass is common and improvement in symptoms following therapy correlates with measurable regression of all disease indicators—primary and metastatic tumors and serum levels of prostatic acid phosphatase and prostate-specific antigen (PSA)—disease in hormone-refractory patients is often restricted to bony sites, which are inherently difficult to evaluate. As a result, many clinical trials reporting efficacy are based either on secondary

*This study was supported in part by grant CA-05826 from the National Institutes of Health, Bethesda, Md.; The Merrell-Dow Research Institute; and The David Cogan and Solid Tumor Service Funds. Howard Scher is the recipient of an American Cancer Society Clinical Oncology Career Development Award.

manifestations of the tumor such as bone turnover visible on scintiscans and elevated serum levels of alkaline phosphatase or acid phosphatase—measurements that are unreliable in hormone-refractory disease—or on subjective criteria such as pain and performance status. This accounts for the wide disparity in reported response rates for "standard agents" such as doxorubicin and *cis*-diamminedichloroplatinum.

No single agent or combination regimen can be recommended as standard therapy for hormone-refractory prostatic cancer. The approach at Memorial Sloan-Kettering Cancer Center (MSKCC) is to use investigational agents as first-line therapy. These agents are evaluated first in a highly selected patient population with disease bidimensionally measurable (in centimeters) across the tumor's diameter and perpendicularly at its widest portion, thus allowing serial monitoring throughout the course of treatment. Measurable disease can include lymph nodes or subcutaneous masses palpable on physical examination; pulmonary masses or peripheral lesions measurable radiologically; hepatomegaly identified by physical examination, sonography, or computerized tomography (CT); or abdominal and pelvic masses identified by CT or sonography (transabdominal or transrectal). Serum acid phosphatase elevations alone cannot be used in place of bidimensionally measurable disease. The response criteria are listed in Table 28–1.

Depending on the extent of the pretreatment evaluation, this group may represent 5% to 15% of patients considered for therapy. Although some investigators have criticized this approach for selecting a group destined to do poorly despite therapy or as not being representative of the majority of patients who never develop measurable lesions, it is the only group in whom reliable leads can be obtained. Other trial end points such as time to progression and overall survival fall outside the realm of these disease-oriented studies.

BIOLOGIC MARKERS

Biologic markers can be divided into two categories: those that reflect the tumor directly, e.g., serum levels of acid phosphatase and PSA, and those that reflect secondary effects of the tumor on the host, e.g., serum alkaline phosphatase and osteocalcin or urinary excretion

TABLE 28–1.
Response Criteria at MSKCC*

Response Level	Criteria
Subjective	Determined by Karnofsky performance status.
Objective	
Complete remission (CR)	Disappearance for 1 mo of all clinical evidence of tumor on physical examination and x-ray and biochemical evaluation plus normalization of acid phosphatase level.
Partial remission (PR)	>50% decrease on physical examination or radiography of the summed products of the perpendicular diameters of all measured lesions; no simultaneous increase in size of any lesion or appearance of any new lesion. *In liver disease:* At least a 50% reduction in the sums of all liver measurements below the costal margin and normalization of liver tests (if abnormal). Serum acid phosphatase level, if elevated, must decrease by more than 50% for 1 mo.
Minor remission (MR)	25%–59% decrease in the summed products of diameters of measured lesions.
Stabilization (STAB)	Less than 25% decrease or increase in tumor size for at least 3 mo.
Progression (PROG)	>25% increase in the sum of all measured lesions or appearance of new lesions. >50% increase in the acid phosphatase level also constitutes progression of disease.

*MSKCC = Memorial Sloan-Kettering Cancer Center.

of hydroxyproline. A distinct difference is observed between patients with hormone-naive and hormone-refractory disease. At first presentation, marker elevations and regression both correlate well with the clinical course and prognosis. However, in hormone-refractory patients, biologic markers are subject to many nontreatment-related changes. In a recent clinical trial, osteocalcin, a marker of bone formation, was elevated in only 47% of subjects; the ratio of hydroxyproline (a breakdown product of collagen that reflects bone turnover) to creatinine (normal, <4.0) was elevated in 77%; and the alkaline phosphatase level was elevated in 91% (Scher et al. 1987). However, all were insensitive as serial indices of response to therapy. Our experience in monitoring prostatic acid phosphatase is similar to that reported by other investigators (Zweig and Ihde 1985): we do not consider it of value as the sole criterion for entry into a clinical trial or to assess response of hormone-refractory disease to therapy.

The value of biologic markers may improve as additional data are obtained for PSA, a 34,000-dalton protein localized to prostatic epithelial cells that is cell-type– and organ-site– specific and is expressed independent of prostatic acid phosphatase (Pontes et al. 1978). At MSKCC, abnormal PSA levels (mean +3 SD or >3.67 ng/ml) were observed in 75% of men with stage B and 93% of those with stage C prostatic cancer (Schwartz et al. 1987). Elevated levels (median, 136 ng/dl; range, no measurable amount to 3,740 ng/dl) have been observed with progressive hormone-refractory disease in 27 of 29 patients (93%).

Data evaluating changes in PSA in response to chemotherapy are limited because few patients achieve objective responses. In a preliminary evaluation of 10 patients with bidimensionally measurable disease treated on chemotherapy programs, decreases of 50% or more in PSA levels were observed in 2 of 2 patients who achieved partial remissions, whereas 8 of 8 with progressive disease demonstrated serial elevations in PSA. If tumor regression by objective response criteria can be shown to correlate with decreases in PSA, a more accurate and reproducible response assessment will be possible.

CHEMOTHERAPY STUDIES

The results of phase II trials in a patient population with bidimensionally measurable disease are listed in Table 28–2. As noted, minimal activity has been observed for cisplatin (Yagoda et al. 1979), zinostatin (formerly neocarzinostatin) (Natale et al. 1980), amsacrine (Natale et al. 1982), doxorubicin (Adriamycin) (Scher et al. 1984), and etoposide (Scher et al. 1986b).

The predominant pattern of prostatic cancer metastatic to bone is osteoblastic rather than osteolytic (Jacobs 1983). This is probably induced by a specific osteoblast growth factor that has been shown to stimulate mitogenesis in rat osteosarcoma and normal osteoblasts in culture (Jacobs and Lawson 1980; Koutsilieris et al. 1986). A series of histomorphometric biopsies at MSKCC revealed that despite active new bone formation in the area of tumor, osteoclast numbers were also increased. Further, a comparison of tumor vs. nontumor sites revealed increased resorptive activity in areas of tumor (Scher et al. 1986a). In clinical trials, dichloromethylene diphosphonate, an agent known to inhibit bone resorption, produced significant pain relief in the absence of antitumor activity (Adami et al. 1985). This suggested the possibility of site-specific therapy for this disease.

Gallium nitrate is an anhydrous salt of the naturally occurring group 3 metal salts that has been shown to be incorporated into hydroxyapatite crystals; this incorporation makes them less soluble and less susceptible to dissolution (Warrell et al. 1984). It inhibits bone resorption without a direct toxic effect to bone cells. In a phase II trial using a continuous-infusion dose schedule in 20 patients with bidimensionally measurable disease, only 2 patients

TABLE 28–2.
MSKCC Chemotherapy Trials in Bidimensionally
Measurable Prostate Cancer*

Agent	No. of Patients	PR (%)	95% CI
Cisplatin	22	12	4–34
Zinostatin (formerly neocarzinostatin)	20	0	0
Amsacrine	18	0	0
Doxorubicin (Adriamycin)	39	5	0–12
Mitoguazone (MGBG)	25	24	11–44
Etoposide (VP-16-213)	20	5	0–24
Gallium nitrate	20	10	2–32
Doxorubicin (weekly)	32	12	1–32
DFMO/MGBG	14	0	0-23

*MSKCC = Memorial Sloan-Kettering Cancer Center; PR = partial response; CI = confidence interval; DFMO = α-difluoromethylornithine.

(10%; 95% confidence limits, 0%–22%) achieved a partial remission. In one, biopsy-proved cervical lymphadenopathy regressed for 5+ months, but the patient developed pulmonary nodules after 1 month; in the second, a postsacral mass with associated osteolytic disease showed healing for 6+ months, but the patient developed epidural bone disease at a distant site. Six patients (30%) showed a greater than 50% decrease in prostatic acid phosphatase levels following treatment. Pain diminished in a total of 7 patients, including 3 with evidence of progressing soft-tissue disease (Scher et al. 1987).

The study suggested that therapy directed to specific metastatic sites can be useful. Although gallium nitrate was not toxic to bone cells, it is possible that other chemotherapeutic agents may improve symptoms by destroying osteoclasts in the area of tumor invasion without direct toxicity to tumor cells (Scher and Yagoda 1987). Further investigations are warranted.

Interest in agents that affect polyamine biosynthesis derived from the observation that polyamine content is elevated in the prostate glands of rodents and humans (Fair et al. 1975; Dunzendorfer and Russell 1978). Alpha-difluoromethylornithine (DFMO) is a specific enzyme-activated irreversible inhibitor of ornithine decarboxylase, the initial enzyme in polyamine biosynthesis that converts ornithine to putrescine. Putrescine then receives a propylamine group from S-adenosylmethionine, a reaction catalyzed by S-adenosylmethionine decarboxylase (SAM-DC), to form spermidine and spermine. The latter is inhibited by mitoguazone (MGBG). A phase II trial of mitoguazone at MSKCC, 500 to 600 mg/m^2 intravenously weekly, produced partial remissions in 6 of 25 (24%; 95% confidence, 8%–42%) adequately treated patients with soft-tissue lesions. In general, responses were of short duration and limited to soft-tissue lesions (Scher et al. 1985).

Based on this experience and the reported synergism between MGBG and DFMO in the treatment of rat prostatic cancers (Herr et al. 1984), a phase II trial of the combination of DFMO and MGBG was initiated. To correlate antitumor activity and in vivo drug effect, biopsies of measurable tumor masses were performed for assays of polyamine levels. Because other investigators using these two agents in combination had encountered toxicity, a phase I study was designed. The dose of DFMO was held constant at 1.5 g/m^2 orally every 6 hours for 14 days, and MGBG at 200 mg/m^2 was administered intravenously on days 4 and 11 of each treatment cycle. In the absence of toxicity, the dose of MGBG was increased by increments of 50 mg/m^2. Dose-limiting toxicity, manifested by weakness, diarrhea, and thrombocytopenia, was reached at a dose of 350 mg/m². There was one toxic death. No antitumor activity was observed in 14 evaluable patients (Scher et al. 1988).

Doxorubicin, 20 mg/m² administered intravenously weekly, has also been evaluated. Although it was well tolerated and produced minimal toxicity, only 12% (95% confidence limits, 1%–32%) of 32 adequately treated patients achieved partial remissions on therapy (see Table 28–2). Currently we are evaluating a synthetic antifolate, trimetrexate, in patients with measurable disease.

DISCUSSION

The results of published investigations make it difficult to recommend a standard therapy for hormone-refractory prostatic cancer. For progress to occur, a better understanding of the basic biology of the disease and an incorporation of these principles into well-designed clinical trials are required. Examples are the recent identification of specific metastatic subclones of the R-3327-G tumor (Isaacs et al. 1986) and the isolation of a specific osteoblast growth factor (Koutsilieris et al. 1986).

Data from animal investigations suggest that androgen-resistant cells are present de novo in established tumors (Isaacs and Coffey 1982). This information provides a rationale for evaluating chemotherapeutic agents in the untreated population. As more patients who have measurable disease are identified before hormonal therapy, more agents can be tested in a shorter period of time, which will allow the more rapid development of effective combination programs. As more experience is gained with PSA determinations, more patients can be entered on clinical trials.

REFERENCES

1. Adami S, Salvagno G, Guarrera G, et al. 1985. Dichloromethylene-disphosphonate patients with prostatic carcinoma metastatic to the skeleton. *J Urol* 134:1152–1155.
2. Dunzendorfer U, Russell D. 1978. Altered polyamine profiles in prostatic hyperplasia and in kidney tumors. *Cancer Res* 38:2321–2324.
3. Eisenberger M, Kennedy P, Abrams J. 1987. How effective is cytotoxic chemotherapy for disseminated prostatic carcinoma? *Oncology* 2:59–69.
4. Fair W, Wehner N, Brorsson U. 1975. Urinary polyamine levels in the diagnosis of carcinoma of the prostate. *J Urol* 114:88–90.
5. Herr H, Kleinert E, Relyea N, et al. 1984. Potentiation of methylglyoxal-bis-guanylhydrazone by alpha-difluoromethylornithine in rat prostate cancer. *Cancer* 53:1294–1298.
6. Isaacs JT, Coffey DS. 1982. Adaptation vs. selection as the mechanism responsible for the relapse of prostatic cancer to androgen therapy as studied in the Dunning R-3327-H adenocarcinoma. *Cancer Res* 42:2353–2358.
7. Isaacs JT, Isaacs WB, Feitz WFJ, et al. 1986. Establishment and characterization of seven Dunning rat prostatic cancer cell lines and their use in developing methods for predicting metastatic abilities of prostatic cancers. *Prostate* 9:261–278.
8. Jacobs S. 1983. Spread of prostatic cancer to bone. *Urology* 21:337–341.
9. Jacobs SC, Lawson RK. 1980. Mitogenic factor in human prostate extracts. *Urology* 16:488–491.
10. Koutsilieris R, Rabbini SA, Goltzman D. 1986. Selective osteoblast mitogens can be extracted from prostatic tissue. *Prostate* 9:109–116.
11. Natale RB, Yagoda A, Watson RC. 1982. Phase II trial of AMSA (4'[9-acridinylamino methanesulfon-m-anisidide]) in prostatic cancer. *Cancer Treat Rep* 66:208–212.
12. Natale RB, Yagoda A, Watson RC, et al. 1980. Phase II trial of neocarcinostatin in patients with bladder and prostatic cancer: Toxicity of a 5 day bolus schedule. *Cancer* 45:2836–2837.

13. Pontes JE, Chu TM, Slack N, et al. 1978. Serum prostatic antigen measurement in localized prostatic cancer: Correlation with clinical course. *J Urol* 128:1216–1219.
14. Scher HI, Yagoda A. 1987. Bone metastases: Pathogenesis, treatment and rationale for use of resorption inhibitors. *Am J Med* 82 (suppl 2A):6–28.
15. Scher H, Ahmed T, Yagoda A, et al. 1985. Methyl glyoxal-bis(guanylhydrazone) in hormone resistant adenocarcinoma of the prostate. *J Clin Oncol* 3:224–227.
16. Scher H, Bansal M, Zackson D, et al. 1986a. Is there a systemic metabolic bone defect in prostatic cancer metastatic to bone? (abstract). *Ninth International Conference on Calcium Regulating Hormones,* p 242.
17. Scher H, Curley T, Geller NL, et al. 1987. Gallium nitrate in prostatic cancer: Evaluation of antitumor activity and effects of bone turnover. *Cancer Treat Rep* 71:887–893.
18. Scher H, Smart-Curley T, Heston WDW, et al. 1988. Phase I-II trial of alpha-difluoromethylornithine (DFMO) [MDL 71,782] and mitoguazone in hormone refractory prostatic cancer (PC) (abstract). *Proc Am Assoc Cancer Res* 29:191.
19. Scher HI, Sternberg C, Heston WDW, et al. 1986b. Etoposide in prostatic cancer: Experimental studies and phase II trial in patients with bidimensionally measurable disease. *Cancer Chemother Pharmacol* 18:24–26.
20. Scher H, Yagoda A, Serber M, et al. 1984. Phase II trial of doxorubicin in bidimensionally measurable prostatic adenocarcinoma. *J Urol* 131:1099–1102.
21. Schwartz MK, Nisselbaum J, Stone N, et al. 1987. A comparison of the Hybritech immunoradiometric and immunoenzymetric assays of prostate specific antigen (PSA) (abstract). *Clin Chem* 33:928.
22. Warrell RP Jr, Bockman RS, Coonley CJ, et al. 1984. Gallium nitrate inhibits calcium resorption from bone and is effective treatment for cancer-related hypercalcemia. *J Clin Invest* 73:1487–1490.
23. Yagoda A. 1983. Response in prostatic cancer: An enigma. *Semin Urol* 1:311–320.
24. Yagoda A, Watson RC, Natale RB, et al. 1979. A critical analysis of response criteria in patients with prostatic cancer treated with cis-diamminedichloride platinum II. *Cancer* 44:1553–1559.
25. Zweig M, Ihde D. 1985. Assessment of serum and enzymatic prostatic acid phosphatase and radioimmune creatinine kinase BB for monitoring response to therapy in metastatic prostatic carcinoma. *Cancer Res* 45:3945–3950.

Chapter 29

Cytotoxic Chemotherapy for Hormone-Refractory Metastatic Prostate Cancer

Christopher J. Logothetis, M.D.

Francisco Dexeus, M.D.

Clayton D. K. Chong, M.D.

Avishay Sella, M.D.

Laury Finn, R.T.

Classic adenocarcinoma of the prostate is very responsive to hormonal therapy; response rates ranging from 50% to 80% have been reported. Patients who respond to hormonal therapy benefit by controlling the symptoms of their disease with a relatively nontoxic therapy. Once hormonal resistance develops, however, currently available therapy includes palliative radiation, cytotoxic chemotherapy, and further hormonal therapy, although the latter is generally considered ineffective.

Cytotoxic chemotherapy of metastatic prostatic carcinoma has produced disappointing results. Although various response rates have been reported and clear symptomatic responses achieved, a dispute remains over whether these agents produce any therapeutic benefit. Randomized trials have failed to document an improved survival rate when chemotherapy is included.

A major factor complicating the treatment of prostatic carcinoma is the poor definition of response criteria. The difficulty in measuring prostatic carcinoma can be attributed to the nature of the disease. Bony metastases are the dominant mode of spread of this tumor, but the bony metastases from prostatic carcinoma are most frequently blastic and therefore ill defined. Tumor biomarkers (acid phosphatase, alkaline phosphatase) are either indirect measurements of disease or can fluctuate spontaneously. The assessment of the result of treatment is further complicated by the very heterogeneous behavior of metastatic prostatic carcinoma and the advanced stage of disease in the patients treated. In addition, patients with metastatic prostatic carcinoma have a relatively high rate of associated medical disorders restricting their ability to tolerate intensive chemotherapy.

Criteria used in the Section of Genitourinary Oncology at The University of Texas M. D. Anderson Cancer Center to evaluate response to treatment of prostatic carcinoma incorporate standard tumor measurements. For patients with visceral disease and measurable soft-tissue masses, the classic 50% reduction of the bidimensional measurements is employed (Table 29–1). To reduce the likelihood that a single drop in the serum acid phosphatase level would be attributed to a spontaneous fluctuation, but yet incorporate responses less than complete normalization of a high serum acid phosphatase, we have used the criterion of a greater than 50% reduction in the baseline level on three subsequent measurements. Bone scans have been considered indirect measurements of disease, and we believe that they only crudely reflect the disease volume. A response on a bone scan requires a reduction in the size or the number of established areas of above-normal uptake. The intensity of the uptake is not considered a response factor. Progression on a bone scan is defined as the development of new metastatic sites or an increase in the size of established sites.

Metastatic prostatic carcinoma has a heterogeneous behavior. Part of its behavior can be related to the volume of metastatic disease and the extent of dissemination. We attempted to group patients into clinical categories determined first by the extent of dissemination and second by the volume of disease at each site. Thus patients with osseous metastases are divided into two large categories (Table 29–2), those with just axial skeleton involvement and those whose disease involves axial skeleton and long bones. The resulting categories were labeled O_1, minimal osseous disease, and O_2, extensive osseous disease. Two similar categories were established for patients with visceral metastases. Those with visceral metastases involving the lung only were categorized V_1, and those whose liver and brain were also involved were categorized V_2. A comparison of the survival rates of the patients who receive chemotherapy reveals that the patients with minimal osseous disease have the highest mean survival rate, followed by those with extensive osseous disease and with visceral disease (Table 29–3).

The chemotherapy regimens employed at UT M. D. Anderson Cancer Center for met-

TABLE 29–1.
Response Criteria for Metastatic Prostatic Carcinoma

Criterion	Response
Visceral disease	>50% reduction
Osseous disease	Improvement on bone scan, no new lesions, healing of lytic metastasis
Serum biomarker levels	CEA,* acid phosphatase, alkaline phosphatase: 50% reduction in 3 subsequent measurements
Performance status	Improvement in Dubrov's performance status

*CEA = carcinoembryonic antigen.

TABLE 29–2.
Clinical Categories of Metastatic Prostate Cancer

Stage	Tumor Involvement
O_1	Axial skeleton
O_2	Epiphyseal + axial skeleton
V_1	Lung parenchyma
V_2	Liver and brain ± lung

TABLE 29–3.
Mean Survival Duration (wk) by Stage and Protocol*†

	Protocol					
	Doxorubicin + Vinblastine		DMF		Vinblastine	
Stage	R	N	R	N	R	N
O_1	45.433	44.21	100.43	47.089	45.325	47.433
O_2	—	48.95	61.533	37.737	64.3	28.22
V_1	30.733	76.3	65.075	26.3	43.233	126.0
V_2	79.7	36.575	33.267	17.75	—	19.3

*See text for explanation of stage.
†DMF = doxorubicin, mitomycin C, 5-fluorouracil; R = responders; N = nonresponders.

astatic prostate cancer include the original combination of doxorubicin (Adriamycin), mitomycin C, and 5-fluorouracil (DMF); Adriamycin and vinblastine; and the most recent combination of vinblastine, Adriamycin, mitomycin C (VAM) (Table 29–4).

Among the 159 patients who were treated for metastatic prostate cancer in the Section of Genitourinary Oncology, only the 128 patients who received the DMF combination, doxorubicin and vinblastine, or vinblastine alone have been followed-up long enough to be compared for survival rate. The patients treated with VAM are compared only for response rates (Table 29–5).

TABLE 29–4.
Chemotherapy Dosages, 1980–1986

No. of Patients	Chemotherapy			
78	Doxorubicin	50	mg/m² Cl* × 1	
	Mitomycin C	5	mg/m² × 2	
	5-Fluorouracil	750	mg/m² × 2	
22	Vinblastine	1.5	mg/m² Cl × 5	
27	Doxorubicin	50	mg/m² Cl × 1	
	Vinblastine	1.5	mg/m² Cl × 5	
32	Adriamycin	50	mg/m² Cl × 1	
	Vinblastine	1.5	mg/m² Cl × 5	
	Mitomycin C	10	mg/m² × 1	

*Cl = course one.

TABLE 29–5.
Comparison of Response Rate by Stage and Protocol*

Stage	Total Patients	Chemotherapy				P Value
		Doxorubicin + Vinblastine	DMF	Vinblastine	VAM	
O_1	70	3/11 (27.3%)	15/34 (44.1%)	4/11 (36.4%)	5/14 (35.71%)	.77707 (NS)
O_2	48	0/6 (0%)	6/25 (24%)	1/6 (16.7%)	5/11 (45.45%)	.19596 (NS)
V_1	19	3/4 (75%)	8/10 (80%)	3/5 (60%)	—	.70751 (NS)
V_2	23	22/6 (33.3%)	3/9 (33.3%)	0/1 (0%)	3/7 (42.86%)	.86186 (NS)
Total	160	8/27 (29%)	32/78 (41%)	8/23 (35%)	13/32 (41%)	
P value		.88810	.02199	.42022	.87766	

*DMF = doxorubicin, mitomycin C, and 5-fluorouracil; VAM = vinblastine, Adriamycin, mitomycin C.

The clinical characteristics of the patients treated between 1980 and 1986 as defined by our staging criteria are outlined (Table 29–6). The largest single category of patients in each study was minimal osseous disease. We also determined the degree of elevation of the serum acid phosphatase, alkaline phosphatase, and carcinoembryonic antigen (CEA) for each of the stages. Carcinoembryonic antigen was elevated most frequently in those patients with visceral disease, although the difference was not statistically significant. The serum alkaline phosphatase level was elevated frequently and over a wide range in patients of all groups, but it was highest in those patients with large-volume osseous disease (O_2). The serum acid phosphatase level was elevated least often among patients with V_2 disease, but patients with visceral disease generally had a higher level of serum acid phosphatase than those with osseous disease.

The survival durations of patients by chemotherapy regimen evaluable for response and by volume of disease revealed that the longest survivors were those patients with O_1 disease who responded to chemotherapy. Patients with O_1 disease who failed to respond to chemotherapy frequently survived longer than equivalent nonresponding, or even responding, patients in the other clinical categories.

We compared the response frequency to the four chemotherapy regimens. The response rates in categories with adequate numbers of patients to compare revealed that the likelihood of response was higher in the mitomycin-containing regimens (DMF, VAM) than in the regimens not containing mitomycin C (see Table 29–5). Patients responding to chemotherapy frequently benefitted by very gratifying relief from their pain. The duration of response for these relatively advanced-stage patients was short.

We reviewed the records of our patients in an attempt to find a subpopulation that may be highly responsive to therapy. Some of our patients had minimal osseous disease (O_1) at the time they developed visceral disease. In addition, some patients with visceral disease had high-volume osseous disease. The difference between these two populations represents, we believe, two subtypes of prostatic carcinoma: a rapidly growing tumor that has a short transit time through the osseous metastatic phase and quickly involves viscera, and tumor that metastasizes from bone to bone and finally, as the end-stage manifestation of further progression, involves viscera. Thirteen patients had minimal osseous disease with visceral involvement, 10 of whom have responded, whereas only 1 of the patients with O_2 disease and visceral involvement has responded to chemotherapy. This difference in survival rate is very significant ($P = .004$) (see Table 29–3).

The results of our experience with cytotoxic chemotherapy for hormonally refractory prostate cancer confirm that mitomycin C-based cytotoxic therapy is effective in palliating almost half the patients with metastatic disease. The patients benefit from relief of pain and some prolongation in survival. We also believe that our data confirm that mitomycin C may

TABLE 29–6.
Chemotherapy Patients

| Stage | Chemotherapy* | | | |
	DMF	Vinblastine	Doxorubicin + Vinblastine	VAM
O_1	34	11	10	14
O_2	25	6	6	11
V_1	10	4	5	—
V_2	9	6	1	7
Total	78	27	22	32

*DMF = doxorubicin, mitomycin C, 5-fluorouracil; VAM = vinblastine, Adriamycin, mitomycin C.

be the most effective cytotoxic agent that we have used in treating metastatic hormone-refractory prostate cancer. The regimens not employing mitomycin C produce a lower response rate than those incorporating mitomycin C.

Chemotherapy for metastatic prostatic carcinoma must, at present, be reserved for those with symptomatic metastases and those with visceral metastases who have an expected very short survival duration. A trial in which chemotherapy is introduced earlier, along with hormonal therapy, is justified. We base this conclusion on our interpretation of this experience; patients with minimum osseous disease have a higher likelihood of responding than patients who have high-volume osseous disease and visceral metastases, which we believe represents further progression of this tumor.

Chapter 30

Approaches to Advanced Prostate Cancer at Stanford University

Frank M. Torti, M.D.

Bert Lum, Pharm.D.

Fuad S. Freiha, M.D.

Richard K. Lo, M.D.

Until recently, the number and quality of chemotherapeutic trials in prostate cancer were limited. Few studies prior to 1973 were randomized comparisons, many were anecdotal case reports, and others reported limited numbers of patients from drug-oriented phase II studies in which few of the specialized examinations required to evaluate patients with prostatic cancer were performed. Recently, however, investigations that systematically evaluate the role of cytotoxic agents in prostatic carcinoma have been completed. It is not the purpose of this chapter to review this literature in detail, but rather to focus on the therapeutic results in advanced disease from the Stanford University and the Northern California Oncology Group (NCOG) trials and on the response criteria used to assess these results (Tables 30–1 and 30–2).

RESPONSE CRITERIA FOR PROSTATIC CARCINOMA

In most solid tumors, response to chemotherapy is easily quantitated by measuring changes in tumor diameter clinically or radiographically. In prostate cancer, measurable disease in the lung, lymph nodes, and soft tissue is uncommon; bone remains the most common clinically apparent site of metastatic spread and the predominant site of symptomatic disease. The skeletal distribution of metastases makes accurate measurement of response difficult. This creates variations in response criteria and patient eligibility requirements for clinical trials. Further, patients with prostatic carcinoma and bone metastasis are frequently excluded from drug-oriented phase II trials because bone is a "nonmeasurable" disease site.

Quantitation of the Primary Prostatic Tumor Nodule

Sequential digital examination of the prostate gland by the same observer may be a useful

TABLE 30–1.
Stanford/NCOG Definitions of Response for Prostatic Cancer*

Category	Definition
Complete response	Complete disappearance of tumor; all sites initially involved must be reevaluated (including bone scan) prior to scoring an overall CR

Partial response	1. Bidimensional tumor
	  a. Prostatic nodule: 75% decrease in the product of the two largest perpendicular diameters by sequential rectal digital examination or rectal ultrasound
	  b. Other than prostate nodule: 50% decrease in the product of the two largest perpendicular diameters of soft-tissue mass, palpable lymph nodes, liver mass, or retroperitoneal mass on computerized tomographic scan, pulmonary nodes, etc.; no evidence of progression on bone scan or bone roentgenograms; no deterioration in pain or Karnofsky performance status (as defined under progression)
	2. Evaluable disease, not bidimensional
	  a. Ureteral obstruction on intravenous pyelogram or ultrasound: complete resolution
	  b. Pleural effusion: complete resolution
	  c. Diffuse interstitial (lymphangitic) disease: complete resolution
	3. Acid phosphatase serum level (evaluable if greater than 2 times normal): 50% reduction

Ancillary response	1. Pain: 20% improvement on pain status scale[†] not attributable to analgesic therapy 2. Alkaline phosphatase serum level (evaluation if greater than 2 times normal): 50% reduction or normalization 3. Karnofsky performance status (evaluable if <80): 20% improvement

Progression	1. Bone scan: >3 new lesions at 6 mo; >3 new lesions at any time of symptomatic progression
	2. Bidimensional disease
	  a. Prostate nodule: 50% increase in the product of the two largest perpendicular diameters of any measurable lesion; appearance of any lesion
	3. Evaluable disease, not bidimensional
	  a. Ureteral obstruction: occurrence of partial or complete ureteral obstruction while on therapy
	  b. Pleural effusion: occurrence of cytologically positive effusion while on therapy
	4. Acid phosphatase serum level: 50% increase over baseline maintained for at least two measurements at least 1 wk apart
	5. Symptomatic measures
	  a. Pain: 20% or greater increase in pain on pain status scale that persists over 3 wks
	  b. Karnofsky performance status: 20% decrease that persists for at least 3 wks and is attributable to tumor
	  c. Use of radiation for pain control during therapy

*NCOG = Northern California Oncology Group; CR = complete response.
†See Table 30–2, Stanford/NCOG Pain Status Scale.

measure of disease activity and appears to parallel other measures of response. Occasionally, local response may occur while bone disease is progressing (Slack et al. 1980). The response of local disease may occur later than response in other disease sites; patients responding to hormonal therapy as evidenced by decreasing acid phosphatase level and bone pain may show little local tumor change at 3 months but demonstrate continuous improvement in nodule size between 3 and 6 months. Anatomical grids displaying the prostate gland in at least two axes are essential in quantitating local response.

In all Stanford/NCOG trials, the criteria for local disease response have been defined more rigorously than conventional response criteria. This is done specifically to avoid the well-known problems of assessing prostatic cancer dimensions by digital rectal examination. Thus, the criterion for partial response in the prostate demands a 75% reduction in area of the involved prostatic nodule. Further, a nodule must be readily measurable before treatment to qualify as a "measurable site." Areas of induration are excluded, although they probably represent cancer tissue, because their margins are too indiscreet to qualify for sequential measurement.

Our experience in the use of rectal ultrasound in measuring changes in the local tumor have been moderately encouraging. This technique can accurately measure prostate volume

TABLE 30–2.
Stanford/NCOG Pain Status Scale

Status (%)	Definition
100	Normal, without pain
90	Able to carry on normal activity, minor pain, no special care
80	Normal activities with effort, some pain, no special care
70	Cares for self, unable to carry on normal activity or do active work due to pain
60	Requires occasional assistance in self-care but can accomplish most of own needs; pain is reason for assistance
50	Requires considerable assistance with personal needs and frequent medical care due to pain
40	Disabled; requires special medical care and assistance due to pain
30	Severely disabled; hospitalization is indicated for pain
20	Hospitalization necessary; active supportive therapy needed for pain control; intravenous narcotics not completely effective
10	Intractable, constant, and completely debilitating pain

and assess stage (periprostatic invasion or seminal vesicle involvement). Response to hormonal therapy has been monitored with ultrasonography with good results. However, the utility of this method in determining chemotherapeutic response or progression has been questioned (Resnick 1981). Recent advances at Stanford and at other institutions in quantifying prostate size and in measuring the extent of localized prostate cancers prior to radical prostatectomy make it likely that the technique involved will be applied more effectively in the future to measure hormonal and chemotherapeutic responses.

Acid Phosphatase

The acid phosphatases are lysosomal enzymes found in glandular epithelium and are present in many body fluids and tissues, including serum, red blood cells, spleen, liver, kidney, and bone, especially in osteoclasts. These enzymes hydrolyze orthophosphoric acid esters in acid environments. Per unit weight, prostatic tissue has 1,000 times the concentration of acid phosphatases of any other tissue, and malignant prostatic tissue has been demonstrated to have less measurable enzyme activity than normal prostate tissue (Yam 1974). The primary role of prostatic acid phosphatases appears to be extracellular; they supply phosphate and catalyze phosphate group activity in spermatozoa (Bodansky 1972). No major metabolic role has been recognized for prostate cells. Prostatic acid phosphatase (PAP) is heterogeneous, with at least two molecular variants (isoenzymes) (Smith and Whitby 1968). Most acid phosphatase-containing tissues have two or more isoenzymes (Bodansky 1972; Lam et al. 1973; Yam 1974; Foti et al. 1977). The acid phosphatase level in the serum of healthy volunteers is primarily from enzyme contributed from red blood cells and platelets. Various substrates and enzyme inhibitors have been used to identify and quantitate enzyme activity attributable to the prostate, but PAP has not been shown to be more useful than serum acid phosphatase. Although serum acid phosphatase levels may be elevated by hemolysis of red cells and release of platelets during clotting and as a result of a number of malignant and nonmalignant diseases, Murphy et al. (1969) found conventional serum acid phosphatase to be as useful as the more specific enzyme assay.

The degree of initial elevation of acid phosphatase is prognostically significant in most series. A comparison between patients, with or without metastases, who present with elevated serum acid phosphatase at diagnosis and patients with normal levels shows that patients with normal serum acid phosphatase levels live longer (Murphy et al. 1969; Nesbit et al. 1951). One exception to this was a study by Ishibe et al. (1974) in which degree of initial elevation of serum acid phosphatase did not correlate with survival following hormonal therapy.

Serum acid phosphatase, when elevated, parallels other measures of response, although imperfectly. Johnson et al. (1976) demonstrated that normalization of serum acid phosphatase correlated with pain relief and decreased tumor size. In their series, 17 of 91 patients achieved a 50% or greater reduction of tumor mass with chemotherapy. In 59% of these 17 responders, serum acid phosphatase levels normalized. As a single-response variable, the reduction or normalization of the serum acid phosphatase level correlates with improved outcome in most series (Byar 1972; Ishibe et al. 1974; Citrin et al. 1983).

The radioimmunoassay (RIA) method for serum acid phosphatase determinations appears to be more sensitive than enzymatic assays, although its lack of specificity has raised questions. The clinical utility of the RIA method for measuring response to treatment has been studied for a limited number of patients with encouraging results (Mahan and Doctor 1979; Vihko et al. 1981; Moon et al. 1983).

Prostate-Specific Antigen (PSA)

Recent work at Stanford (Stamey et al. 1987) and at other institutions has shown that volume of prostatic tissue has a higher degree of correlation with prostate-specific antigen (PSA) than with PAP. In addition, after radical prostatectomy, PSA disappears more completely than acid phosphatase. Whether the improved diagnostic accuracy of PSA over acid phosphatase in localized disease also holds true for metastatic disease is currently being investigated in prospective trials at Stanford.

STANFORD/NCOG TRIALS

In the initial Stanford/NCOG trial, 37 patients with hormonally refractory prostatic carcinoma entered a randomized trial comparing doxorubicin (Adriamycin) and Adriamycin plus cisplatin. Sites of disease at entrance into study are shown in Table 30–3. All patients had failed prior hormonal treatment. Mean Karnofsky performance status (76%, Adriamycin group vs. 75%, combination group), percent of patients who had prior palliative irradiation (40%, Adriamycin vs. 35% combination), and hemoglobin levels of less than 12 g/dl (30% Adriamycin vs. 24% combination) were roughly equivalent in the two treatment groups. More patients treated with Adriamycin than with the combination had an elevated serum acid phosphatase level at study entry (90% vs. 65%). Measurable bidimensional tumors were present in 13 patients in 16 sites in the Adriamycin arm and in 10 patients in 11 sites in the combination arm.

Partial responses were seen in 1 of 13 patients in the Adriamycin arm and 2 of 10 patients in the combination arm. Improvement in Karnofsky performance status of 20% or greater was rarely observed with either treatment (7% Adriamycin vs. 8% combination). Acid phosphatase levels normalized or improved by 50% in 39% of patients who received Adriamycin and 27% of patients who received the combination. The overall response rate by National Prostatic Cancer Project criteria was 53% for Adriamycin and 59% for Adriamycin plus cisplatin. Myelotoxicity and gastrointestinal toxicity were severe, particularly in the combination arm, and required discontinuation of treatment for some patients who were responding. Moderate renal dysfunction (creatinine value, 2.0–3.0 mg/dl) occurred only in the combination arm at an incidence of 23%. Time to progression and survival duration were similar for the two treatment groups. In this small group of 37 patients, the combination of cisplatin and Adriamycin showed no benefit over Adriamycin alone in response rate, response duration, or survival and was difficult to administer in this patient population.

TABLE 30–3.
Sites of Disease at Study Entry: 3-Weekly vs. Weekly Adriamycin Trials

Site	Trial (No. of Patients Positive/Total No. Evaluated)					
	3-Weekly				Weekly Adriamycin	
	Adriamycin		Adriamycin + cisplatin			
	No.	%	No.	%	No.	%
Prostate: measurable tumor	5/20	25	7/17	41	8/25	32
Bone	20/20	100	13/17	77	24/25	96
Lymph nodes						
Peripheral	1/18	6	2/17	12	2/25	8
Pelvic or paraortic	2/17	12	2/14	14	4/17	24
Pulmonary nodules	3/20	15	0/16	0	1/25	4
Mediastinal mass	1/20	5	0/16	6	2/25	8
Pleural effusion	3/20	15	1/16	6	3/25	12
Liver	2/20	10	1/15	7	1/25	4
IVP*/ureteral obstruction	5/18	28	6/15	40	1/17	6
Soft tissue	2/17	12	1/15	7	1/25	4

*IVP = intravenous pyelogram.

These results contrast with those subsequently obtained by our same group of investigators in a study using weekly Adriamycin. Twenty-five patients with endocrine-refractory prostatic carcinoma were treated with Adriamycin, 20 mg/m^2, administered weekly. Doses were modified according to leucocyte and platelet counts (Table 30–4). All patients had had prior hormonal therapy (68% had had two or more prior hormonal maneuvers), and 21 (84%) had received prior therapeutic or palliative irradiation. Median Karnofsky performance status at the time of entry was 70. Hemoglobin was less that 12.0 g/dl in 15 patients. Bidimensional tumors were present in 12 patients in 19 disease sites. Four of the 12 patients (33%) responded in 8 of the 19 sites (42%), and 3 of 8 patients had a 75% decrease in prostatic nodule size. In 10 of 20 evaluable patients, the Karnofsky performance status improved by 20% or more, and in 67% (14 of 21), pain improved markedly. A greater than 50% reduction or normalization of serum acid phosphatase occurred in 19% and of serum alkaline phosphatase in 53%. The overall response rate by National Prostatic Cancer Project criteria was 84%. Gastrointestinal toxicity and alopecia were minimal, and myelosuppression was not life threatening in any patient.

TABLE 30–4.
Dose Reduction for Weekly Adriamycin

Leukocytes (Cells/µl)	Platelets (Cells/µl)			
	>150,000	100,000–149,000	75,000–99,999	<75,000
3,500	100*	100	50	0
3,000–3,499	100	75	50	0
2,500–2,999	50	0	0	0
<2,500	0	0	0	0

*Values represent percentage of calculated dose.

Our strategy has been to build on the reproducible responses and acceptable toxicity of the weekly Adriamycin protocol. In recently completed trials, which are still undergoing final analysis, we investigated the use of weekly Adriamycin plus methotrexate and of weekly doxorubicin plus difluoromethylornithine (DFMO) to treat advanced endocrine-refractory disease.

REFERENCES

1. Bodansky O. 1972. Acid phosphatase. *Adv Clin Chem* 15:43–147.
2. Byar DP. 1972. Treatment of prostatic cancer: Studies by the Veterans Administration Cooperative Urological Research Group (VACURG). *Bull NY Acad Med* 48:751–766.
3. Citrin DL, Elson P, DeWys WD. 1983. Treatment of metastatic prostate cancer: An analysis of response criteria in patients with measurable soft tissue disease (abstract). *Proc Am Soc Clin Oncol* 2:142.
4. Foti AG, Herschman H, Cooper JF. 1977. Isozymes of acid phosphatase in normal and cancerous human prostatic tissue. *Cancer Res* 37:4120–4124.
5. Ishibe T, Usui T, Nihira H. 1974. Prognostic usefulness of serum acid phosphatase levels in carcinoma of the prostate. *J Urol* 112:237–240.
6. Johnson DE, Prout GR, Scott WW, et al. 1976. Clinical significance of serum acid phosphatase levels in advanced prostatic carcinoma. *Urology* 8:123–126.
7. Lam KW, Li O, Li CY, et al. 1973. Biochemical properties of human prostatic acid phosphatase. *Clin Chem* 19:483–487.
8. Mahan DE, Doctor BP. 1979. A radioimmune assay for human prostatic acid phosphatase levels in prostatic disease. *Clin Biochem* 12:10–17.
9. Moon TD, Vessella RL, Eickhoff M, et al. 1983. Acid phosphatase for monitoring prostatic carcinoma: Comparison of radioimmunoassay and enzymatic techniques. *Urology* 22:16–19.
10. Murphy GP, Raynoso G, Kenny GM, et al. 1969. Comparison of total and prostatic fraction serum acid phosphatase levels in patients with differentiated and undifferentiated prostatic carcinoma. *Cancer* 23:1309–1314.
11. Nesbit RM, Baum WC, Mich AA. 1951. Serum phosphatase determination in diagnosis of prostatic cancer: A review of 1150 cases. *JAMA* 145:1321ff.
12. Resnick MI. 1981. Noninvasive techniques in evaluating patients with carcinoma of the prostate. *Urology* 17(suppl 3):25–30.
13. Slack NH, Mittleman A, Brady MF, et al. 1980. The importance of the stable category for chemotherapy treated patients with advanced and relapsing prostate cancer. *Cancer* 46:2393–2402.
14. Smith JK, Whitby LG. 1968. The heterogeneity of prostatic acid phosphatase. *Biochim Biophys Acta* 151:607–618.
15. Stamey TA, Yang N, Hay AR, et al. 1987. Prostate-specific antigen as a serum marker for adenocarcinoma of the prostate. *N Engl J Med* 317:909–916.
16. Vihko P, Lukkarinen O, Kontturi M, et al. 1981. Effectiveness of radioimmunoassay of human prostate-specific acid phosphatase in the diagnosis and follow-up of therapy in prostatic carcinoma. *Cancer Res* 41:1180–1183.
17. Yam LT. 1974. Clinical significance of the human acid phosphatase: A review. *Am J Med* 56:604–616.

Chapter 31

Management of Hormone-Resistant Prostate Cancer: Experience at Royal Prince Alfred Hospital*

D. Raghavan, M.B.B.S., Ph.D., F.R.A.C.P.

B. Pearson, M.B.B.S., F.R.C.S., F.R.A.C.S.

G. Coorey, M.B.B.S., F.R.C.S., F.R.A.C.S.

M. Rosen, M.B.B.S., F.R.C.S., F.R.A.C.S.

T. Farebrother, M.B.B.S., F.R.A.C.S.

P. Bilenkij, M.B.B.S., F.R.A.C.S.

J. Rogers, M.B.B.S., F.R.C.S., F.R.A.C.S.

Metastatic prostate cancer that has relapsed after initial hormonal manipulation remains a major problem in management, since the median duration of patient survival in most reported series is less than 10 months (Torti et al. 1983; Raghavan and Lange 1985; Scher and Sternberg 1985; Tannock 1985). The patients are elderly, and a variety of intercurrent disorders and age-related metabolic abnormalities render them less able to tolerate aggressive treatment programs. In this chapter, we report our experience in managing this complex problem, emphasizing our attempt to develop relatively nontoxic approaches to treatment without losing efficacy.

PATIENTS AND METHODS

Patients with relapsed, metastatic prostate cancer underwent a thorough staging program, including a detailed history and physical examination, the measurement of circulating tumor marker levels (including prostatic acid phosphatase, serum alkaline phosphatase, and prostate-

*Supported in part by grants from Merrion Rawlinson Cancer Trust and New South Wales Women's Bowl for Others Club.

specific antigen), a full hormonal profile (including luteinizing hormone, follicle-stimulating hormone, and circulating androgens), baseline radionuclide bone scan, bone x-rays, and chest x-ray. Selected patients also had computed tomographic (CT) scanning of abdomen and pelvis. Patients with baseline hematologic abnormalities or with a history of increasing blood transfusion requirements underwent a bone marrow biopsy. Of particular importance, fluctuations of tumor marker levels were assessed monthly for the first 3 months as predictors of response (Mackintosh et al. in press).

After treatment, patients were monitored regularly with physical examination, detailed history, and measurement of tumor markers. In most programs, repeat bone scans were performed at 3-, 6-, and 12-month intervals, and other investigations were repeated as indicated. Indices of quality of life, including symptoms of disease, treatment, weight, and performance status (by Eastern Cooperative Oncology Group [ECOG] criteria) and analgesic requirements were documented at each visit.

The characteristics of patients with hormone-resistant prostate cancer treated in a series of recent institutional protocols are summarized in Table 31–1. Their features are typical of

TABLE 31–1.
Patient Characteristics (n = 134)

Characteristic	Treatment[*]			
	AG[†]	MEG[‡]	DAN[§]	MITOX[‖]
No.	34	43	19	38
Age (yr)				
Mean	65	71	68	67.6
Range	53–79	52–81	59–77	50–77
ECOG[‖] status				
0–1		16	6	21
2–3		27	9	17
4		0	4	0
Metastatic sites				
Bone	34	39	19	34
Prostate	21	33	—	28
Nodes	1	5	—	3
Lung	1	5	—	2
Liver	2	1	—	3
Marrow	0	2	—	3
Other	2	0	—	0
Prior treatment				
Radiotherapy	—	24	—	21
Estrogens	10	34	13	20
Orchidectomy	28	23	18	29
Chemotherapy	0	6	3	0

*AG = aminoglutethimide; MEG = megestrol acetate; DAN = danazol; MITOX = mitoxantrone; ECOG = Eastern Cooperative Oncology Group.
†Data from Harnett PR, Raghavan D, Caterson I, et al. 1987. Aminoglutethimide in advanced prostatic carcinoma. *Br J Urol* 59:323–327.
‡Data from Crombie C, Raghavan D, Page J, et al. 1987. Phase II study of megestrol acetate for metastatic carcinoma of the prostate. *Br J Urol* 59:443–446.
§Data from Cole RM, Raghavan D, Caterson I, et al. 1986. Danazol treatment of advanced prostate cancer: Clinical and hormonal effects. *Prostate* 9:15–20.
§Data from Cole RM, Raghavan D, Caterson I, et al. 1986. Danazol treatment of advanced prostate cancer: Clinical and hormonal effects. *Prostate* 9:15–20.
‖Data from Raghavan et al. (unpublished data).

patients with this disease, apart from a weighting towards an ambulant status. Most patients were advanced in age and had a performance status of 2-3; the dominant sites of disease were bone and prostate gland.

The details of the regimens of treatment are summarized in Table 31–2. In this consecutive series of trials, single agents were assessed for efficacy and toxicity. Objective response was defined according to the criteria of the National Prostatic Cancer Project (NPCP) (Slack et al. 1984), with the exception that stable disease per se was not regarded as *"objective response."* Prior to treatment, all patients gave fully informed consent in accordance with the principles espoused in the Declaration of Helsinki and the guidelines of the National Health and Medical Research Council of Australia.

RESULTS

The objective responses after treatment with a series of single agents are summarized in Table 31–3. Objective evidence of tumor mass reduction as classified by NPCP criteria occurred infrequently. This was consistent with the pattern of bone-dominant disease and

TABLE 31–2.
Treatment Regimens

Drug	Dosage	Route	Cycle	Trial Status
Salvage hormones				
Aminoglutethimide	250 mg 4 ×/day			
+ cortisone acetate	25 mg A.M.	Oral	Continuous	Completed
	12.5 mg P.M.			
± fludrocortisone	0.1 mg daily			
Megestrol acetate	40 mg 4 ×/day	Oral	Continuous	Completed
Danazol	200 mg 4 ×/day	Oral	Continuous	Completed
Cytotoxics				
Mitoxantrone	12–14 mg/m²	IV	Every 3 wk	Completed
Cyclophosphamide	100 mg/m²	Oral	Daily for 2 wk then 2-wk gap and recommence	Ongoing
Carboplatin	150 mg/m²/day	IV	Daily × 3; 1-mo cycle	Ongoing
Mitomycin C	10–15 mg/m²	IV	Every 5–6 wk	Ongoing

TABLE 31–3.
Objective Response

Drug	Response* CR	PR	SD	PD	No. Evaluated	No. Treated
Aminoglutethimide	0	1	6	27	34	34
Megestrol acetate	0	1	7	35	43[†]	43
Danazol	0	0	3	16	19	19
Mitoxantrone	0	0	23	15	38	38[‡]
Cyclophosphamide	←———Ongoing———→				15	15
Carboplatin	←———Ongoing———→				14	14
Mitomycin C	←———Ongoing———→				7	7

*CR = complete response; PR = partial response; SD = stable disease; PD = progressive disease.
[†]28 received drug for ≥6 weeks.
[‡]Treated as part of multicenter trial (Raghavan et al. unpublished data 1988).

the paucity of bidimensionally measurable deposits. When mitoxantrone was evaluated, the removal of the requirement for the serum level of prostatic acid phosphatase to return to normal (in the NPCP and European Organization on Research and Treatment of Cancer [EORTC] studies) was associated with a substantial redefinition of objective response rate (Table 31–4).

In each of the salvage hormonal protocols, subjective improvement was demonstrated in up to one third of the patients (Cole et al. 1986; Crombie et al. 1987; Harnett et al. 1987). The evaluation of mitoxantrone showed that 50% of the patients had a reduction of symptoms (especially pain), accompanied by an improved performance status (34%) and increased weight (42%). These results correlated, in fact, with stabilization of disease: 42% of the treated patients achieved stable disease for 6 months or longer.

The toxicity of the salvage hormonal treatments was less than that reported for combination cytotoxic regimens (Table 31–5). However, in the trial of aminoglutethimide, depres-

TABLE 31–4.
Mitoxantrone for Prostate Cancer: Variability of Response Rate, Depending on Criteria of Response

Response	Classification*			
	NPCP[†]	EORTC[‡]	NCOG[§]	MDAH[‖]
CR	0	0	0	0
PR	0	0	10	7
SD	23	23	13	16
PD	15	15	15	15

*NPCP = National Prostatic Cancer Project; EORTC = European Organization on Research and Treatment of Cancer; NCOG = Northern California Oncology Study Group; MDAH = The M. D. Anderson Cancer Center; CR = complete response; PR = partial response; SD = stable disease; PD = progressive disease.
[†]Data from Slack et al. 1984.
[‡]Data from Schroeder FH. 1984.
[§]Data from Torti et al. 1983.
[‖]Data from Logothetis et al. 1983.

TABLE 31–5.
Toxicity of Salvage Hormonal Therapy*[†]

Toxicity	AG (n = 34)	MEG (n = 43)	DAN (n = 19)
Depression	10	—	—
Rash	7	—	—
Nausea/vomiting	4	5	—
Raised liver function tests	2	5	—
Tumor flare	1	3	7
Drowsiness	4	—	—
Lassitude	3	—	—
Gynecomastia	—	4[‡]	—
Postural hypotension	3	—	—
Thromboembolic disorders	—	2[‡]	—
Peripheral edema	—	2	—
Cardiac	—	2	—
Fits	—	1	—
Emotional lability	1	—	—
Confusion	1	—	—

*Modified from Cole et al. 1986; Crombie et al. 1987; Hartnett et al. 1987.
[†]AG = aminoglutethimide; MEG = megestrol acetate; DAN = danazol .
[‡]Concomitant estrogens.

sion and lassitude reduced its utility as a palliative agent (Harnett et al. 1987). Megestrol acetate, in contrast, was well tolerated (Crombie et al. 1987), but occasional tumor flare reactions were a cause for concern, mandating the need for careful monitoring of treatment.

The pattern of toxicity for mitoxantrone is summarized in Table 31–6. It, too, was well tolerated in general; the major toxicity was myelosuppression. Of interest, an unusual pattern of nail and nail bed changes was documented—thickening and ridging of the nails with associated subungual hemorrhages. Clinical cardiotoxicity did not present a problem in this elderly patient group, although serial ejection fractions were not monitored routinely in all instances.

TABLE 31–6.
Toxicity From Mitoxantrone in 38 Patients

Side Effect	WHO* Grade		
	0	1–2	3–4
Leukopenia	17	12	9
Thrombocytopenia	35	2	1
Nausea/vomiting	12	23	3
Stomatitis	36	2	0
Alopecia	23	14	1
Infection	35	0	3
Cardiac[†]	35	2	1
Eyes (conjunctivitis)	35	3	0
Nail changes	32	6	0
Anorexia	30	4	0
Diarrhea	36	1	0
Pruritis	36	1	0

*WHO = World Health Organization.
[†]Ejection fraction evaluations were not routinely performed.

DISCUSSION

In a series of single-arm, noncomparative phase II studies, we have demonstrated that effective palliation can be achieved for patients with hormone-resistant prostate cancer without the toxicity associated with combination cytotoxic regimens. Aminoglutethimide and megestrol acetate can yield occasional objective partial responses, although the side effects of depression and lassitude limit the clinical utility of the former drug (Crombie et al. 1987; Harnett et al. 1987). By contrast, we believe that danazol has no role to play in the management of this disease because it lacks activity and tends to cause tumor flare reactions (Cole et al. 1986).

Mitoxantrone is active against hormone-resistant prostate cancer. Although the objective response rate varies from 0% to 50% depending on the classification employed, we have demonstrated subjective improvement in 50% of treated patients accompanied by objectively stable disease in 42%. Although, in general, there are important limitations to the relevance of "stable disease" (Tannock 1985; Raghavan 1988), its coincidence with a reduction of symptoms and an improvement in weight and performance status suggest a real benefit for up to half the patients treated with mitoxantrone. The median survival of 10 months is disappointingly short, but it is comparable to the figures achieved with other single-agent and combination cytotoxic regimens (Logothetis et al. 1983; Torti et al. 1983; Tannock 1985; Raghavan 1988).

However, the true relevance of cytotoxic chemotherapy remains to be proved in the management of hormone-resistant prostate cancer. Accordingly, we are initiating a multi-center randomized trial to compare the use of cytotoxic chemotherapy with a "best supportive care" and salvage hormone regimen.

Acknowledgments

We are grateful for the support from our urological colleagues, who referred patients for treatment according to these protocols. The assistance of Mrs. Barbara Reschke (Department of Urology, The University of Texas M. D. Anderson Cancer Center at Houston) in the preparation of this manuscript is gratefully acknowledged.

REFERENCES

1. Cole RM, Raghavan D, Caterson I, et al. 1986. Danazol treatment of advanced prostate cancer: Clinical and hormonal effects. *Prostate* 9:15–20.
2. Crombie C, Raghavan D, Page J, et al. 1987. Phase II study of megestrol acetate for metastatic carcinoma of the prostate. *Br J Urol* 59:443–446.
3. Harnett PR, Raghavan D, Caterson I, et al. 1987. Aminoglutethimide in advanced prostatic carcinoma. *Br J Urol* 59:323–327.
4. Logothetis CJ, Samuels M, von Eschenbach AC, et al. 1983. Doxorubicin, mitomycin-C, and 5-fluorouracil (DMF) in the treatment of metastatic hormone refractory adenocarcinoma of the prostate, with a note on the staging of metastatic prostate cancer. *J Clin Oncol* 1:368–379.
5. Mackintosh J, Simes J, Raghavan D. (In press). Prostate cancer with bone metastases: Serum alkaline phosphatase (SAP) as a predictor of response, and the significance of the SAP "flare." *Br J Urol*
6. Raghavan D. 1988. Non-hormone chemotherapy for prostate cancer: Principles of treatment and application to the testing of new drugs. *Semin Oncol* 15:371–389.
7. Raghavan D, Lange PH. 1985. Endocrine aspects of genito-urinary neoplasia, in Shearman RP (ed): *Clinical Reproductive Endocrinology*. New York, Churchill Livingstone, Inc, pp 727–752.
8. Scher HI, Sternberg CN. 1985. Chemotherapy of urologic malignancies. *Semin Urol* 3:239–280.
9. Schroeder FH. 1984. Treatment response criteria for prostatic cancer. *Prostate* 5:181–191.
10. Slack NH, Brady MF, Murphy GP, et al. 1984. Stable versus partial response in advanced prostate cancer. *Prostate* 5:401–415.
11. Tannock IF. 1985. Is there evidence that chemotherapy is of benefit to patients with carcinoma of the prostate? *J Clin Oncol* 3:1013–1021.
12. Torti FM, Aston D, Lum B, et al. 1983. Weekly doxorubicin in endocrine-refractory carcinoma of the prostate. *J Clin Oncol* 1:477–482.

Chapter 32

Prostatic Cancer: Commentary

Andrew C. von Eschenbach, M.D.

Douglas E. Johnson, M.D.

Christopher J. Logothetis, M.D.

In 1941, Huggins and Hodges revolutionized the therapy of cancer by demonstrating the endocrine dependence of prostate cancer (Huggins et al. 1941). The knowledge that orchiectomy and estrogen therapy could deprive prostatic cancer cells of the stimulating effect of circulating androgens gave physicians a weapon with which they could dramatically relieve symptoms and lengthen patients' survivals. Skeptics maintain that this was the last major advance in the treatment of systemic prostate cancer.

Despite impressive tumor responses, disease eventually relapsed in almost all patients, and attention was then focused on alternative therapies. For the last 45 years, urologic oncology has been preoccupied with finding effective therapy for those patients whose tumors no longer respond to orchiectomy or to estrogens and with improving the results that initial therapy with orchiectomy and estrogens can achieve. Much that has been learned and much that is hoped for has been presented in this volume.

At the outset, Gleason (Chapter 22) provided very important information regarding the relationship between tumor grade and a patient's response to estrogen therapy. He corrected a common misconception regarding the results of the Veterans Administration Cooperative Urological Study by stating that endocrine therapy does significantly improve the survival rate of patients by reducing their cancer death rate. This effect is most emphatic in those patients whose primary tumor has a Gleason score of 6, 7, or 8. This conclusion reflects the fact that patients with scores of 2, 3, 4, and 5 do not die of prostate cancer, and therefore the real effect of therapy is obscured by death from other causes. At the other extreme, patients whose tumors have a Gleason score of 9 or 10 usually have disease that is poorly responsive to endocrine therapy. These data make an important statement about therapy: they underscore the need to employ endocrine therapy readily for those patients who will benefit and to continue the search for nonendocrine systemic therapy that is effective against those clones of cells that are not sensitive to hormones.

Given the fact that prostate cancer cells respond to androgen deprivation, Zincke (Chapter 27) captures our interest by proposing that a favorable impact on survival occurs when the primary prostate cancer is controlled by radical prostatectomy and microscopic residual or metastatic disease is controlled by adjuvant endocrine therapy. The data he offers on the 5-year survival rate of patients with stage D_1 disease are impressive. It is important to note that an analysis of tumor ploidy by DNA flow cytometry demonstrates that those patients whose primary tumor contains a diploid pattern have very favorable outcomes, whereas patients with tetraploid or aneuploid tumors do poorly. This finding raises concern about whether an observed favorable outcome is a result of therapy or of the natural history of the disease. Nevertheless, Zincke's data call for carefully designed prospective randomized trials to evaluate the effect of primary tumor control by surgery or radiation therapy plus endocrine manipulation for patients with microscopic or surgically resected metastatic disease.

To provide initial therapy for patients with more extensive disease, the use of luteinizing hormone-releasing hormone (LH-RH) agonists is now established as a suitable alternative to surgical castration or the use of estrogens. Results of studies in which either leuprolide or buserelin were used have confirmed that these agents are capable of producing anorchid levels of serum testosterone. Subjective and objective regressions and survival rates are comparable to those achieved by standard therapy. It is lamentable, although not surprising, that the effect of these agents on survival is not superior to that of standard therapy, but they still have an important place in our therapeutic repertoire. They are expensive at present, and one must be cautious regarding the possibility of an initial tumor flare, but they are otherwise safe and easy to administer. Their freedom from side effects is a significant advantage over estrogens, and their ease of administration compared to surgical castration is a decided benefit. Combining the LH-RH agonists with an antiandrogen has not provided any significant advantage in patient survival rate, although the time to relapse may be lengthened (Schroeder et al. 1987; Schulze et al. 1987).

The lack of significant benefit of total androgen ablation as initial therapy is also demonstrated in the chapter by Johnson et al. (Chapter 25) on the use of megestrol acetate and minidose estrogen. Although this regimen was extremely effective in achieving androgen ablation, the resulting survival statistics were not significantly better than historical results of trials using orchiectomy or estrogens, and the side effects, including cardiovascular complications and adrenal insufficiency, were significant.

However, there may be a role for adrenal androgen suppression in patients who relapse following standard endocrine therapy, as pointed out by Babaian et al. (Chapter 26) in their report on ketoconazole. Patients whose disease is progressing despite orchiectomy and estrogen may find that further androgen suppression significantly relieves their symptoms, especially pain, and also provides objective responses manifested by a decline in serum levels of acid phosphatase.

This finding reopens the discussion of the nature of androgen sensitivity of prostate cancer. It seems apparent that tumor cells are extremely heterogeneous with regard to their dependence on androgens (Isaacs and Kyprianou 1987). Although the majority of tumor cells respond when circulating androgens are reduced to anorchid levels, some tumor cells may be able to survive and perhaps even prosper with a slightly lower androgen level. This is the population of cells that accounts for the secondary response to therapies such as ketoconazole, which suppresses weak adrenal androgens, or for the reported increase in duration of response that occurs with initial total androgen ablation. Most unfortunately, there are still other tumor cells that are not at all dependent on androgen for survival; even if all circulating androgens are removed, these cells behave like other tumor cells of somatic origin and continue to divide and grow. Regrettably, then, no form of endocrine therapy will ever prove to be curative for the vast majority of patients with advanced prostatic cancer (D. Coffey, personal comunication, 1987).

Thus, despite initial dramatic responses and lengthened tumor-free survivals, the processes of clonal selection and expansion will eventually result in the reemergence of a tumor that is not androgen dependent. The time interval for its emergence is a function of the magnitude of the initial regression of the endocrine-sensitive tumor mass, the volume of endocrine-insensitive tumor cells, and, finally, the growth rate of the endocrine-unresponsive tumor. Thus, the most logical strategy for producing "cures" in advanced prostate cancer is to achieve total permanent eradication of all tumor cells by combining endocrine therapy and chemotherapy.

This strategy, however, is dependent on the availability of effective chemotherapy—and unfortunately, no chemotherapy programs exist that are capable of achieving sustained complete remissions of prostate tumors. Reliance on endocrine therapy and fear of employing high-dose chemotherapeutic drugs in elderly, often debilitated, patients with prostate cancer have created great barriers to the development of chemotherapy for this disease. In the 1970s, the National Prostate Cancer Project fostered the search for effective single agents. Tumor response to single agents has thus far been only modest, and it seems evident that no single currently available agent is capable of significantly affecting prostate tumors. This observation has fueled a continued search for new single agents and stimulated an effort to use modestly effective drugs in combination in hope that a synergistic or additive effect can be achieved.

Scher and colleagues (Chapter 28) have pointed out many of the problems in evaluating the effectiveness of chemotherapy trials for prostate cancer because only 5% to 15% of presentations offer bidimensional measurable lesions in which to assess response. This situation underscores the need to develop unique strategies for evaluating response in patients whose metastases are almost exclusively osteoblastic bone lesions. Perhaps new markers such as prostate-specific antigen will serve as indicators of tumor eradication.

To limit entry into phase II trials only to those patients with bidimensional disease provides a reliable population for assessing magnitude of response but severely limits accrual. Nevertheless, the search for effective drugs must proceed. Using new drugs that attempt to exploit the unique metabolic properties of prostate cancer cells such as high levels of polyamine synthesis seems appropriate, although the initial results with alpha-difluoromethylornithine (DFMO) and mitoguazone (MGBG) reported by Scher et al. are disappointing: no antitumor activity was seen among 14 evaluable patients in a phase II trial.

Ongoing trials of new single agents continue (Raghavan et al., Chapter 31), while combination programs are employed for palliation and in hopes of increasing survival. In evaluation of such programs, Logothetis et al. (Chapter 29) have pointed out that the rates and durations of response vary with different metastatic presentations. Tumor burden and the site of metastasis are important features affecting a patient's outcome. This knowledge about the biology of the tumor and heterogeneity in metastatic sites is important in planning treatment. It is also essential to categorize patients according to these factors when comparing the results of various chemotherapeutic programs.

The important conclusion is that responses do occur. Although they are disappointing in magnitude and duration, they provide a basis for future progress.

Advances in the treatment of systemic prostatic cancer have been made, but the search for "curative" therapy continues. There is reason for hope, however. Effective therapies are being developed, and perhaps, when they are applied aggressively and in combination, they will lead to progress.

REFERENCES

1. Huggins C, Stevens RE Jr, Hodges CV. 1941. Studies on prostatic cancer II: The effects of castration on advanced carcinoma of the prostate gland. *Arch Surg* 43:209–223.
2. Isaacs JT, Kyprianou N. 1987. Development of androgen independent tumor cells and their implication for the treatment of prostate cancer. *Urol Res* 15:133–138.

3. Schroeder FH, Lock TM, Chadha DR, et al. 1987. Metastatic cancer of the prostate managed with buserelin versus buserelin plus cyproterone acetate. *J Urol* 137:912–918.
4. Schulze H, Isaacs J, Senge T. 1987. Inability of complete androgen blockade to increase survival of patients with advanced prostatic cancer as compared to standard hormonal therapy. *J Urol* 137:909–911.

Chapter 33 _____

Chemotherapy for Advanced Squamous Carcinoma of the Male External Genital Tract and Urethra

Francisco H. Dexeus, M.D.

Christopher J. Logothetis, M.D.

Hikmet Sipahi, M.D.

Few trials of chemotherapy for squamous cell carcinoma of the penis have been published because of its rarity in the United States and Europe. Some of the published reports describe chemotherapy for the primary lesion, while others discuss metastatic disease. In primary tumors, bleomycin has produced response rates of 29% to 73% and a number of complete responses (Blum et al. 1973). The best responses have occurred in patients with small, well-differentiated tumors. For patients with metastatic disease, bleomycin, methotrexate, and cisplatin have been reported to be active as single agents (Ahmed et al. 1984). No phase II studies of combination chemotherapy for metastatic disease have been published.

In this chapter, we report our experience with combination chemotherapy for patients with unresectable or metastatic squamous cell carcinoma of the penis and, because the histology, pattern of spread and treatment given were similar, for two cases of squamous carcinoma of the urethra and one of the scrotum.

PATIENTS

Between June 1981 and August 1987, we administered chemotherapy to 14 men who had squamous cell carcinoma of the penis, scrotum, or urethra. Patient characteristics are summarized in Table 33–1. In all cases, the pathologic material was reviewed and graded according to the tumor-grading system of Broder: grade 1, well-differentiated; grade 2, moderately well-differentiated; and grade 3, poorly differentiated. All patients had inoperable disease because of local invasion from the tumor, fixed regional lymph nodes, or distant metastasis. Five patients had an infection in the local recurrence or lymph node metastasis.

TABLE 33–1.
Patient Characteristics: Penile-Genital Squamous Cell
Carcinoma (n = 14)

Characteristics	No. of Patients
Age (yr)	
Median, 64	
Range, 37–82	
Origin	
Penis	9
Urethra	2
Multifocal (glans and urethra)	2
Scrotum	1
Tumor grade	
1	3
2	9
3	2
Prior treatment	
Biopsy only	6
Surgery	8
Radiotherapy	3
Chemotherapy	1
Site of disease at presentation	
Local disease (penis, adjacent skin, perineum, pubic bone)	3
Regional lymph nodes	3
Local disease and inguinal nodes	4
Distant metastasis	4
Lung	3
Skin	1

TREATMENT

Chemotherapy consisted primarily of cyclophosphamide, bleomycin, and cisplatin (CBP) (Table 33–2). Courses were repeated every 3 to 4 weeks.

For patients with locally advanced disease or with regional lymph node metastasis without

TABLE 33–2.
Chemotherapy Protocols*

Intra-arterial CBP (8 patients)
  Cyclophosphamide, 500–650 mg/m² IV day 1.
  Bleomycin, 15–35 mg/m² over 24–48 hr by continuous infusion IA.
  Cisplatin, 75–100 mg/m² over 2 hr IA.
Intravenous CBP (5 patients†)
  Cyclophosphamide, 500–650 mg/m² IV day 1.
  Bleomycin, 15 mg IV by continuous infusion daily for 5 days.
  Cisplatin, 20 mg/m² IV daily days 1 to 5.
Intravenous FAMP (1 patient)
  5-Flourouracil, 750 mg/m² IV days 1 and 2.
  Doxorubicin (Adriamycin) 25 mg/m² IV days 1 and 2.
  Mitomycin C, 5 mg/m² IV days 1 and 2.
  Cisplatin, 100 mg/m² IV day 2.

*IA = intra-arterially; IV = intravenously.
†One of these five patients did not receive bleomycin.

distant spread (10 patients), we administered intra-arterial chemotherapy when possible. However, two of these patients could not receive intra-arterial chemotherapy because of severe arteriosclerosis. Bilateral iliac arteriography was performed via the femoral arteries. The arterial catheters were then left in place for chemotherapy infusion in the internal iliac arteries, anterior divisions of the internal iliac arteries, or the medial circumflex branch of the common femoral arteries, depending on the tumor location and arterial supply. When blood flow to the gluteal regions was significant, the superior gluteal artery was embolized with a steel coil and an absorbable gelatin sponge (Gelfoam). Verification of appropriate catheter position and arterial distribution was done with nuclear scans using technetium-99m microaggregates. Thereafter, bleomycin and cisplatin were infused via the arterial catheters, the latter drug with concomitant intravenous forced mannitol and saline diuresis. The doses of bleomycin and cisplatin were divided between the two arterial catheters according to the relative proportion of blood supply to the tumor by each artery, as determined by the nuclear scan. Cyclophosphamide was infused intravenously because of its necessary activation by the liver.

For patients with distant metastasis, all drugs were infused intravenously. One patient received an alternate intravenous chemotherapy regimen: 5-fluorouracil, Adriamycin, mitomycin C, and cisplatin (FAMP).

We used the standard criteria in determining response. Duration of response was calculated from the date of initiation of the protocol.

RESULTS

Six of the 14 patients (43%) responded: one completely, four partially, and one with a minor response (Table 33–3). The median duration of response was 4 months (range, 2–45+ months). Of particular note is one patient who had fixed inguinal lymph node metastasis: he received five courses of intra-arterial chemotherapy and three of intravenous chemotherapy, achieving a clinical complete response of the penile lesion and inguinal nodes. However, at follow-up urethroscopy, two superficial urethral lesions were observed. These were carcinoma in situ and were removed. This patient did not receive any further therapy and remains alive without evidence of disease at nearly 4 years. Tumors in 5 of the 6 responding patients were grade 2, and the other was a grade 3. None of the 5 patients who had infected tumors

TABLE 33–3.
Response to Chemotherapy
_____

Intra-arterial CBP (8 patients)
   Complete response
      1 patient with fixed inguinal nodes, alive without disease at 45 mo.
   Partial response
      1 patient with perineal recurrence, 5 months' duration.
Intravenous CBP (5 patients)
   Partial response
      2 patients with fixed inguinal nodes, 4 and 6 months' duration.
   Minor response
      1 patient with pulmonary metastasis, 3.5 months' duration.
Intravenous FAMP (1 patient)
   Partial response
      1 patient with pulmonary metastasis, 2 months' duration.

*CBP = cyclophosphamide, bleomycin, cisplatin; FAMP = 5-fluorouracil, Adriamycin, mitomycin, cisplatin.
_____

responded. The median survival duration for all patients from initiation of chemotherapy was 6 months (range, 2–45+ months). For responders the median survival was 11 months (range, 2–45+ months), and for nonresponders it was 4 months (range 2–10 months).

Thirty-eight courses of chemotherapy were given, 21 intra-arterially and 17 intravenously. Three courses were associated with mucositis. Fourteen courses were complicated by fever due to infection; five were associated with neutropenia, and nine were not. Two patients had a decrease in forced vital capacity of 12% and 25%, respectively. In two patients, the serum creatinine level rose permanently, 0.4 and 1.0 mg/100 ml, respectively. One toxic death occurred as a consequence of pneumonia in the patient who received FAMP chemotherapy.

DISCUSSION

Experience in chemotherapy for metastatic squamous carcinoma of the penis or urethra is limited, but the most active agent appears to be methotrexate (Garnick et al. 1979; Ahmed et al. 1984); the response rate is 61% for the 13 treated patients described in the literature. The median duration of response, however, was short (3 months). Similarly, bleomycin has produced responses in 21% of patients (3 of 14), again of short (3 months) duration. Cisplatin was effective in 25% of patients (3 of 12), who achieved a median duration of response of 7 months.

We attempted to improve on the response rate and duration of response by combining cyclophosphamide, bleomycin, and cisplatin, chemotherapeutic agents with nonoverlapping toxicities. We observed two responses, one complete, among eight patients treated intra-arterially. Four of the 5 patients with local infection in the tumor received intra-arterial therapy, but none responded. Four of 6 patients treated intravenously (3 with CBP and 1 with FAMP) responded, although there were no complete responses with intravenous therapy.

Because of the small number of patients, we cannot make a statement about the relative merits of intra-arterial vs. intravenous chemotherapy. Patients with advanced squamous cell carcinoma of the penis often present with locally advanced unresectable disease without distant metastasis. In this setting it is reasonable to consider intra-arterial chemotherapy because of the existence of a limited and defined vascular supply.

The median duration of response with our combination chemotherapy regimens is not essentially different from that reported with single agents, although patient populations might be quite dissimilar. Five of our patients had infection in the local recurrence or lymph node metastasis at initiation of chemotherapy, and none of these 5 responded. Other possible prognostic factors that could influence response to chemotherapy, such as performance status, prior therapy, tumor grade, and tumor burden, have not yet been defined.

CONCLUSION

We observed 6 responses among 14 patients with squamous cell carcinoma of the penis, urethra, and scrotum. One patient given intra-arterial chemotherapy achieved a durable complete response; no patient with an infected recurrence responded. We believe further studies of combinations of known active agents are indicated, and perhaps intra-arterial chemotherapy should be considered for selected patients.

REFERENCES

1. Ahmed T, Sklaroff R, Yagoda A. 1984. Sequential trials of methotrexate, cisplatin and bleomycin for penile cancer. *J Urol* 132:465–468.
2. Blum RH, Carter SK, Agre K. 1973. A clinical review of bleomycin: A new antineoplastic agent. *Cancer* 31:903–914.
3. Garnick MB, Skarin AT, Steele GD Jr. 1979. Metastatic carcinoma of the penis: Complete remission after high dose methotrexate chemotherapy. *J Urol* 122:265–266.

Chapter 34

Genitourinary Sarcomas in Adults: Characteristics and Chemotherapy

Nicholas E. J. Papadopoulos, M.D.

Robert S. Benjamin, M.D.

Genitourinary sarcomas in adults are rare tumors that represent less than 1% of all genitourinary malignancies. Because of their rarity, investigators have been unable to devise a reliable interinstitutional staging system, and clinicians have not yet identified a treatment protocol that offers predictable long-term survival.

At The University of Texas M. D. Anderson Cancer Center, we have retrospectively analyzed 84 cases of genitourinary sarcomas treated here between 1944 and 1985. To be included in the group analyzed, the cases were required to meet certain specific criteria. First, the origins of the tumors had been established to be in the genitourinary tract by clinical, surgical, or pathologic criteria. Second, the pathologic diagnosis (if made by an outside source) had been reviewed by a pathologist at UT M. D. Anderson Cancer Center. All patients included were at least 16 years old. Two forms of genitourinary sarcoma were excluded from review: carcinosarcomas of the kidney and sarcomas of the female genital tract.

CLINICAL AND PATHOLOGIC FEATURES

Primary Sites

Sarcomas arose from four primary locations, the kidney, bladder, prostate, and paratesticular tissue. Paratesticular tissue was the most common site of origin, followed in order by the prostate, bladder, and kidney (Fig 34–1).

The greatest difficulty in determining site of origin lies in distinguishing between a sarcoma that arises primarily in a retroperitoneal structure and one that involves a structure secondarily. In the past, only clinical evidence was available, and it is often unclear. Even with modern radiologic techniques such as computed tomography (CT) and angiography, it is still difficult to determine, for example, whether a renal mass is intracapsular or extracapsular, as illustrated by the case discussed later in this chapter.

Histologic Varieties

The most common histologic variety among our patients was leiomyosarcoma (Fig 34–

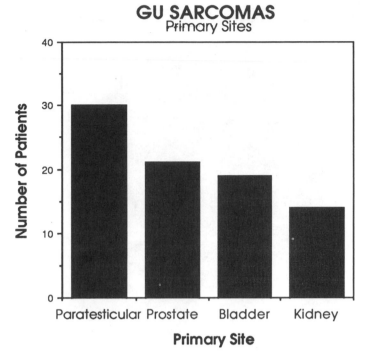

FIG 34–1.
Primary sites of genitourinary sarcomas.

2). Rhabdomyosarcoma occurred next most frequently, followed by a variety of tumors that we have grouped under "other." The majority of these were unclassified sarcomas; next most frequent were malignant fibrous histiocytomas and liposarcomas. We found one case each of Ewing's sarcoma (Papadopoulous et al. 1983), fibrosarcoma, hemangiopericytoma, neurofibrosarcoma (Johnson et al. 1985), and synovial sarcoma (Fig 34–3).

Primary leiomyosarcomas occurred fairly frequently in the kidney, bladder, and prostate. Two were of paratesticular origin. Interestingly, we identified one case of leiomyosarcoma of the prostate coexisting with a low-grade prostatic adenocarcinoma. Rhabdomyosarcomas were predominantly paratesticular in origin, followed by prostate and bladder sites. This series contained no case of kidney rhabdomyosarcoma.

Origins of the "other" sarcomas were as diverse as the tumors themselves, although the most common site of origin was paratesticular. The five liposarcomas and the neurofibrosarcoma arose in paratesticular tissue, and the Ewing's sarcoma lesion was located in the region between the corpus cavernosum and the spermatic cord. The synovial sarcoma, hemangiopericytoma, and fibrosarcoma were primary in the kidney; the latter arose from the kidney capsule. We also identified one case of carcinosarcoma of the prostate and three cases of bladder carcinosarcoma.

Epidemiologic Features

Genitourinary sarcomas occur during all decades of life (Fig 34–4). Overall, the age distribution is bimodal: rhabdomyosarcomas occur most often in younger patients, whereas leiomyosarcomas and the other types occur most often in older persons.

Rhabdomyosarcomas are among the most common forms of childhood solid tumors. Since

GU SARCOMAS HISTOLOGY

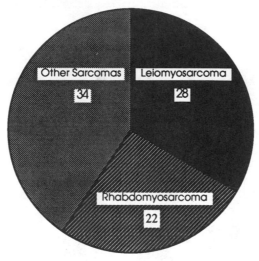

FIG 34–2.
Histologic types of genitourinary sarcomas seen at M. D. Anderson Cancer Center.

GU SARCOMAS - OTHER HISTOLOGIES

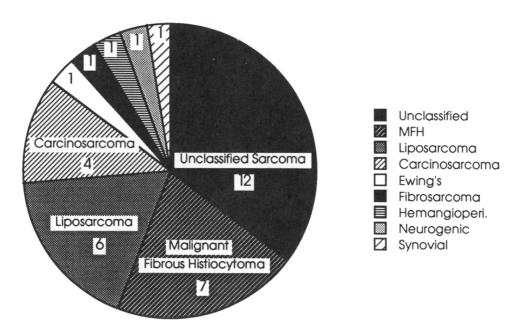

FIG 34–3.
Frequency distribution according to histologic type for the 34 patients with "other" sarcomas.

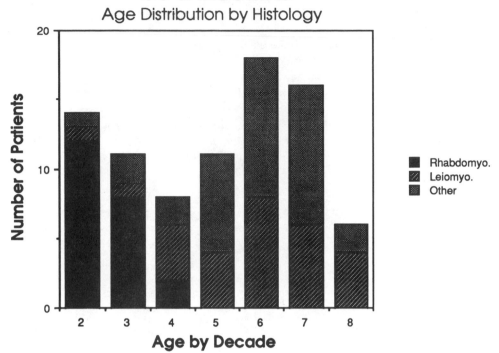

FIG 34–4.
Distribution of genitourinary sarcomas by age of patients and cell types.

our review is limited to persons at least 16 years old, the bars shown in the second decade of life (see Fig 34–4) represent tumors in young adults between 16 and 19 years of age. The oldest patient with rhabdomyosarcoma in this series was 32 years old. When a patient much above this age is diagnosed as having a rhabdomyosarcoma, the validity of the histologic diagnosis should be questioned and the tumor analyzed further. Swartz and colleagues (1985) from our institution have reported an interesting case of leiomyosarcoma of the bladder in a 19-year-old woman in conjunction with a sibling who had osteogenic sarcoma and a family with a history of congenital bone defects.

Our study revealed no specific male-female predilection for sarcoma of the bladder and kidney, although the kidney sarcomas occurred slightly more often (57%) in men. This finding is in contrast to previous reports.

Metastatic Potential

The likelihood of genitourinary sarcomas metastasizing varies according to histologic type (Fig 34–5,A through C). Patients with rhabdomyosarcomas are likely to present with metastatic disease involving the retroperitoneum, lung, and bone marrow, whereas patients with leiomyosarcomas usually do not have metastases at diagnosis. The other varieties frequently present with metastatic disease, although those with paratesticular primaries do so less often. Well-differentiated liposarcomas develop local recurrences; interestingly, a history of herniorrhaphy has often preceded diagnosis. Paratesticular malignant fibrous histiocytomas and unclassified sarcomas can be seen evolving along with retroperitoneal and more distant metastatic disease.

Prognostic Factors Related to Survival

The 5-year survival rate of all patients with genitourinary sarcomas is slightly over 40%; the 11-year survival rate is slightly over 20% (Fig 34–6). Analysis has identified only three important prognostic factors: the presence of metastasis at the time of diagnosis, histologic tumor type, and site of the primary tumor.

The presence of metastasis at diagnosis seems to be the most significant prognostic factor. The survival curve for patients without metastatic disease shows a steady reduction up to 11 years. Histologic type of disease does not influence the survival rate of these patients to the same extent as does the location of the primary disease site (Fig 34–7,A and B). In fact, patients with sarcomas of paratesticular origin but no metastases have a singularly better survival rate than patients with kidney primaries. There is no statistically significant difference

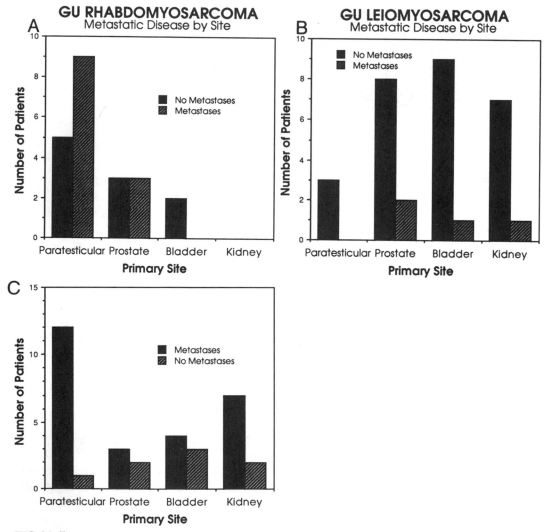

FIG 34–5.
Frequency of metastatic disease by cell type and site of the primary tumor: **A**, rhabdomyosarcoma; **B**, leiomyosarcoma; **C**, other genitourinary sarcomas.

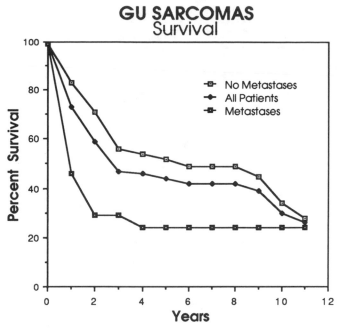

FIG 34–6.
Survival rates of patients with genitourinary sarcomas.

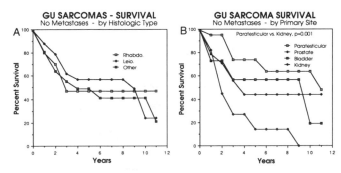

FIG 34–7.
The influence of histologic type of disease (**A**) and site of primary tumor (**B**) on the survival of patients without metastatic disease at diagnosis.

in survival rate, however, between patients with paratesticular sarcomas and those with primary tumors of the prostate or bladder.

When a patient presents with metastatic disease, both the histologic type and the location of the primary tumor influence the survival rate. Among this group of patients, those with rhabdomyosarcomas (Fig 34–8) and with paratesticular primary tumors (Fig 34–9) have a better survival rate than other patients. In fact, the survival rate of patients with primary paratesticular sarcomas plus metastases is as good as the survival rate of their counterparts without metastasis at diagnosis.

THE ROLE OF CHEMOTHERAPY

At UT M. D. Anderson Cancer Center, we have used two basic chemotherapeutic

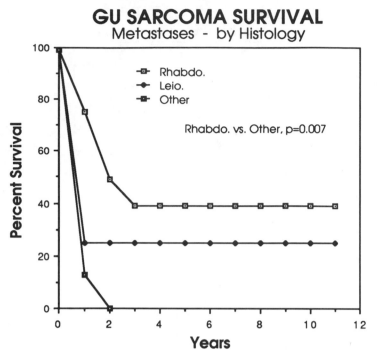

FIG 34–8.
The influence of histologic type of disease on survival of patients with metastasis at diagnosis. Rhabdo. = rhabdomyosarcoma; Leio. = leiomyosarcoma.

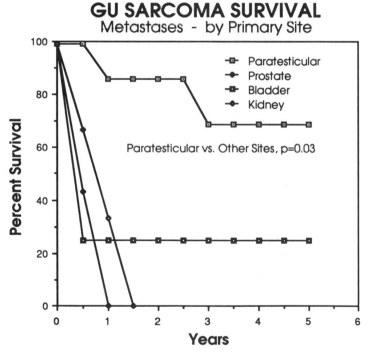

FIG 34–9.
The influence of site of primary tumor on survival of patients with metastasis at diagnosis.

regimens most frequently. The first combines vincristine, dactinomycin (actinomycin D), and cyclophosphamide (VAC) at various dosages, and the second is a combination of doxorubicin (Adriamycin) and, most often, dacarbazine (DTIC)—with or without cyclophosphamide and vincristine. We have used chemotherapy as the primary treatment and also in an adjuvant or neoadjuvant role.

Regimens Using Vincristine, Actinomycin D, and Cyclophosphamide

The VAC regimen has produced partial remissions but no complete responses (CRs). Two of 3 patients with rhabdomyosarcoma achieved partial remissions of 3- and 6-months' duration, and 2 of 6 patients with leiomyosarcoma achieved 9- and 10-month partial remissions (Table 34–1).

We have used VAC as adjuvant therapy for 6 patients, 5 with rhabdomyosarcoma and 1 with bladder leiomyosarcoma. Four of the rhabdomyosarcomas were paratesticular in origin. Disease has progressed in 2 of the latter at 11- and 12-month follow-ups; the other 2 patients remain free of disease, 1 at 172 months and the other at 15 months. The fifth patient had primary prostatic rhabdomyosarcoma; he received radiation therapy to the primary lesion followed by adjuvant VAC chemotherapy and remains disease free at 72 months. A final patient had leiomyosarcoma of the bladder and documented peritoneal seeding at the time of partial cystectomy. This patient remains free of disease at 156 months.

Regimens Containing Adriamycin and Dacarbazine (A-DIC)

Both partial and complete remissions have been achieved with the Adriamycin and dacarbazine (A-DIC) regimens. Among patients with rhabdomyosarcomas (Table 34–2), 6 of 9 patients responded, 4 with a CR; 2 of these who had a paratesticular primary tumor remain free of disease at 108 and 96 months, but the other 2, 1 with a paratesticular primary and 1 with a prostatic primary, have relapsed at 13 and 10 months, respectively. The other two responses were partial; that of a patient with a paratesticular primary tumor lasted 6 months. The other partial responder had a bladder primary; he received primary chemotherapy and was rendered free of disease surgically; he remains disease free at 59-months' follow-up.

TABLE 34–1.
Response to VAC Chemotherapy*

Sarcoma Type	No. of Patients	CR (%)	CR + PR (%)
Rhabdomyosarcoma	3	0	67
Leiomyosarcoma	6	0	33
Total	9	0	44

*VAC = vincristine, actinomycin D, cyclophosphamide.

TABLE 34–2.
Response to A-DIC Chemotherapy Regimens*†

Sarcoma Type	No. of Patients	CR (%)	CR + PR (%)
Rhabdomyosarcoma	9	44	67
Leiomyosarcoma	9	11	78
Other	8	0	50
Total	26	19	65

*A-DIC = Adriamycin and dacarbazine.
†Some patients received cyclophosphamide and/or vincristine in addition to A-DIC.

Six of 9 patients with prostatic leiomyosarcomas responded to chemotherapy (see Table 34–2). One achieved a CR of 10 months' duration; the other five remissions were partial, lasting 4, 6, 6, 9, and 12 months. Four partial remissions (PRs) also occurred among eight patients with sarcomas of other sites or histologic types: three were in patients with a kidney primary (leiomyosarcoma, malignant fibrous histiocytoma, synovial sarcoma) lasting 8, 9, and 9 months, respectively, and the other, lasting 9 months, occurred in a patient with an unclassified paratesticular tumor.

A regimen containing A-DIC was used adjuvantly in four patients. Two had paratesticular primaries; one remains free of disease at 20 months, and the other relapsed in 6 months. Two patients with kidney primary tumors have relapsed at 10 and 11 months. A final patient with paratesticular rhabdomyosarcoma and metastatic disease in the lungs was salvaged with two thoracotomies and postoperative chemotherapy in which an A-DIC regimen was used; he remains free of disease at 72 months.

Miscellaneous Regimens

Over the years, we have tried a number of different chemotherapy combinations in our attempts to treat successfully our patients with sarcomas. In that group, treatment has produced definite, but varied, responses. One patient who had prostatic carcinosarcoma received vinblastine, dactinomycin, and cyclophosphamide preoperatively and had a definite response; he remains without any evidence of disease at 36 months. Another with metastatic leiomyosarcoma of the bladder received lomustine (methyl-CCNU), dactinomycin, and bacille Calmette-Guérin and achieved a CR of 156 months' duration. In a patient with prostatic leiomyosarcoma, local perfusion therapy using phenylalanine mustard and nitrogen mustard produced a 6 months' partial response. Procarbazine and radiation therapy for lung lesions in a patient with a primary kidney sarcoma produced a minor response. Frequent low doses of intralesional methotrexate with leucovorin rescue produced some response in a patient with leiomyosarcoma.

CASE ILLUSTRATION

The importance of thorough clinical, radiographic, and pathologic evaluation and of definitive chemotherapy is illustrated by the case of a 70-year-old man who presented with a 1-month history of left flank pain. A CT scan disclosed a hydronephrotic kidney thought to be produced by an extrarenal retroperitoneal mass (Fig 34–10,A and B). An angiogram revealed that the mass was pushing the kidney upwards, bowing the renal artery (Fig 34–11). A needle biopsy established the pathologic diagnosis of leiomyosarcoma.

The patient received three preoperative courses of chemotherapy with cyclophosphamide, Adriamycin, and DTIC and showed a definite response (Fig 34–12). He then underwent surgical resection of the mass and a left nephrectomy. A subsequent pathologic diagnosis confirmed the needle-biopsy determination: the patient had leiomyosarcoma of the kidney, completely contained within the renal capsule. We administered chemotherapy to maximum benefit, and he remains free of disease at 30 months' follow-up.

This case illustrates two important points. The first is the difficulty of distinguishing the true origin of a retroperitoneal tumor; this tumor could have arisen from the kidney or involved the kidney secondarily. The second is that neoadjuvant chemotherapy has a definite and valuable role in treating a patient with a genitourinary sarcoma.

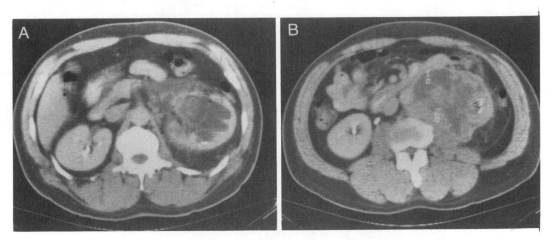

FIG 34–10.
Computed tomographic scan showing a hydronephrotic kidney (**A**) resulting from a large retroperitoneal tumor (**B**).

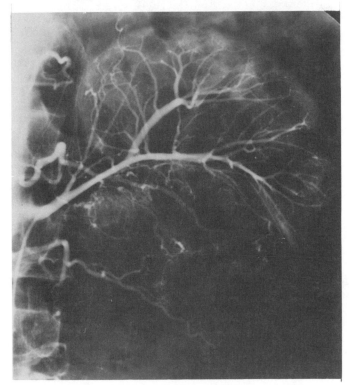

FIG 34–11.
A renal arteriogram showing only a displaced renal artery from an extrarenal mass.

CONCLUSION

Genitourinary sarcomas are very rare tumors that occur in a variety of histologic types, in a variety of locations, and with individual patterns of metastasis. They have a poor but variable prognosis; the prognosis of paratesticular sarcomas, even with metastases, is the

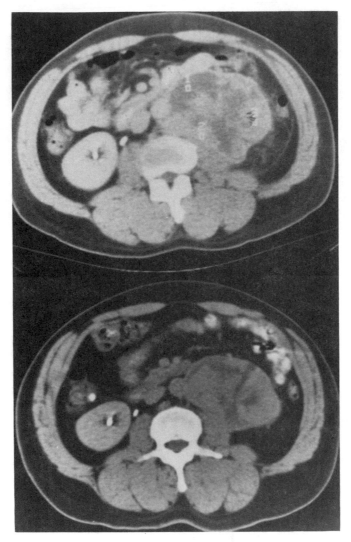

FIG 34–12.
Computed tomography. *Top*, a large retroperitoneal leiomyosarcoma before chemotherapy. *Bottom*, tumor mass is reduced after three courses of chemotherapy.

best, because chemotherapy is most effective against sarcomas arising in this site.

Chemotherapy plays an integral part in the treatment of sarcomas. We recommend that chemotherapy include both Adriamycin and dacarbazine, with or without cyclophosphamide. The Adriamycin should be administered over 48 to 96 hours by continuous infusion through a central venous catheter at a dose of 60 to 90 mg/m². In small round cell sarcomas (rhabdomyosarcomas and soft-tissue Ewing's sarcoma), vincristine is a potent agent and should be added, along with cyclophosphamide, to the A-DIC regimen.

With the possible exception of low-grade sarcomas, such as well-differentiated liposarcoma, if the histologic type can be determined prior to definitive surgery, chemotherapy should be administered before surgery to aid in resection and to establish tumor responsiveness.

REFERENCES

1. Johnson DE, Kaesler KE, Mackay BM, et al. 1975. Neurofibrosarcoma of spermatic cord. *Urology* 5:680–683.
2. Papadopoulos NEJ, Ayala A, Plager C, et al. 1983. Extraskeletal Ewing's sarcoma: Natural history and management suggestions (abstract). *Proceedings of the 19th Annual Meeting of the American Society of Clinical Oncology,* 238.
3. Swartz DA, Johnson DE, Ayala AG, et al. 1985. Bladder leiomyosarcoma: A review of 10 cases with 5-year follow-up. *J Urol* 133:200–202.

Chapter 35

Germ Cell Tumors: Clinically Relevant Advances

Christopher J. Logothetis, M.D.

Jae Y. Ro, M.D.

For clinicians to treat effectively patients with germ cell tumors of extragonadal or gonadal origin, they need to understand the unique pathologic features that predict for survival, response to therapy, and likelihood of metastases. Also essential for the clinician treating and studying germ cell tumors is an understanding of the relationship between tumor histology, site of origin, stage, and secretion of biomarkers. Major advances in understanding these relationships have occurred since effective therapy was introduced into the clinic 15 years ago.

For the pathologic evaluation of patients with germ cell tumors, we at The University of Texas M. D. Anderson Cancer Center currently employ the modification of the initial Dixon and Moore classification proposed by the World Health Organization (WHO) (Table 35–1). It is our belief that patients with germ cell tumors should be categorized, first, by site of origin (gonadal or extragonadal), and second, by the two major histologic subtypes, seminoma and nonseminomatous germ cell tumors (NSGCT). Tumors in each of these categories and major histologic subtypes are associated with unique clinical behaviors that influence both the selection of therapy and the results.

Testicular neoplasms only constitute 1% to 2% of all cancers in males, but they are virtually all malignant (Krain 1973). The majority (90%) are of germinal origin, and these have attracted the most interest.

Determining the correct histologic diagnosis and extent of tumor and recognizing the histologic variables that affect prognosis are critical to selecting the initial treatment and determining the need for and type of additional therapy. Therefore, the pathologist must initially carefully screen the specimen to determine whether it is a seminoma or an NSGCT. The need for further analysis is determined by the information necessary for the clinician to provide correct and effective treatment.

SEMINOMAS

Forty to 50% of all testicular germ cell tumors are seminomas. Ninety percent of these are of the "typical" or classic variety; the remainder are variants, including spermatocytic

TABLE 35–1.
WHO* Classification of Testis Tumors

A. Tumors of one histologic type
  1. Seminoma
  2. Spermatocytic seminoma
  3. Embryonal carcinoma
  4. Yolk sac tumor (embryonal carcinoma, infantile type; endodermal sinus tumor)
  5. Polyembryoma
  6. Choriocarcinoma
  7. Teratomas
    a. Mature
    b. Immature
    c. With malignant transformation
B. Tumors of more than one histologic type
  1. Embryonal carcinoma and teratoma (teratocarcinoma)
  2. Choriocarcinoma and any other types (specify type)
  3. Other combinations (specify)

*World Health Organization.

seminoma, anaplastic seminoma (Mostofi and Price 1983), and the recently described seminoma containing syncytiotrophoblastic giant cells (Nochomovitz et al. 1977), an additional variant of questionable significance.

It is generally agreed that, stage by stage, typical and anaplastic seminomas do not behave differently in response to therapy or in degree of tumor dissemination, although anaplastic seminomas tend to occur more frequently at higher stages. Spermatocytic seminoma is a rare histologic subtype that occurs in elderly men. It is a tumor of low metastatic potential, and some authors recommend orchiectomy only as the appropriate therapy.

The most obvious clinical trait of seminomas is their low metastatic potential. Seventy-five percent of patients with seminoma present with clinical stage I disease. This is in contrast to NSGCTs; 50% to 70% of patients with these tumors, depending on the series reported, present at outset with distant metastases.

The only important variables prognostic for outcome of patients with seminoma are bulk of metastases and degree of tumor dissemination. Clinical staging of seminomas, therefore, is important. Seminomas predominantly spread via nodal metastases; visceral metastases are unusual, and when they occur they are equally distributed between lung and bone. The high frequency of osseous involvement is a trait unique to seminoma among germ cell tumors (Fossa et al. 1987; Logothetis et al. 1987a).

Selection of therapy for patients with distant metastases from seminoma is determined by the sites of metastases. No controversy exists when patients have disease above the diaphragm or involving viscera. Although the therapy for disease confined to the abdomen frequently incorporates radiation therapy, patients with disease extension above the diaphragm or metastases to viscera require chemotherapy as their primary therapeutic modality. When disease is confined to the abdomen, however, the volume of the retroperitoneal disease determines whether radiation therapy is likely to achieve a cure or whether these patients should receive chemotherapy (Bosl et al. 1983). Dispute remains in the literature as to the volume of disease in the retroperitoneum that predicts for likelihood of relapse.

The staging system currently employed at UT M. D. Anderson Cancer Center is a simple one (Table 35–2). This simple staging system does not meticulously evaluate the degree of tumor dissemination within viscera because it has been shown that patients with retroperitoneal seminoma have an overwhelmingly high likelihood of achieving a complete remission,

TABLE 35–2.
Staging Classification for Seminoma

Stage I	Disease confined to testis
Stage II	Retroperitoneal disease only*
	A. ≤9.9cm
	1. ≤5 cm
	2. >5 cm ≤9.9 cm
	B. ≥10 cm
Stage III	Supradiaphragmatic or visceral disease
	A. Nodal involvement only
	B. Visceral involvement

*Measurements by computed tomography.

independent of the number of sites of involvement (Stanton et al. 1985; Logothetis et al. 1987). The staging system does, however, meticulously measure the volume of retroperitoneal disease by using computerized tomography (CT). It allows for appropriate comparison of data between institutions and facilitates studies whose purpose is to define the correct therapeutic approach for patients with disease confined to the retroperitoneum.

Unlike their role in NSGCT, serum biomarkers are believed not to have great importance in the prognosis of seminoma. This is in part related to the relatively low frequency of seminoma and the lack of experience using the markers. In addition, the sensitivity of this disease to chemotherapy and radiation therapy makes the evaluation of serum tumor markers superfluous.

It is generally agreed that patients who have pathologically confirmed pure seminoma but an elevated serum level of alpha-fetoprotein (AFP) must be treated as if they had non-seminomatous germ cell tumors. The degree of elevation of the serum beta-human chorionic gonadotropin (β-HCG) and serum lactic dehydrogenase (LDH) does not predict for response to therapy, as it does in NSGCT, but does reliably predict for the persistence of disease. The initial studies that reported relatively low frequencies of elevated serum β-HCG have left the erroneous impression in the literature that seminoma is a germ cell tumor that only rarely has elevated markers. This impression is a result of the low stage of tumors incorporated in the initial studies. In some series, the β-HCG level has been reported elevated in more than 50% of patients with higher-volume disease.

NONSEMINOMATOUS GERM CELL TUMORS

In tumors designated as NSGCT, histologic type plays a paramount role in predicting for response to therapy, necessity of surgery, and distant metastasis. In addition, the clinical stage of disease in patients with metastases predicts for likelihood of response to therapy. It is generally recognized that volume of disease, as reflected by the degree of serum biomarker elevation and the number of sites of metastases, also predicts for response and survival (Bosl et al. 1983; Stoter et al. 1987). The interrelationship between the three—histologic type, degree of serum biomarker elevation, and sites of metastases—has become readily apparent.

The role of the pathologist in evaluating patients with NSGCT is determined in part by the stage of disease. Following initial pathologic classification, the clinician requires specific information with which to assign a prognostic category and determine the therapeutic approach. For patients with clinical stage I disease, the pathologist must determine the likelihood of distant metastases developing despite the apparent confinement of the disease to the body of the testis. Recent reports have indicated that, when the primary tumor contains embryonal carcinoma and the lymphatics or vessels are invaded, patients are at an extremely high risk for developing later distal visceral metastases (Javadpour and Young 1986; Dewar et al. 1987; Dunphy et al. 1988). Thorough clinical evaluation of patients with stage I disease requires the use of modern radiologic techniques (CT scan of the abdomen and pelvis), a chest x-ray, and determination of the serum biomarker levels. The routine use of bipedal lymphangiography remains disputed.

For clinical stage II disease, the pathologist's role differs. Metastases have already occurred, and appropriate therapy must be selected. Various forms of treatment have been proposed, as determined by the volume of retroperitoneal disease. It is generally recognized that patients with higher-volume retroperitoneal disease are more likely to develop distant visceral metastases. At UT M. D. Anderson Cancer Center, the histologic type of the primary tumor also influences the selection of therapy.

We have, therefore, developed a staging system for patients with clinical stage II disease that requires meticulous assessment of the retroperitoneum with bipedal lymphangiography and CT (Table 35–3). The staging system is precise and detailed enough to allow reliable comparison between series and to facilitate the development of the least morbid therapeutic approach without sacrificing the extremely high cure rate presently achieved. We have arbitrarily included in the clinical stage II classification patients who have persistently elevated serum biomarkers after undergoing orchiectomy but not a retroperitoneal lymph node dissection.

Determining the likelihood of requiring surgery is an important part of the clinical evaluation of patients with stage II disease. Experience at UT M. D. Anderson Cancer Center reflects experience throughout the country in treating patients with distant metastases from NSGCT. Chemotherapy is least likely to eradicate disease completely in those patients with a high proportion of teratomatous elements in the primary tumor. Such patients require surgery in addition to chemotherapy.

Selecting therapy appropriately for patients with clinical stage II NSGCT requires meticulous histologic evaluation for the presence of histologic subtypes that predict for relapse in the retroperitoneum or for the likelihood of persistent retroperitoneal disease following chemotherapy. Although patients with clinical stage II disease are extremely likely to be cured with chemotherapy and surgery, they continue to suffer significant morbid side effects from their treatment. By incorporating pathologic evaluation in the clinical staging system, as we propose, we believe unwarranted morbidity can be eliminated while a high cure rate is maintained.

TABLE 35–3.
UT M. D. Anderson Cancer Center Classification of Clinical Stage II NSGCT*†

Clinical Stage‡	Criteria
II$_A$	Rising levels of serum biomarkers (AFP and β-HCG) after orchiectomy
II$_B$	Retroperitoneal mass <2 cm maximum diameter
II$_C$	Retroperitoneal mass ≥2 cm and <5 cm in maximum diameter
II$_D$	Retroperitoneal mass ≥5 cm and <10 cm maximum diameter

*NSGCT = nonseminomatous germ cell tumors; AFP = alpha-fetoprotein; β-HCG = beta - human chorionic gonadotropin.
†All tumors measured by computed tomography.
‡Biopsy proof of retroperitoneal disease is required when patients have normal levels of serum biomarkers.

DISSEMINATED GERM CELL TUMORS

Patients with germ cell tumors disseminated to sites other than the retroperitoneum (stage III) require an evaluation different from that which suffices for patients with stages I and II NSGCT. Those who have distant visceral metastases continue to be threatened by their tumor and do not achieve the overwhelmingly high cure rate of patients with stages I and II disease. It is imperative that the pathologist and the clinician initially define the likelihood of achieving a complete remission with the combination of surgery and chemotherapy before they begin treatment. This they can do by evaluating the prognostic variables that affect the outcome of stage III disease to select appropriate treatment and maximize the likelihood of achieving a complete remission. The most important predictors of survival for patients with distant metastases are bulk of disease and degree of dissemination of tumor (Samuels et al. 1975). Patients with low-stage, low-volume disease should be the subjects of attempts at reducing the intensity of chemotherapy, whereas those patients with high-volume disease should be the subjects of efforts to further intensify the chemotherapy.

The pathologist's role in the evaluation of patients with distant metastases differs from his role in evaluating patients with stages I and II disease. For stage III, after the initial diagnosis and histologic characterization of the tumor have been made and chemotherapy has been administered, the pathologist is called on to evaluate tissue that has been removed for examination. It is imperative that this tissue be evaluated meticulously for persistence of immature teratoma, viable carcinomatous elements, or, as recently has been reported by Ulbright et al. (1984, 1986), the presence of sarcomatoid elements, which predict for a very poor chance of survival. Investigators agree that, in the absence of viable carcinoma in the retroperitoneum, further chemotherapy is not justified. In this situation patients are expected to have a disease-free survival rate of 90% or more. When elements of immature teratoma or sarcomatoid elements remain, however, patients deserve more intense postoperative chemotherapy. Patients with mature teratoma as defined by the pathologist require close followup for late but infrequent relapses and, most important, for adequate resection of residual tumors.

A clinical staging system for patients with disseminated germ cell tumors must incorporate recent knowledge about both histology and serum biomarkers. The experience of UT M. D. Anderson Cancer Center and that of Memorial Sloan-Kettering Cancer Center and the Netherlands Group all suggest that the degree of elevation of the serum β-HCG is an important variable for patients with disseminated germ cell tumors: a high serum level predicts an unfavorable outcome (Bosl et al. 1983; Stoter et al. 1987). It is very clear, therefore, that degree of elevation of this serum biomarker must be included in newly developed staging systems. The staging system currently used at UT M. D. Anderson Cancer Center incorporates accurate measurements of retroperitoneal disease, categorizing patients with greater than 10-cm retroperitoneal metastases into stage III disease (Table 35–4). Disease is arbitrarily categorized as stage III when tumors, by most physicians' definition, are clearly unresectable with a curative intent and cannot be encompassed adequately with radiation therapy portals.

EXTRAGONADAL GERM CELL TUMORS

Extragonadal germ cell tumors represent challenging clinical problems. They have unique features that justify their segregation from the majority of apparent germ cell tumors.

The major clinical dilemma confronting clinicians treating patients with extragonadal germ cell tumors is separating them from those with occult primary testicular tumors and those with nongerminal tumors arising in extragonadal sites that mimic extragonadal germ cell tumors. Making this distinction is important because, if patients with occult primary testicular germ cell tumors or nongerminal extragonadal tumors are included in a clinical series, they will greatly skew the outcome of studies. Therefore a staging classification that aids in making such a separation is necessary.

The staging classification for extragonadal germ cell tumors currently employed at UT M. D. Anderson Cancer Center (Table 35–5) allows for such a segregation. It has been noted that extragonadal anterior mediastinal germ cell tumors are likely to be germinal tumors of true extragonadal origin. They are not accompanied by abnormal testicular findings, whereas primary retroperitoneal germ cell tumors are frequently associated with carcinoma in situ of the testis and, of equal importance, occult primary testicular tumors (Daugaard et al. 1987). By separating patients with tumors that demonstrate pathologic features diagnostic for germinal origin but occur in sites not recognized as primary sites of metastasis from primary testicular tumors (anterior mediastinum, brain, presacral area) from those who have germinal tumors that arise in the retroperitoneum and represent the first site of metastasis from germinal tumors, we can quickly establish two broad categories. The prognosis for patients with anterior mediastinal germ cell tumors is significantly worse than that for patients with

TABLE 35–4.
Modification of Samuels' Staging Criteria

Stage	Criteria
III-A	Disease confined to supraclavicular nodes.
III-B$_1$	Either one or more elevated biomarkers, or gynecomastia, unilateral or bilateral; both may be present; no demonstrable mass.
III-B$_2$	Minimal pulmonary disease up to five nodules in each lung field; the largest diameter of any single lesion no greater than 2.0 cm (total tumor volume does not exceed 40 cm^{3*}).
III-B$_3$	Advanced pulmonary disease: presence of any mediastinal or hilar mass, neoplastic pleural effusion, or intrapulmonary mass greater than 40 cm^3.
III-B$_4$	Advanced abdominal disease, defined as abdominal mass greater than 10 cm†.
III-B$_5$	Visceral disease (excluding lung), most often liver but also gastrointestinal tract and brain.

*Based on each nodule being spherical; volume of sphere is 1/6 of the diameter cubed.
†Abdominal mass measured by computed tomography; hydronephrosis is no longer included in the staging system.

TABLE 35–5.
UT M.D. Anderson Staging System for Extragonadal Germ Cell Tumors

1. True extragonadal germ cell tumors
   a. Pineal
   b. Anterior mediastinum
   c. Presacral teratoma
   d. Unusual sites*
2. Probable germ cell tumors of extragonadal origin
   Retroperitoneal tumors
3. Poorly differentiated tumors at all sites when accompanied by elevated levels of serum biomarkers (β-HCG, AFP)†

*Liver, prostate, cerebral hemispheres.
†AFP = alpha-fetoprotein; β-HCG = beta-human chorionic gonadotropin.

primary retroperitoneal tumors (Garnick et al. 1983). This difference in prognosis further confirms the need for separating patients into distinct categories.

Patients with extragonadal nongerminal tumors appear to be sensitive to, but not to be cured by, chemotherapy; they clearly need to be distinguished from patients with germinal tumors. Accordingly, the occult teratoma syndrome (Fox et al. 1979), the name given to a cautionary diagnosis, was proposed by investigators to assure that patients with germ cell tumors were not mistaken for those with nongerminal tumors and therefore failed to receive the benefit of vinblastine-bleomycin-platinum–based chemotherapy. Since that time, Hainsworth et al. (1987) have carried this diagnosis further and have confirmed some of our findings. In this third category is a group of patients whose tumors have clinical features compatible with germinal origin but pathologic features that are not. In our experience, these patients have a high response rate to cisplatin-based chemotherapy but ultimately are not cured of their disease. At autopsy a large portion of them are found to have occult primary tumors (nongerminal) (Logothetis et al. 1986). In such instances, pathologists greatly aid treatment by distinguishing between categories of patients.

CONCLUSION

Appropriate integration of the knowledge gained by meticulous pathologic review of patients with germ cell tumors and the incorporation of clinical data as manifested by response to surgery and chemotherapy will improve the treatment and, we hope, the survival rates of patients with germinal tumors. In addition, an understanding of the pathologic and clinical features of germinal tumors as they apply to treatment will make it possible for investigators at various institutions to interpret the clinical results and appropriately compare data.

REFERENCES

1. Bosl GJ, Geller NL, Cirrincione C, et al. 1983. Multivariate analysis of prognostic variables in patients with metastatic testicular cancer. *Cancer Res* 43:3403–3407.
2. Daugaard G, von der Maase H, Olsen J, et al. 1987. Carcinoma-in-situ testis in patients with assumed extragonadal germ-cell tumours. *Lancet* 1:528–530.
3. Dewar JM, Spagnolo DV, Jamrozik KD, et al. 1987. Predicting relapse in stage I non-seminomatous germ cell tumours of the testis (letter). *Lancet* 1:454.
4. Dunphy CH, Ayala AG, Swanson DA, et al. 1988. Stage I nonseminomatous and mixed germ cell tumors of the testis: Clinicopathologic study of 93 cases. *Cancer* 62:1202–1206.
5. Fossa SD, Borge L, Aass N, et al. 1987. The treatment of advanced metastatic seminoma: Experience in 55 cases. *J Clin Oncol* 5:1071–1077.
6. Fox RM, Woods RL, Tattersall MHN. 1979. Undifferentiated carcinoma in young men: That typical teratoma syndrome. *Lancet* 1:1316–1318.
7. Garnick MB, Canellos GP, Richie JP. 1983. Treatment and surgical staging of testicular and primary extragonadal germ cell cancer. *JAMA* 250:1733–1741.
8. Hainsworth JD, Wright EP, Gray GF Jr, et al. 1987. Poorly differentiated carcinoma of unknown primary site: Correlation of light microscopic findings with response to cisplatin-based combination chemotherapy. *J Clin Oncol* 5:1275–1280.
9. Javadpour N, Young JD Jr. 1986. Prognostic factors in nonseminomatous testicular cancer. *J Urol* 135:497–499.
10. Krain LS. 1973. Testicular cancer in California from 1942 to 1969: The California Tumor Registry experience. *Oncology* 27:45–51.
11. Logothetis CJ, Samuels ML, Ogden SL, et al. 1987a. Cyclophosphamide and sequential cisplatin for

advanced seminoma: Long-term follow-up in 52 patients. *J Urol* 138:789–794.

12. Logothetis CJ, Samuels ML, Selig DE, et al. 1986. Cyclic chemotherapy with cyclophosphamide, doxorubicin, and cisplatin plus vinblastine and bleomycin in advanced germinal tumors: Results with 100 patients. *Am J Med* 81:219–228.

13. Logothetis CJ, Swanson DA, Dexeus FH, et al. 1987b. Primary chemotherapy for clinical stage II nonseminomatous germ cell tumors of the testis: A follow-up of 50 patients. *J Clin Oncol* 5:906–911.

14. Mostofi FK, Price EB. 1988. Tumors of the male genital system, in *Atlas of Tumor Pathology,* series 2, fascicle 8. Washington, DC, Armed Forces Institute of Pathology, pp 7–84.

15. Nochomovitz LE, DeLa Torre FE, Rosai J. 1977. Pathology of germ cell tumors of the testis. *Urol Clin North Am* 4:359–378.

16. Samuels ML, Johnson DE, Holoye PY. 1975. Continuous intravenous bleomycin (NSC-125066) therapy with vinblastine (NSC-49842) in stage III testicular neoplasia. *Cancer Chemother Rep* 59:563–570.

17. Stanton GR, Bosl GJ, Whitmore WF, et al. 1985. VAB-6 as initial treatment of patients with advanced seminoma. *J Clin Oncol* 3:336–339.

18. Stoter G, Sylvester R, Sleijfer DT, et al. 1987. Multivariate analysis of prognostic factors in patients with disseminated nonseminatous testicular cancer: Results from a European Organization for Research on Treatment of Cancer multiinstitutional phase III study. *Cancer Res* 47:2714–2718.

19. Ulbright TM, Goheen MP, Roth LM, et al. 1986. The differentiation of carcinomas of teratomatous origin from embryonal carcinoma: A light and electron microscopic study. *Cancer* 57:257–263.

20. Ulbright TM, Loehrer PJ, Roth LM, et al. 1984. The development of non-germ cell malignancies within germ cell tumors: A clinicopathologic study of 11 cases. *Cancer* 54:1824–1833.

Chapter 36

Cisplatin-Based Chemotherapy for Metastatic Pure Seminoma

Clayton D.K. Chong, M.D.

Christopher J. Logothetis, M.D.

Although seminoma constitutes approximately 50% of all germ cell tumors, it is rarely encountered by the chemotherapist. Seminoma has a low metastatic potential, and patients usually present with either stage I or stage II disease. Such patients are highly curable with radiation therapy (Thomas et al. 1982; Schultz et al. 1984; Vaeth et al. 1984). When seminomas do metastasize, they differ from mixed germ cell tumors in the metastases distribution: their metastatic spread is predominantly nodal (Calman et al. 1979). Viscera are usually invaded directly rather than hematogenously. This pattern also differs from that of nonseminomatous germ cell tumors, which have a high frequency of hematogenous metastasis.

In the initial experience of Samuels et al. (1980) using vinblastine/bleomycin combination chemotherapy for germ cell tumors, none of the patients with pure seminoma achieved a complete remission. Treatment with alkylating agents produced regular responses, although usually they were palliative (Whitmore et al. 1977; Calman et al. 1979). When cisplatin was first introduced, striking responses occurred among patients with pure seminoma (Einhorn and Williams 1980). Since then, chemotherapy for seminoma has evolved so that at present it consists of cisplatin-based combinations with or without alkylating agents (Vugrin and Whitmore 1984; Friedman et al. 1985; Loehrer et al. 1987). These chemotherapy programs are similar to those used for nonseminomatous germ cell tumors (NSGCT) and produce identical toxicities.

Factors that complicate the treatment of seminoma include the relatively advanced ages of the patients (those with seminoma are almost a decade older than those with NSGCT) and the frequent history of prior irradiation. Irradiated patients have an exhausted bone marrow, making them candidates for highly toxic reactions to chemotherapy. Vinblastine/bleomycin-based chemotherapy regimens, for example, are reported to be associated with a high rate of fatal bleomycin pulmonary toxicity in patients who have pure seminoma (Samuels et al. 1976). Prior mediastinal radiotherapy may be partly responsible for these patients' higher rate of pulmonary toxicity.

CYCLOPHOSPHAMIDE AND SEQUENTIAL CISPLATIN

A regimen that avoids the use of bleomycin and is not severely myelosuppressive, while incorporating two of the agents most active against seminoma, has been used at The University of Texas M. D. Anderson Cancer Center. This is the combination of cyclophosphamide and weekly sequential cisplatin. The chemotherapy regimen consists of cyclophosphamide, 1 g, on day 1 followed by cisplatin, 100 mg/m², on days 2, 9, and 16. Figure 36–1 summarizes the chemotherapy schema. The dose of cisplatin is adjusted downward for patients with renal dysfunction or peripheral neuropathy.

Fifty-two patients received this regimen for a metastatic pure seminoma between 1977 and 1984 at UT M. D. Anderson Cancer Center (Samuels and Logothetis 1983). Of these 52 patients, 22 had received, and failed, previous treatments: 14 had failed radiation therapy, 4 chemotherapy, and 4 the combination of chemotherapy and radiation therapy. The clinical presentations of these 52 patients are documented in Table 36–1. As previously noted, the dominant mode of spread is nodal, with visceral spread occurring most frequently by direct tumor invasion. Hematogenous spread did occur and involved lung, liver, and bone at an equal frequency. The frequency of bone metastasis is different from that seen with NSGCT, from which bone metastases are extremely unusual.

Table 36–2 lists the complicating factors attributed to the tumor at presentation for chemotherapy. Hypercalcemia, which we have not encountered among patients with NSGCT, was present in three patients. Most of the other complications were attributed to direct contiguous invasion of viscera adjacent to the tumor.

The complications from cyclophosphamide and weekly sequential cisplatin chemotherapy are displayed in Table 36–3. Most were related to the neurotoxicity of cisplatin: a clinical hearing loss in 13%, tinnitus in 19%, and painful dysesthesia in 8%. Although prolonged myelosuppression occurred, this was not as severe as the myelosuppression associated with the acutely toxic regimens for NSGCT. Most typical was transient bone marrow hypoplasia. Infectious complications of treatment were rare, owing to the lack of both severe myelosuppression and severe mucositis.

Forty-eight patients (92%) remained alive and disease free from 70 to 541 weeks. Forty-four (85%) of the patients achieved complete remission with chemotherapy only. An additional four patients (8%) were salvaged with further treatment—chemotherapy for one and radiation therapy for the other three. Patients who relapsed within the initial area of high-volume

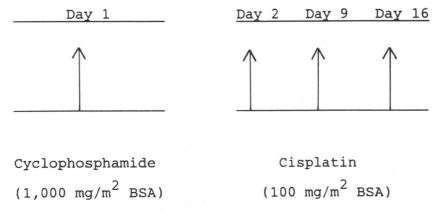

FIG 36–1.
Regimen of cyclophosphamide and sequential cisplatin chemotherapy used at M. D. Anderson Cancer Center for pure seminoma. The initial sequence consists of cyclophosphamide and three weekly pulses of cisplatin. Subsequent sequences, administered at 6-week intervals, include two pulse doses of weekly cisplatin (day 2 and day 9). Each dose of cisplatin is delivered with prehydration plus simultaneous forced mannitol diuresis. *BSA* = body surface area.

TABLE 36–1.
Distribution of Advanced Seminoma at
Presentation: UT M.D. Anderson Cancer Center

Metastatic Site(s)	Patients Involved	
	No.	%
Testicular primary		
Nodal metastasis		
Supraclavicular	1	2
Para-aortic <10 cm	7	14
Para-aortic >10 cm	9	17
Total	17	33
Visceral metastasis		
Lung	6	12
Bone	5	10
Liver	2	4
Direct visceral invasion*	8	15
Total	20	38
Extragonadal primary†		
Abdominal	9	
Anterior mediastinal	6	
Total	15	29
Total	52	

*Gastrointestinal tract (5), bladder (1), kidney (2), pericardial (2), chest wall (2). Three patients had visceral invasion at multiple sites.
†Superior vena cava syndrome (4), inferior vena cava syndrome (3).

TABLE 36–2.
Tumor Complications at Presentation: UT M.D.
Anderson Cancer Center (n = 52)

Complication	Patients Affected	
	No.	%
Ureteral obstruction	4	8
Paraparesis (epidural deposit)	2	4
Superior vena cava syndrome	4	8
Inferior vena cava syndrome	3	6
Bowel obstruction	3	6
Gastrointestinal tract bleeding	2	4
Myocardial invasion	1	2
Respiratory failure	3	6
Pericardial invasion	3	6
Chest wall invasion	2	4
Hypercalcemia	3	6

disease were salvaged with radiation therapy, but patients who relapsed with disseminated disease were rarely salvaged.

Rarely (in two patients) a pure seminoma was transformed to NSGCT, either by adopting new cell types or by secreting alpha-fetoprotein. Both patients had failed chemotherapy containing vinca alkaloids prior to their referral to UT M. D. Anderson Cancer Center.

Figure 36–2 is a Kaplan-Meier survival plot of all 52 patients treated with cyclophosphamide and sequential cisplatin. The most important predictor of failure for this regimen was the prior receipt of major chemotherapy. Prior radiation therapy, extragonadal origin, or secretion of beta-human chorionic gonadotropin did not predict a likelihood of relapse after cyclophosphamide and weekly sequential cisplatin (Table 36–4).

TABLE 36–3.
Complications of Cyclophosphamide and Sequential Cisplatin for Advanced Seminoma

Complication	Patients Affected	
	No.	%
Infection		
Culture-negative fever	7	13*
Bacteremia	2	4[†]
Renal toxicity		
Transient (>0.4% rise)	11	21
Persistent (>0.4% rise)	2	4
Neurotoxicity		
Painful dysesthesia	4	8
Tinnitus	10	19
Hearing loss	7	13

*One patient suffered a leukopenic fever with each course of chemotherapy.
[†]Tumor invaded the gastrointestinal tract in all patients with bacteremia.

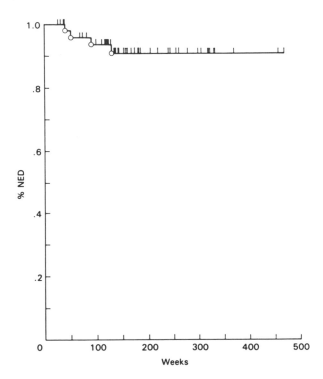

FIG 36–2.
Kaplan-Meier survival plot of 52 patients who received cyclophosphamide and sequential cisplatin for advanced seminoma. *NED* = no evidence of disease.

Our experience in treating advanced seminoma at UT M. D. Anderson Cancer Center since the introduction of cisplatin confirms that seminoma is highly curable. We have achieved an 88% complete-response rate with our cyclophosphamide and sequential cisplatin program. As important as the high response rate, however, is the relative absence of toxicity as compared to NSGCT programs when they are used to treat seminoma. The major side effect of cyclo-

TABLE 36–4.
Predictors of Complete Remission

Predictive Factor	Affected Patients (No.)	Disease-Free Patients	
		No.	%
Previous treatment			
Radiation therapy	14	14	100
Chemotherapy*	4	2	50
Radiation + chemotherapy	4	2	50
Clinical presentation			
Visceral invasion†	8	6	75
Nodal presentation	17	15	88
Extragonadal primary	15	12	80
Elevated serum β-HCG‡	34	30	88

*Major therapy including vinca alkaloids.
†Includes patients with hematogenous metastasis.
‡β-HCG = beta-human chorionic gonadotropin.

phosphamide and sequential cisplatin is neurotoxicity, which, at present, is unavoidable.

Our data differ from those of other investigators, in that we have found a low frequency (4%) of NSGCT transformation. Tumor volume, prior radiation therapy, and delay in initiation of therapy did not adversely affect the treatment outcome. As previously noted, prior exposure to chemotherapy was the most important predictor of therapy failure.

CONCLUSION

Before treatment, patients with seminoma require a meticulous pathologic review to be sure that their disease is pure seminoma. In addition, their serum levels of alpha-fetoprotein should be normal. After pure seminoma is confirmed, we believe these patients should receive seminoma-specific therapy.

The regimen of cyclophosphamide and weekly sequential cisplatin has proved to be superior to conventional combination chemotherapy employed for NSGCT and causes less morbidity. Patients with seminoma, because of their relatively advanced ages and prior radiation therapy, may be uniquely prone to develop myelosuppression and pulmonary toxicity. Consequently, the use of combination chemotherapy that is severely myelosuppressive is contraindicated.

We believe cyclophosphamide and weekly sequential cisplatin is the treatment of choice for patients with metastatic pure seminoma. With this program, we have achieved a high cure rate—one superior to most reported with combination therapy.

REFERENCES

1. Calman FMB, Peckham MJ, Hendry WF. 1979. The pattern of spread and treatment of metastases in testicular seminoma. *Br J Urol* 51:154–160.
2. Einhorn LH, Williams SD. 1980. Chemotherapy of disseminated seminoma. *Cancer Clin Trial* 3:307–313.
3. Friedman CL, Garnick MB, Stomper PL, et al. 1985. Therapeutic guidelines and results in advanced seminoma. *J Clin Oncol* 3:1325–1332.
4. Loehrer PJ, Birch R, Williams SD, et al. 1987. Chemotherapy of metastatic seminoma: The Southeastern

Cancer Study Group experience. *J Clin Oncol* 5:1212–1220.

5. Samuels ML, Logothetis CJ. 1983. Follow-up study of sequential weekly pulse-dose cisplatinum for far-advanced seminoma (abstract). *Proc Am Soc Clin Oncol* 2:137.

6. Samuels ML, Johnson DE, Holoye PY, et al. 1976. Large-dose bleomycin therapy and pulmonary toxicity: A possible rate of prior radiotherapy. *JAMA* 235:1117–1120.

7. Samuels ML, Logothetis CJ, Trindade A, et al. 1980. Sequential weekly pulse-dose cisplatin for far-advanced seminoma (abstract). *Proc Am Soc Clin Oncol* 21:423.

8. Schultz HP, von der Maase H, Rorth M, et al. 1984. Testicular seminoma in Denmark 1976–1980: Results of treatment. *Acta Radiol [Oncol]* 23:263–270.

9. Thomas GM, Rider WD, Pembo AJ. 1982. Seminoma of the testis: Results of treatment and patterns of failure after radiation therapy. *J Radiol Oncol Biol Phys* 8:165–174.

10. Vaeth M, Schultz HP, von der Maase H, et al. 1984. Prognostic factors in testicular germ cell tumours: Experiences from 1058 consecutive cases. *Acta Radiol [Oncol]* 23:271–285.

11. Vugrin D, Whitmore WF Jr. 1984. The VAB-6 regimen in the treatment of metastatic seminoma. *Cancer* 53:2422–2424.

12. Whitmore WF, Smith A, Yagoda A, et al. 1977. Chemotherapy of seminoma. *Recent Results Cancer Res* 60:244–249.

Chapter 37 _____

The Treatment of Advanced Seminoma: The Memorial Sloan-Kettering Cancer Center Experience, 1978–1986*

George J. Bosl, M.D.

BACKGROUND

The traditional treatment for patients with seminoma has been radiation. In patients with clinical stage I and early stage II disease (retroperitoneal adenopathy <5 cm), radiotherapy is curative for 75% to 90% of those patients who remain disease free. Relatively low doses of radiation are required, and toxicity is generally tolerable and transient.

For chemotherapy, the experience with seminoma has paralleled that with nonseminomatous germ cell tumors (NSGCT). The introduction of high-dose cisplatin (≥100 mg/m² per cycle of therapy) into systemic therapy led to cures for both NSGCT and seminoma. Early results with combinations of cyclophosphamide and cisplatin (Vugrin and Whitmore 1981) and cisplatin, vinblastine, and bleomycin (PVB) (Einhorn and Williams 1980) demonstrated that the majority of patients with seminoma could be rendered disease free despite extensive prior radiation therapy.

In 1979, the VAB-6 regimen was initiated at Memorial Sloan-Kettering Cancer Center (MSKCC) (Table 37–1). Its activity against both seminoma and NSGCT was recognized early in the trial (Vugrin et al. 1981). Since patients with seminomas, however, had usually received prior radiation therapy, the increased myelosuppression often resulted in difficulty when the full dosage of chemotherapy was administered.

Through 1981, chemotherapy results for seminoma were largely limited to patients with stage III disease at diagnosis (a rare presentation) and those who relapsed after initial radiotherapy for either clinical stage I–II or extragonadal seminoma. Experience with untreated patients who had bulky stage II (retroperitoneal adenopathy ≥5 cm) and extragonadal pre-

*This work was supported in part by grant CA-05826 and contract CA-07337 from the National Cancer Institute.

TABLE 37–1.
The VAB-6 Treatment Program for Germ Cell Tumors*

Agent	Dosage	Route	Specification
Vinblastine	4.0 mg/m^2	IV	Day 1
Dactinomycin (actinomycin D)	1.0 mg/m^2	IV	Day 1
Cyclophosphamide	600 mg/m^2	IV	Day 1
Bleomycin	30 U	IV	Day 1
Bleomycin	20 U/m^2	IV	Days 1–3, by continuous infusion
Cisplatin	120 mg/m^2	IV	Day 4, with mannitol diuresis

*Repeated every 4 weeks for three cycles; no bleomycin in third cycle.

sentations was anecdotal. In addition, since mature teratoma was rarely observed at operation, the indications for operation after chemotherapy were unclear.

Several factors led to a change in the management of seminoma at MSKCC. First, our experience with extragonadal seminoma treated with surgery, radiation, or both was unsatisfactory. Martini et al. (1974), in reporting the MSKCC experience with extragonadal germ cell tumors, found that only 3 of 10 patients with these tumors survived. The experience of others indicated that about 50% of patients with extragonadal seminoma relapse after radiotherapy and require systemic therapy (Abell et al. 1965; Sterchi and Cordell 1975).

Second, when Ball et al. (1982) reviewed their experience with radiation therapy for patients with seminoma, they were able to correlate the likelihood of relapse in patients with stage II disease with the size of retroperitoneal disease. When disease was larger than 5 cm, the likelihood of relapse approached 50%. Moreover, the disease-free survival rate distributions were similar for patients with retroperitoneal disease larger than 5 cm and larger than 10 cm. Similar relapse rates were reported by others (Doornbos et al. 1975; Dosoretz et al. 1981). These data do differ from those of Thomas and Herman (1984), but even in their experience, 24 of 46 patients (52%) who had retroperitoneal disease measuring 10 cm or more relapsed and required secondary treatment with either further radiation or systemic chemotherapy.

Third, we were concerned about the extent of myelosuppression after radiotherapy and impressed with our initial success using chemotherapy in untreated patients who had extragonadal or bulky stage II disease (Jain et al. 1984; Stanton et al. 1985). Most previously untreated patients with seminoma had achieved a complete remission (CR) and very few relapsed, implying that only one treatment modality was necessary to achieve cure. In addition, residual seminoma was rare at operation after VAB-6. Thus a treatment plan that minimized the number of modalities used to effect a cure became the goal of our seminoma treatment studies. All previously untreated patients with bulky ($\geq$5 cm) stage II disease or extragonadal seminoma were subsequently included in prospective germ cell tumor chemotherapy studies, along with those who had stage III disease and those relapsing after radiation therapy. These results have been described in greater detail elsewhere (Motzer et al. 1988).

RESULTS OF TREATMENT

Patient Characteristics

Between January 1979 and July 1986, we treated 62 patients who had seminoma with VAB-6 (45 patients), etoposide and cisplatin (EP) (15 patients), or VAB-6 alternating with EP (2 patients) (Table 37–2). By definition, no patient could be included who had an above-

TABLE 37-2.
Patients with Seminoma: Characteristics and
Results of Treatment*

		%
Patients		
Total no.	62	
No. evaluable for response	60	
Primary site (N = 62)		
Testis		71
Extragonadal		28
Unknown		1
Increased tumor marker serum levels (N = 62)		
HCG		18
LDH		84
Prior treatment (N = 60)		
None		73
Radiotherapy ± chemotherapy		27
CR (N = 60)		88
Relapse from CR		11
Alive and free of disease (N = 62)		85

*HCG = human chorionic gonadotropin; LDH = lactate dehydrogenase; CR = complete response.

normal serum level of alpha-fetoprotein (AFP). Most patients had elevated serum levels of lactate dehydrogenase (LDH), and a minority had elevated serum levels of human chorionic gonadotropin (HCG).

Response

Two patients were not evaluable for response; both had a solitary distant metastatic site treated before they began systemic therapy. Both are alive and disease free.

Of the remaining 60 patients, 53 (88%) achieved a CR, including 98% of those patients who were previously untreated and 81% of those who had received some prior treatment. Eighty percent of those receiving VAB-6 and 100% of those receiving EP achieved a CR. Three additional patients achieved partial responses (PR), which have endured for longer than 20+ months. Each had achieved a nearly complete regression of disease and normal tumor marker values with VAB-6.

Four patients failed to respond to therapy, and an additional 6 relapsed from CR. Three of those relapsing achieved a second CR. Seven patients have died of their disease, and 2 patients died in CR (both with a myocardial infarction). Thus, overall, 9 patients died. Therefore, of 62 patients treated for metastatic or locally advanced seminoma, 53 (86%) achieved a durable disease-free state. The median follow-up is 39+ months.

Prognostic Factors

A variety of clinical variables were analyzed for their impact on survival. The only statistically significant prognostic variable was the presence of an increased level of HCG at the time of diagnosis ($P = .05$). Neither the primary site (testis vs. extragonadal; $P = .36$), nor prior therapy (none vs. some; $P = .22$), nor increased level of LDH at diagnosis (normal vs. elevated; $P = .08$), nor chemotherapy regimen (VAB-6 vs. EP; $P = .15$) (Motzer et al. 1988) was correlated with survival.

Surgery

The first 41 patients achieving CR were divided into three groups: those with no radiographically apparent residual disease, those with a residual mass smaller than 3 cm, and those with a residual mass of 3 cm or more. Twenty-nine underwent either exploratory laparotomy, exploratory thoracotomy, or liver biopsy in an attempt to define the nature of possible residual disease. Those not undergoing operation either refused surgery or had no disease evident after chemotherapy.

Seventeen patients had no radiographic residual disease after chemotherapy. Nine of these underwent surgery; residual viable seminoma was found in none, but 2 subsequently relapsed. Among the other 8 patients, who were only observed, none have relapsed (Motzer et al. 1987).

Twenty-four patients had a residual mass, 20 of whom underwent an operation. Thirteen of the 20 (65%) had a mass greater than or equal to 3 cm, of whom 5 had viable residual germ cell tumor (4 seminoma and 1 mature teratoma). Seven patients with masses less than 3 cm had no residual viable tumor at surgery, and none has relapsed. Among the 4 patients who were only observed, one had a mass larger than 3 cm; this patient subsequently had biopsy-proved progressive seminoma and achieved a second CR with EP therapy. The remaining 3 patients remain free of disease. Thus, of 14 patients with residual masses larger than 3 cm, 6 (43%) had residual tumor (Motzer et al. 1987). No patient had intraoperative hemorrhage, and none died as a result of surgery.

DISCUSSION

It is evident that advanced seminoma responds as well to cisplatin-based chemotherapy as does NSGCT. A high proportion of CRs should be expected. We can draw several conclusions from these results.

Etoposide and cisplatin as two-drug therapy is as effective as and less toxic than VAB-6. Only one patient who received EP has relapsed. These results are the same as those observed in our larger randomized trial of VAB-6 vs. EP (Bosl et al. 1986) and discussed in Bosl and Geller, Chapter 44 of this volume. Myelosuppression, emesis, and renal magnesium wasting were all less severe with EP. Thus, EP is excellent therapy for patients with advanced seminoma.

Patients with bulky stage II (retroperitoneal adenopathy ≥5 cm) or extragonadal seminoma should be considered for initial chemotherapy rather than radiotherapy. The overwhelming majority of previously untreated patients in these two groups in our series achieved a CR and required no irradiation, thus limiting the number of treatment modalities necessary to achieve a cure. Although prior treatment failed to alter the proportion of patients surviving in our series, the effect of prior treatment on survival was striking in the recent report of Loehrer et al. (1987). Among the 62 patients treated, 78% of those previously untreated, 72% of those who had received radiation only to the abdomen or mediastinum, and 42% of those whose irradiation encompassed both the abdomen and mediastinum achieved a CR. Moreover, thrombocytopenia was worse in those previously irradiated, a finding similar to our own results (Stanton et al. 1985; Loehrer et al. 1987). Although these data are difficult to compare, and relapse after radiation therapy may imply inherent treatment resistance, they also imply that prior treatment may influence subsequent survival. In addition, even if subsequent survival is not affected, those patients relapsing after radiation therapy must undergo a second treatment modality (usually chemotherapy) to achieve cure; therefore they experience greater toxicity, including treatment-related death (Loehrer et al. 1987).

Patients with advanced seminoma can be considered good risks. After January 1983, all patients with advanced seminoma were entered into our "good-risk" study. Of 29 patients with seminoma prospectively allocated to ongoing studies, 26 (90%) remain free of relapse. Even among patients with increased values of HCG prior to treatment, two thirds were cured. Obviously, the criteria for "poor-risk" seminoma have not yet been defined.

Finally, surgery after chemotherapy for seminoma is not routinely necessary. An attempted complete retroperitoneal lymph node dissection may result in massive hemorrhage and death (Friedman et al. 1985). Because of the dense fibrosis overlying the great vessels after chemotherapy for seminoma, a retroperitoneal lymphadenectomy is not possible and should not be attempted. In addition, residual mature teratoma is rare, thereby eliminating one justification for adjunctive surgery. In our experience, the size of the residual mass (if one is present) correlates with the likelihood of residual viable germ cell tumor. Of 41 patients who achieved CR, 14 (34%) had a residual mass of at least 3 cm and 6 had viable tumor. Surgery can therefore be limited to a select patient population, sparing the majority of patients a surgical procedure. Radiotherapy could be administered to all patients with residual masses of 3 cm or more, but this would result in unnecessary irradiation for the majority of patients with residual masses.

CURRENT RECOMMENDATIONS

As a result of our experience treating patients with advanced seminoma at MSKCC, we can make the following three recommendations. First, cisplatin-based chemotherapy should be considered not only for all patients with stage III and relapsing seminoma, but also for those with bulky stage II (retroperitoneal adenopathy ≥5 cm) or extragonadal presentations. Second, EP as two-drug therapy is as efficacious as combinations of three or more drugs and is less toxic. And third, further intervention after chemotherapy can be limited to those patients who have residual masses of 3 cm or more. We currently favor excising such masses in the mediastinum or retroperitoneum and administering radiation therapy only to those with viable residual seminoma.

REFERENCES

1. Abell MR, Fayos JV, Lampe I. 1965. Retroperitoneal germinoma without evidence of testicular involvement. *Cancer* 18:273–290.
2. Ball D, Barrett A, Peckham MJ. 1982. The management of metastatic seminoma testis. *Cancer* 50:2289–2294.
3. Bosl GJ, Leitner S, Bajorin D, Geller NL, et al. 1988. A randomized trial of etoposide + cisplatin versus vinblastine + cyclophosphamide + bleomycin + cisplatin + dactinomycin in patients with good-prognosis germ cell tumors. *J Clin Oncol* 6:1231–1238.
4. Doornbos JF, Hussey D, Johnson DE. 1975. Radiotherapy for pure seminoma of the testis. *Radiology* 116:401–404.
5. Dosoretz DE, Shipley WU, Blitzer PH, et al. 1981. Megavoltage irradiation for pure testicular seminoma: Results and patterns of failure. *Cancer* 48:2184–2190.
6. Einhorn LH, Williams SD. 1980. Chemotherapy of disseminated seminoma. *Cancer Clin Trials* 3:307–313.
7. Friedman E, Garnick MB, Stomper P, et al. 1985. Therapeutic guidelines and results in advanced seminoma. *J Clin Oncol* 3:1325–1332.
8. Jain KK, Bosl GJ, Bains MS, et al. 1984. The treatment of extragonadal seminoma. *J Clin Oncol* 2:820–827.

9. Loehrer PJ, Birch R, Williams SD, et al. 1987. Chemotherapy of metastatic seminoma: The Southeastern Cancer Study Group experience. *J Clin Oncol* 5:1212–1220.
10. Martini N, Golbey RB, Hajdu ST, et al. 1974. Primary mediastinal germ-cell tumors. *Cancer* 33:763–769.
11. Motzer RJ, Bosl GJ, Geller NL, et al. 1988. Advanced seminoma: The role of chemotherapy and adjunctive surgery. *Ann Intern Med* 108:513–518.
12. Motzer R, Bosl GJ, Geller NL, et al. 1987. Residual mass: An indication for further therapy in patients with advanced seminoma following systemic chemotherapy. *J Clin Oncol* 5:1064–1070.
13. Stanton GF, Bosl GJ, Whitmore WF. 1985. VAB-6 as initial treatment of patients with advanced seminoma. *J Clin Oncol* 3:336–339.
14. Sterchi M, Cordell AR. 1975. Seminoma of the anterior mediastinum. *Ann Thorac Surg* 19:371–377.
15. Thomas GM, Herman JG. 1984. The role of radiation in the management of seminoma. *Prog Clin Biol Res* 153:91–102.
16. Vugrin D, Whitmore WF. 1981. Chemotherapy of disseminated seminoma with combination of cis-diamminedichloroplatinum (II) and cyclophosphamide. *Cancer Clin Trials* 4:423–427.
17. Vugrin D, Herr HW, Whitmore WF, et al. 1981. VAB-6 combination chemotherapy in disseminated cancer of the testis. *Ann Intern Med* 95:59–61.

Chapter 38

The Role of Radiotherapy in Advanced Abdominal Metastases From Testicular Seminoma[*]

Gunar K. Zagars, M.D.

It has been recognized for well over a decade that those patients with stage II testicular seminoma whose abdominal metastases are bulky (stage IIB) have a relatively poor prognosis, with long-term survival rates on the order of 60% to 70% (Doornbos et al. 1975; Cionini et al. 1978; Thomas et al. 1982). This finding came in an era when radiation therapy was the only potentially curative treatment available for these patients, and by the mid1970s it seemed that radiotherapy had reached its maximal therapeutic utility in this disease. Not surprisingly, newly discovered platinum-based chemotherapy regimens were widely embraced as potential solutions for the problem of the patient with bulky abdominal seminoma (Einhorn 1982). Today, a decade later, opinions are strongly polarized: some authorities hold the view that platinum-based chemotherapy alone is the optimal treatment for these patients (Friedman et al. 1985; Peckham et al. 1985; Schuette et al. 1985; Gregory and Peckham 1986), whereas others, emphasizing the biologic, radiobiologic, and technologic advances in radiotherapy, maintain that irradiation is still the optimal treatment (Green et al. 1983; Smalley et al. 1985; Thomas 1985; Laukkanen et al. 1988).

Several factors have led to this present state of controversy. First, and most significantly, stage IIB seminoma is very rare; many large centers report patient accruals either in radiotherapy series (Smalley et al. 1985; Thomas 1985; Gregory and Peckham 1986; Zagars and Babaian 1987) or in chemotherapy reports (Friedman et al. 1985; Peckham et al. 1985; Schuette et al. 1985; Stanton et al. 1985) that average only one or two new patients per year. Second, there is no agreement on what constitutes bulky abdominal metastasis, and intercomparison of results among different series is hampered by the discordance in staging patients. Third, many of the radiotherapy series against which modern chemotherapy is judged include patients, accrued many years ago, who were treated without the benefits of sensitive imaging techniques, without knowledge of tumor markers, and even in some cases without megavoltage irradiation.

At The University of Texas M. D. Anderson Cancer Center, a policy decision was made in 1978 to use platinum-based chemotherapy for patients with bulky abdominal me-

[*]This study was supported in part by grant CA-06294 awarded by the National Cancer Institute, U.S. Department of Health and Human Services, Bethesda, Md.

tastases from testicular seminoma. Prior to this, radiation therapy was the recommended treatment for all patients with stage II disease. This chapter contains a review of our experience with radiation for stage II seminoma and, based on the results, an objective criterion for subdividing stage II disease into a prognostically favorable IIA category and a less favorable IIB category. In light of the recent experience with cisplatin chemotherapy (Logothetis et al. 1987), we conclude by reappraising the potential role of radiotherapy for stage IIB disease.

MATERIALS AND METHODS

Between January 1960 and December 1982, 48 patients with stage II testicular seminoma received radiation as definitive postorchiectomy treatment. The diagnosis of pure seminoma was confirmed by the Department of Pathology at UT M. D. Anderson Cancer Center in every case. Stage II was defined as disease involvement of the retroperitoneal, iliac, or inguinal nodes without clinical-radiographic evidence of hematogenous metastases or supradiaphragmatic nodal involvement. Spermatic cord involvement was not a criterion for stage II.

Bipedal lymphangiography was performed on 34 patients (71%), excretory urography on 43 (90%). Abdominal computed tomography (CT) was not routine but was performed with increasing frequency during the last 5 years included in this review. The 14 patients who did not have a lymphangiogram were assigned to stage II on the basis of laparotomy findings, a palpable abdominal mass, CT scan, or a deviated ureter and hydronephrosis. All patients had chest x-rays, but lung and mediastinal tomograms were not routinely performed. Other patient and pathologic characteristics, including serum markers, have been previously reported and will not be reiterated (Zagars and Babaian 1987).

Eleven patients had a palpable abdominal mass, and 37 patients did not. To better quantify the volume of abdominal disease, we have retrospectively reviewed all available lymphangiograms and CT scans and measured the largest diameter of retroperitoneal disease. This information was available for 36 patients (75%).

All patients were treated either with cobalt teletherapy or with 6-MeV linear accelerator photons using techniques previously described (Doornbos et al. 1975; Zagars and Babaian 1987). Patients without a palpable abdominal mass generally received radiation to the para-aortic and ipsilateral pelvic regions to a dose of 25 Gy in 15 fractions over 3 weeks followed by a supplementary dose of 5 to 15 Gy to sites of initial gross disease. All 11 patients with palpable abdominal masses received initial whole-abdomen irradiation to a mean dose of approximately 25 Gy followed by an additional 10 to 15 Gy to sites of initial bulk. Forty-four of the 48 patients (92%) also received prophylactic mediastinal irradiation.

Routine follow-up consisted of a physical examination, chest x-ray, abdominal x-ray, serum marker measurements, and routine blood studies every 3 months for 3 years, then every 6 months until 5 years and yearly thereafter. Patients with large abdominal masses were evaluated more frequently during the first year. Survival and progression-free survival rates were calculated using the actuarial product-limit method, and tests of statistical significance were done with the log-rank method (Desu 1980). We use the term "progression-free" survival rather than "disease-free" survival, since it is common for a large seminoma mass to leave a residual post-treatment abnormality that makes the definition of the time of complete remission difficult. In this review, a patient was scored as progression-free so long as his disease decreased in volume and did not begin to enlarge and no new areas of disease appeared. The duration of follow-up for all surviving patients ranged from 27 to 300 months (median, 74 months).

RESULTS

For all 48 patients, uncorrected actuarial survival rates were 85% at 5 years and 81% from 10 to 20 years. The survival rate corrected for intercurrent–disease-related death was 90% from 2 to 20 years, and no patient died of seminoma after 2 years postirradiation. The progression-free survival rate was 88% from 2 years to 20 years. Time to disease progression (equivalent to relapse) varied from zero (never achieving a clear disease-free status) to 20 months, with an average time to progression of 5.2 months and a median of 3 months.

We have previously reported a prognostic-factor analysis in which the only significant factor was the presence of a palpable abdominal mass (Zagars and Babaian 1987). In 37 patients without a palpable abdominal mass, the 5-year progression-free survival rate was 95%; disease progressed in only two patients. This result was not statistically significantly different from the result achieved with stage I disease. Of the 11 patients with a palpable abdominal mass, 4 relapsed, yielding a 5-year progression-free survival rate of 64%, which is significantly inferior to the result achieved in patients without a palpable mass ($P = .003$). Two of the four patients with palpable abdominal disease who relapsed did so in the abdomen. One of these failed in the upper abdomen at an unusually low and wide gap between the abdominal and mediastinal fields, and one had a true in-field recurrence that proved to be choriocarcinoma. No tumor marker values were obtained for this patient. The two remaining relapses were supradiaphragmatic, one in the supraclavicular fossa and one in the lungs. Of the 2 patients without palpable abdominal disease who relapsed, 1 failed with disseminated embryonal carcinoma (no marker studies had been performed), and 1 failed in a para-aortic area shielded from radiation by an excessively large kidney shield. None received platinum-based chemotherapy.

For the 36 patients in whom radiographs were available to measure disease, the largest tumor dimension ranged from 1.0 cm to 22.0 cm. Table 38–1 summarizes the sizes and tabulates disease progression by size. The difference between relapse rates in patients with a mass smaller than 10 cm (1 of 28) and patients with a mass of 10 cm or larger (4 of 8) is highly significant ($P < .01$ by Fisher's exact test). Furthermore, in only 1 of 28 patients with a mass smaller than 10 cm was the disease palpable, compared to palpability in 6 of 8 patients with masses of at least 10 cm. This difference is also statistically significant.

DISCUSSION

This study strongly suggests that an objective criterion distinguishing between favorable and unfavorable stage II seminoma is a retroperitoneal metastasis less than 10 cm vs. one greater than or equal to 10 cm in its largest dimension. Unlike the report from the Royal Marsden Hospital (Ball et al. 1982), our study does not reveal a high relapse rate of patients

TABLE 38–1.
Largest Dimension of Abdominal Disease vs. Relapses

Size Range (cm)	Total No. of Patients	No. Relapsing
<2	4	0
≥2–<5	14	1
≥5–<10	10	0
≥10	8	4

with masses measuring between 5 and 10 cm in diameter. The 10-cm criterion was also found to be valid by the Norwegian Radium Hospital group (Evenson et al. 1985). Thus, we recognize a favorable stage IIA subgroup of patients whose abdominal metastases measure less than 10 cm and for whom radiotherapy remains the treatment of choice. Stage IIB is defined as abdominal disease measuring equal to or greater than 10 cm, and the role of radiation for this subgroup of patients is controversial.

Proponents of primary radiation therapy for patients with bulky abdominal metastases point out that most reported radiotherapy studies have included a majority of patients treated without the benefits of sensitive imaging techniques and modern radiation technologies (Green et al. 1983; Smalley et al. 1985; Laukkanen et al. 1988). In our series all but one of the patients with bulky abdominal disease were treated prior to 1978. From the radiotherapist's viewpoint, the major problems posed by bulky abdominal disease are the likelihood of inadvertently failing to irradiate some intra-abdominal disease, the likelihood of extranodal relapse even if nodal disease is controlled, and the likelihood of failing to recognize nonseminomatous elements if serum markers are not elevated. The latter problem is now readily solved. The relative importance of the former two problems is illustrated in Table 38–2. From this table it appears that hematogenous dissemination, especially to the lungs, is the major reason for treatment failure. One would, therefore, expect only modest therapeutic gains to follow from further enhancement of eradication of intra-abdominal disease.

Two recent reports on the use of modern image-guided radiation showed excellent progression-free survival rates for patients with stage IIB disease (Green et al. 1983; Smalley et al. 1985), but the report from the Royal Marsden Hospital was less enthusiastic, showing 4 relapses among 14 patients (Gregory and Peckham 1986). Moreover, the question of prophylactic mediastinal irradiation has not been satisfactorily resolved. Patients with bulky abdominal seminoma tend to relapse in the mediastinum unless this receives elective treatment. It has been projected that as many as 50% of patients treated only with abdominal irradiation will relapse (Thomas 1985). Such a high relapse rate seems unacceptable, even if patients who fail can be salvaged. However, the use of prophylactic mediastinal treatment has usually hampered subsequent chemotherapy should this be needed (Friedman et al. 1985; Peckham et al. 1985). Thus, a plan of initial radiotherapy for stage IIB seminoma, reserving chemotherapy for salvage of failing patients, raises a number of problems for which there are no clear-cut solutions.

The alternative approach of cisplatin chemotherapy for stage IIB seminoma is based on the well-documented sensitivity of this tumor to such treatment. Many studies have documented the efficacy of cisplatin-based chemotherapy in advanced seminoma. However, it is

TABLE 38–2.
Sites of First Relapse in Stage IIB Seminoma: Orchiectomy and Radiation Therapy Including Mediastinal Treatment in Most

	No. Relapsed	Site Mediastinum, Supraclavicular	Abdomen, Pelvis	Hematogenous*	Author
	7	1	2	4	Cionini et al. 1978
	4	0	3	1	Dosoretz et al. 1981
	9	1	2	6	Ball et al. 1982
	6	1	1	4	Huben et al. 1984
	6	0	0	6	Willan and McGowan 1985
	4	1	2	1	Present series
Total	36	4	10	22	

*15/22 (68%) in lung.

difficult to evaluate the ultimate outcome in the subgroup of patients with stage IIB disease treated only with chemotherapy. For example, the reports of Schuette et al. (1985), Peckham et al. (1985), and Fossa et al. (1987) together describe 52 patients with bulky abdominal metastases, but approximately half of all these patients received radiation following chemotherapy. Since radiation is curative in up to two thirds of patients with stage IIB disease, it is likely that the excellent results attributed to chemotherapy also partly reflect the beneficial effects of irradiation. Thus, the arguments as to which modality is superior continue.

The important question now is, however, not which single modality is better, but rather, how do we integrate two reasonably efficacious treatments into a scheme that improves therapeutic outcome. The findings of several reports dealing with cisplatin chemotherapy appear to suggest a rational plan for integrating the two modalities. At least three studies (Peckham et al. 1985; Motzer et al. 1987; Zagars and Babaian 1987; Logothetis et al. 1987) report that relapse following chemotherapy appeared in almost all cases in initially involved retroperitoneal sites. Residual masses are not uncommon after the completion of chemotherapy, and relapse, if it occurs, usually stems from viable tumor cells remaining within such residua. Relapse of patients in whom the mass has completely resolved is uncommon. The incidence of viable tumor within residual masses can be estimated from surgical data and from relapse rates; representative figures are: 3 of 12 (25%) (Fossa et al. 1987), 4 of 14 (29%) (Peckham et al. 1985); 6 of 14 with a residuum ≥3 cm (43%) (Motzer et al. 1987). When viable tumor is present in residual masses, it is initially microscopic; dense fibrotic tissue constitutes the bulk (Peckham et al. 1985). The substantial incidence of tumor within residual postchemotherapy masses, the usually small volume of viable tumor, and the known radiosensitivity of seminoma argue strongly for a policy of radiation consolidation for such patients. In our experience (Zagars and Babaian 1987; Logothetis et al. 1987), 3 of 4 patients who relapsed by regrowth of their initial bulky disease after chemotherapy were successfully salvaged by radiation. This implies that relapse would have been prevented if these 3 patients had received postchemotherapy radiation and suggests that the fatally progressive disease in the fourth patient might have been prevented had he received early radiation.

CONCLUSION

Radiation therapy and platinum-based chemotherapy are both relatively effective in the management of stage IIB testicular seminoma. Neither modality alone will cure all patients. There appears to be a complementarity in the virtues and limitations between these modalities, exemplified in the hematogenous metastatic failure pattern following radiation on the one hand and the "within-bulk" regional failure pattern following chemotherapy on the other. This suggests a complementary role for the two modalities and constitutes the rationale for our current multimodal approach to stage IIB seminoma, consisting of orchiectomy, platinum-based chemotherapy, and radiation therapy to residual masses.

REFERENCES

1. Ball D, Barrett A, Peckham MJ. 1982. The management of metastatic seminoma testis. *Cancer* 50:2289–2294.
2. Cionini L, Ciatto S, Pitroli L, et al. 1978. Radiotherapy of seminoma of the testis: Report on 129 patients. *Tumori* 64:182–192.

3. Desu ET. 1980. *Statistical Methods for Survival Data Analysis.* Belmont, Calif, Lifetime Learning Publications.
4. Doornbos JF, Hussey DH, Johnson DE. 1975. Radiotherapy for pure seminoma of the testis. *Radiology* 116:401–404.
5. Dosoretz DE, Shipley WU, Blitzer PH, et al. 1981. Megavoltage irradiation for pure testicular seminoma: Results and patterns of failure. *Cancer* 48:2184–2190.
6. Einhorn LH. 1982. Radiotherapy in seminoma: More is not better. *Int J Radiat Oncol Biol Phys* 8:235–248.
7. Evenson JF, Fossa SD, Kjellevold K, et al. 1985. Testicular seminoma: Analysis of treatment and failure for stage II disease. *Radiother Oncol* 4:55–61.
8. Fossa SD, Borge L, Aass N, et al. 1987. The treatment of advanced metastatic seminoma: Experience in 55 cases. *J Clin Oncol* 5:1071–1077.
9. Friedman EL, Garnick MB, Stomper PC, et al. 1985. Therapeutic guidelines and results in advanced seminoma. *J Clin Oncol* 3:1325–1332.
10. Green N, Booth E, George FW, et al. 1983. Radiation therapy in bulky seminoma. *Urology* 21:467–469.
11. Gregory C, Peckham MJ. 1986. Results of radiotherapy for stage II testicular seminoma. *Radiother Oncol* 6:285–292.
12. Huben RP, Williams PD, Pontes E, et al. 1984. Seminoma at Roswell Park, 1970 to 1979: An analysis of treatment failures. *Cancer* 53:1451–1455.
13. Laukkanen E, Olivotto I, Jackson S. 1988. Management of seminoma with bulky abdominal disease. *Int J Radiat Oncol Biol Phys* 14:227–233.
14. Logothetis CJ, Samuels ML, Ogden S, et al. 1987. Cytoxan and sequential cisplatin for advanced seminoma: Long-term follow-up in fifty-two patients. *J Urol.* 138:789–794.
15. Motzer R, Bosl G, Heelan R, et al. 1987. Residual mass: An indication for further therapy in patients with advanced seminoma following systemic chemotherapy. *J Clin Oncol* 5:1064–1070.
16. Peckham MJ, Horwich A, Hendry WF. 1985. Advanced seminoma: Treatment with cis-platinum-based combination chemotherapy or carboplatin (JM8). *Br J Cancer* 52:7–13.
17. Schuette J, Niederle N, Scheulen ME, et al. 1985. Chemotherapy of metastatic seminoma. *Br J Cancer* 51:467–472.
18. Smalley SR, Evans RG, Richardson RL, et al. 1985. Radiotherapy as initial treatment for bulky stage II testicular seminomas. *J Clin Oncol* 3:1333–1338.
19. Stanton GF, Bosl GJ, Whitmore WF, et al. 1985. VAB-6 as initial treatment of patients with advanced seminoma. *J Clin Oncol* 3:336–339.
20. Thomas GM. 1985. Controversies in the management of testicular seminoma. *Cancer* 55:2296–2302.
21. Thomas GM, Rider WD, Dembo AJ, et al. 1982. Seminoma of the testis: Results of treatment and patterns of failure after radiation therapy. *Int J Radiat Oncol Biol Phys* 8:165–174.
22. Willan BD, McGowan DG. 1985. Seminoma of the testis: A 22-year experience with radiation therapy. *Int J Radiat Oncol Biol Phys* 11:1769–1775.
23. Zagars GK, Babaian RJ. 1987. The role of radiation in stage II testicular seminoma. *Int J Radiat Oncol Biol Phys* 13:163–170.

Chapter 39

Optimizing Therapy in Bulky Stage II Seminoma

Gillian M. Thomas, M.D.

Postorchidectomy radiation therapy constituted the mainstay of curative therapy in testicular seminoma until the advent of cisplatin-based chemotherapy. Recognizing the sensitivity of seminoma to cisplatin, either as a single agent or in combination with other agents such as vinblastine, bleomycin, or etoposide, has raised new questions as to what constitutes optimal therapy for patients with bulky disease still confined to the abdomen and retroperitoneum.

Advocates of chemotherapy believe that all such patients should receive initial chemotherapy followed possibly by consolidation radiation therapy or that radiation therapy or surgery should be used for residual masses (Samuels and Logothetis 1983; Simon et al. 1983; Vugrin and Whitmore 1984). Some advocates of radiation therapy recommend initial infradiaphragmatic (Thomas 1985) or infradiaphragmatic and supradiaphragmatic irradiation (Smalley et al. 1985) and have demonstrated cures of the majority of patients with this approach.

The challenge in treating these patients is not to advocate a modality-oriented therapy, but rather to exploit the advantages of both treatment modalities so that the individual patient has the highest chance of cure while sustaining the least possible treatment-related morbidity.

PATIENT POPULATION

The definitions of "advanced" or "bulky" stage II seminoma have varied, and as yet there is no universally accepted definition of the extent of disease that constitutes the entity. Prior to the advent of radiologic tests such as bipedal lymphography and computed tomographic (CT) scanning, which can assess the size of retroperitoneal adenopathy with some accuracy, stage II disease was divided simply into nonpalpable (stage IIA) and palpable (stage IIB) masses (Thomas et al. 1982). The division of stage II arose because it was recognized that, after initial radiation therapy, prognosis was related to bulk of retroperitoneal disease (Thomas et al. 1982). At that time, when tumor marker status was unknown, the 5-year actuarial survival rates of patients with stage IIA and IIB disease were, respectively, 87% and 62%.

A more precise definition of "bulk" has come from CT scanning of the retroperitoneum. Although no attempt has been made to correlate nodal retroperitoneal disease volume or even two-dimensional measurements with outcome, the maximal transverse diameter of node masses has been correlated with outcome (Ball et al. 1982). Table 39–1 shows a comparison

TABLE 39–1.
Comparison of the Incidence of Relapse by Bulk of Abdominal Disease as Defined by the Staging Systems of the PMH and RMH*

Staging System	No. of Patients	Relapses		% Alive Disease Free
		No.	%	
PMH IIA (nonpalp)	40	3	8	87
RMH IIA (<2 cm)	32	3	9	78
RMH IIB (2–5 cm)	11	2	18	82
PMH IIB (palp)	46	24	39	62
RMH IIC (>5 cm)	23	9	52	57

*PMH = Princess Margaret Hospital; RMH = Royal Marsden Hospital; nonpalp = nonpalpable; palp = palpable (Ball et al. 1982; Thomas et al. 1982).

of the Royal Marsden Hospital (RMH) staging system based on CT-measured transverse diameters and the old Princess Margaret Hospital (PMH) system. It appears that IIA disease defined by the PMH system behaves in a fashion similar to RMH disease IIA or IIB, i.e., node masses up to 5 cm in diameter. Patients with palpable masses (PMH IIB) have an outcome similar to that of patients staged IIC in the RMH system, i.e., those with masses in excess of 5 cm. The RMH did not find a worse prognosis for patients with masses in excess of 10 cm as compared to those with masses of 5 to 10 cm (Ball et al. 1982).

Bulky disease as defined for this chapter refers to disease originally classified as PMH IIB or, where CT scanning is available, to masses equal to or greater than 5 cm. Bulky pure seminoma is a rare entity. As diagnostic methods improve, its apparent frequency is falling. Between 1958 and 1975 at the PMH, it was diagnosed in 10% of patients (46/444); between 1976 and 1981, it was identified in only 3% (5/176) (Thomas et al. 1982; Thomas 1985).

RADIATION THERAPY

Historically, the use of postorchidectomy radiation therapy for bulky seminoma produced survival rates of approximately 65% whether radiation was administered infradiaphragmatically or infradiaphragmatically and supradiaphragmatically (Doornbos et al. 1975; Ball et al. 1982; Thomas et al. 1982). Although these results are now considered inadequate, the studies do reaffirm the exquisite radiosensitivity of seminoma and confirm that even masses of greater than 10 cm can be controlled with modest-dose radiation therapy. Detailed analysis of the irradiated PMH population between 1958 and 1976 (Thomas et al. 1982) and a subsequent understanding of the significance of elevated serum levels of alpha-fetoprotein (AFP) and beta-subunit of human chorionic gonadotropin (β-HCG) (Thomas 1985) defined information important for therapy decision making in subsequent patients:

1. The original population whose survival rate after radiation therapy was 62% must have included some patients with occult nonseminomatous germ cell elements. If β-HCG and AFP level determinations had been available, these patients would have been identified. Clearly radiation is inappropriate and inferior as a first therapy for such patients, and they would now receive initial chemotherapy.

2. Patients with bulky disease do not die because of uncontrolled abdominal disease. Failure may occur because extra-abdominal disseminated disease is more likely to be present or to occur rapidly after initial radiation in bulky vs. nonbulky stage II disease (Thomas et

al. 1982). Figure 39–1 shows the predicted outcome following initial radiation therapy for bulky stage II disease, based on the retrospective analysis of the 46 patients treated in the original series (Thomas et al. 1982).

Between 1977 and 1981, seven patients presented with bulky stage II histologically "pure" seminoma. Two of 7 had elevated serum AFP levels and were therefore considered to have nonseminomatous elements present. The remaining 5 AFP-negative patients were treated with primary infradiaphragmatic radiation to a total tumor dose of 35 Gy. As predicted from the model (see Fig 39–1), 3 of 5 were cured and required no further therapy, whereas the remaining 2 developed mediastinal or distant metastases. They were cured subsequently with salvage cisplatin-containing combination chemotherapy.

Controversies in Radiation Therapy

Uncertainties exist about the way in which initial radiation therapy should be applied: (1) what constitutes an optimal dose and volume if initial retroperitoneal irradiation is to be

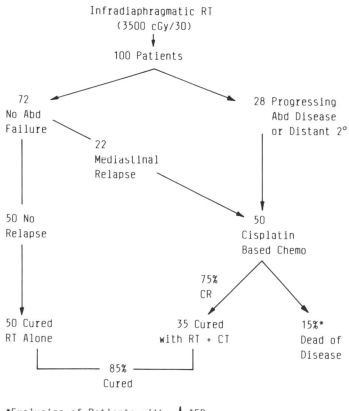

FIG 39–1.
Recommended sequential treatment and its expected results in patients with stage IIB bulky seminoma, marker status unknown. Data based on the results and patterns of failure after radiotherapy and the expected salvage rates resulting from use of cisplatin-containing chemotherapy for relapsing patients. *RT* = radiotherapy; *Abd* = abdominal; distant 2° = distant secondaries; chemo, CT = chemotherapy; AFP = alpha-fetoprotein; DOD = dead of disease.

used, and (2) should the supradiaphragmatic nodal areas (mediastinum and supraclavicular fossae) be irradiated?

Radiation Dose and Volume

By more precisely defining the extent of retroperitoneal disease, CT scanning reduces the risk of "geographic miss" with the irradiation volume. Disease should be more adequately encompassed than when CT was unavailable. Previously, radiation fields were often enlarged to treat the entire width of the abdomen to avoid the possibility of missing tumor. It is unlikely that treatment of the entire peritoneal cavity is necessary unless intraperitoneal tumor is known to be present. Volumes are usually extended superiorly to the top of the tenth thoracic vertebra to include the cisterna chyli and retrocrural areas, which are potential sites of nodal involvement. When retroperitoneal disease is bulky, there is a risk of retrograde spread of disease into the pelvic nodes. The irradiation volume is therefore extended inferiorly to include the pelvic nodes bilaterally.

Unlike epithelial tumors, seminoma is exquisitely radiosensitive. The dose of radiation required to produce local control of even very large tumor masses is comparatively low. Tumor masses up to 5 cm (PMH IIA disease) were controlled in 87% of patients with doses of 25 Gy in 20 fractions (Thomas et al. 1982). The evidence that larger masses of seminoma require radiation doses in excess of 30 Gy for control is inconclusive. Difficulties in the interpretation of dose-control data include (1) a lack of precise preradiation tumor measurements (Thomas et al. 1982); (2) local failure due to geographic miss of tumor with the irradiation volume rather than tumor underdosage; (3) incorrect interpretation of the significance of residual masses visualized on CT scans. In the majority of patients, these masses do not contain disease (Loehrer et al. 1987) and cannot be used as evidence for radiation failure.

Table 39–2 shows abdominal failure rates in three published series. Lester et al. (1986) have interpreted their data to support the benefit of using higher doses of radiation for treating bulkier disease. The abdominal failure rate was 0% (0/7) and 33% (4/12) for doses greater and less, respectively, than 30 Gy. By contrast, Ball et al. (1982) had a 36% (5/14) abdominal failure rate using 30 to 40 Gy. We also were unable to demonstrate increased control with doses in excess of 30 Gy for stage IIB or IIC disease. Unfortunately, the important variable of tumor diameter could not be controlled for in the analysis. Thus, patients treated with higher doses could have had larger masses. Although a dose-control curve may exist for seminoma, it is probably quite shallow compared to that for epithelial tumors. Until more conclusive dose-control data are available,we have elected to use a tumor dose of 35 Gy in 25 to 30 fractions in treating bulky disease.

Supradiaphragmatic Irradiation

In the past, we have strongly advocated omission of prophylactic mediastinal irradiation

TABLE 39–2.
Radiation Dose-Control Data for Seminoma

Author	Disease Stage	Dose (Gy)	Abdominal Control %	Abdominal Control No.
Ball et al. 1982	IIA, B, C	30–40	64	9/14
Thomas et al. 1982	IIB, C	≤30	63	20/32
		>35	57	8/14
Lester et al. 1986	IIA, B, C	<30	67	8/12
		>30	100	7/7

(PMI), even for bulky disease (Thomas et al. 1982; Thomas 1985). Despite the increased risk of mediastinal relapse in stage IIB vs. IIA disease, we could not demonstrate that PMI improved survival rates. Smalley et al. (1985), in contrast, have reported a 100% survival rate for 16 patients, all with stage II disease in excess of 5 cm in diameter. The patients were treated with infradiaphragmatic and supradiaphragmatic radiation, and two relapsing patients were salvaged with further radiation therapy. A survey of the literature overall suggests that, although PMI may prevent mediastinal relapse, it cannot prevent the development of distant metastases in all patients. If chemotherapy is required for relapse, supradiaphragmatic and infradiaphragmatic irradiation may compromise tolerance of curative chemotherapy and increase potential toxicity substantially. Therefore, if radiation is chosen as the primary postoperative treatment modality, we use infradiaphragmatic radiation only.

CHEMOTHERAPY

The chemosensitivity of seminoma is no longer in question. The precise likelihood of curing bulky abdominal seminoma with any of the cisplatin-containing chemotherapy regimens that have been employed is difficult to extract from the literature. Unfortunately, most series have not reported separately on this specific patient subset. Series have included those with marker elevations only, those with extra-abdominal nodal or visceral disease, combinations thereof, those with recurrent disease, as well as those with bulky abdominal disease only (Einhorn and Williams 1980; Samuels and Logothetis 1983; Simon et al. 1983; Vugrin and Whitmore 1984; Van Oosterom et al. 1986; Loehrer et al. 1987). A literature survey indicates 82% of patients treated with regimens containing cisplatin are disease free (Loehrer et al. 1987). Bulky abdominal disease is classified as "moderate" disease extent under the Indiana staging system. The overall complete response rate to cisplatin-based chemotherapy in this group was 81%. Friedman et al. (1985) report five out of five patients with stage IIB disease treated only with cisplatin, vinblastine, bleomycin (PVB) to be disease free. The morbidity associated with the use of cisplatin is not trivial, and in fact a 10% mortality was observed when various cisplatin-containing regimens were used (Loehrer et al. 1987).

Cisplatin-containing chemotherapy will not cure 100% of patients. Loehrer et al. (1987) summarized data showing that 10% of patients with radiologically identified residual masses after chemotherapy have persistent disease. Unfortunately, the percentage of patients who were not surgically evaluated after chemotherapy is unknown. It is not possible to estimate from the literature the number who will relapse in extra-abdominal sites after cisplatin-based chemotherapy.

CONCLUSIONS: RADIATION THERAPY OR CHEMOTHERAPY INITIALLY?

Optimal initial therapy has not yet been established. Biases exist for radiation or chemotherapy depending on the expertise and orientation of the oncologist making the initial treatment decision. It is likely that cure rates will be similar whichever modality is employed initially. Cisplatin-based chemotherapy may cure more patients initially, leaving fewer patients requiring salvage therapies such as radiation, surgery, or further chemotherapy. This approach, however, is potentially more toxic than initial infradiaphragmatic irradiation. Initial radiation therapy is less toxic and more easily tolerated, but an estimated 35% of patients will require salvage chemotherapy (Thomas 1985).

Because seminoma is a rare entity, no single center can test which initial therapy will result in a better therapeutic ratio. An intergroup study comparing initial radiation therapy vs. initial bleomycin, etoposide, and cisplatin, with subsequent therapy used only for progressive disease, should provide an answer to this question.

Our preference, outside of this study, is to recommend initial radiation therapy for the majority of patients. Selection factors in addition to tumor size may well be important influences on the choice of initial therapy, however. Individual patient and tumor characteristics may be present that potentially increase the morbidity of one treatment modality compared to that of the other. If tumor masses significantly encroach on relatively radiosensitive organs such as the liver or both kidneys, which would necessitate irradiating these organs in doses close to tolerance, primary chemotherapy might be selected. Similarly, oncologists with a chemotherapy bias should evaluate the potential morbidity of cisplatin-containing regimens and choose initial radiation therapy if factors are present that could exacerbate the risk of morbidity.

Until definitive data are available, these rare patients with bulky seminoma should be entered on the available study. By pooling data, we will be able to identify individual characteristics that predict the therapy most likely to be associated with the most favorable cure-morbidity ratio.

REFERENCES

1. Ball D, Barrett A, Peckham J. 1982. The management of metastatic seminoma testis. *Cancer* 50:2289–2294.
2. Doornbos JF, Hussey DH, Johnson DE. 1975. Radiotherapy of pure seminoma of the testis. *Radiology* 116:401–404.
3. Einhorn LH, Williams SD. 1980. Chemotherapy of disseminated seminoma. *Cancer Clin Trials* 3:307–313.
4. Friedman EL, Garnick MB, Stomper PC, et al. 1985. Therapeutic guidelines and results in advanced seminoma. *J Clin Oncol* 3:1325–1332.
5. Lester SG, Morphis JG, Hornbach NB. 1986. Testicular seminoma: Analysis of treatment results and failures. *Int J Radiat Oncol Biol Phys* 12:353–358.
6. Loehrer PJ, Birch R, Williams SD, et al. 1987. Chemotherapy of metastatic seminoma: The Southeastern Cancer Study Group experience. *J Clin Oncol* 5:1212–1220.
7. Samuels ML, Logothetis CJ. 1983. Follow-up study of sequential weekly pulse-dose cisplatinum for advanced seminoma (abstract). *Proc Am Soc Clin Oncol* 2:137.
8. Simon SD, Srougi M, Goes GM. 1983. Treatment of advanced seminoma with vinblastine, actinomycin-D, cyclophosphamide, bleomycin and cis-platinum (abstract). *Proc Am Soc Clin Oncol* 2:132.
9. Smalley SR, Evans RG, Richardson RL, et al. 1985. Radiotherapy as initial treatment for bulky stage II testicular seminoma. *J Clin Oncol* 3:1333–1338.
10. Thomas GM. 1985. Controversies in the management of testicular seminoma. *Cancer* 55:2296–2302.
11. Thomas GM, Rider WD, Dembo AJ, et al. 1982. Seminoma of the testis: Results of treatment and patterns of failure after radiation therapy. *Int J Radiat Oncol Biol Phys* 8:165–174.
12. Van Oosterom AT, Williams SD, Cortes-Funes H, et al. 1986. Treatment of advanced seminomas with chemotherapy, in Jones WG, Ward AM, Anderson CK (eds): *Germ Cell Tumour II*. Elmsford, NY, Pergamon Press, pp 229–233.
13. Vugrin D, Whitmore W. 1984. The VAB-6 regimen in the treatment of metastatic seminoma. *Cancer* 53:2422–2424.

Chapter 40

M.D. Anderson Experience With Surveillance for Clinical Stage I Disease

David A. Swanson, M.D.

Douglas E. Johnson, M.D.

Until relatively recently, patients with nonseminomatous germ cell tumors of the testis (NSGCTT) who had no demonstrable distant metastases routinely underwent retroperitoneal lymphadenectomy (Whitmore 1979). Although it is therapeutic for some patients who have limited disease in the retroperitoneal lymph nodes, lymphadenectomy is only a staging procedure for the vast majority of patients (Babaian and Johnson 1980). In fact, when patients undergo a thorough clinical workup, have normal serum levels of alpha-fetoprotein (AFP) and beta-human chorionic gonadotropin (β-HCG), and have no evidence of metastases, retroperitoneal lymphadenectomy should reveal pathologically normal lymph nodes in approximately 80%. This fact, along with a better appreciation of the natural history of germ cell tumors and the advent of reliably effective chemotherapy for metastatic disease, led Peckham and colleagues in 1979 to adopt a policy of close surveillance only—no further treatment after orchiectomy—for patients with stage I disease (Peckham et al. 1982).

At The University of Texas M. D. Anderson Cancer Center, we began a protocol investigating orchiectomy alone (surveillance) for patients with clinical stage I NSGCTT in October 1981. The first 100 consecutive patients have now been monitored until relapse or, if continuously free of disease, for a median of 33 months. The results permit us to estimate the expected rate of relapse and help us to identify prognostic variables that appear to influence that rate. We herein report our results and discuss the implications for management of stage I NSGCTT.

PATIENTS AND PROTOCOL

From Oct 1, 1981, through July 16, 1986, 100 patients were entered into the surveillance protocol. Eleven patients had undergone radical inguinal orchiectomy for the primary tumor at UT M. D. Anderson Cancer Center, but for all others we reviewed the outside slides, requesting blocks of tissue if necessary. Only six patients who had clinical stage I tumors seen during this time span underwent a staging retroperitoneal lymphadenectomy, all of whom had pathologically negative lymph nodes. Four patients who lived in South America and one almost 2,000 miles away could not return for the interval follow-ups required by protocol, and the radiographic workup of 1 patient was inadequate because of an allergy to contrast material.

Before entering the protocol, all patients underwent a complete physical examination, complete blood count, serum multiple analysis (SMA-12), serum biomarker analysis (AFP and β-HCG), chest x-ray (posterior-anterior and lateral without tomograms), computed tomograms (CT) of the abdomen and pelvis, and bipedal lymphangiogram. Acceptance required them to have no definite evidence of metastatic disease and serum biomarker levels within normal limits. The absence of elevated biomarkers, even before orchiectomy, did not preclude entry. One patient was not given a lymphangiogram because of contrast allergy but was considered adequately evaluated otherwise.

The protocol stipulated that patients undergo periodic evaluations at 2-month intervals the first year, every 3 months the second and third years, and every 6 months the fourth and fifth years; we recommend annual checkups after 5 years. Each follow-up visit included a pertinent physical examination, evaluation of serum AFP and β-HCG, chest x-ray, and plain film of the abdomen as long as sufficient contrast material from the lymphangiogram remained in the retroperitoneal lymph nodes to permit evaluation. A CT scan of the abdomen and pelvis was repeated at 6 and 12 months.

RESULTS

Histology

No patient had gross or histologic evidence of tumor involving the spermatic cord. In only one patient was tumor histologically evident outside the tunica albuginea; it had microscopically invaded the rete testis. Very few tumors comprised pure histologic cell types. Nine were pure embryonal carcinoma, one was pure endodermal sinus tumor (EST), and five were mature teratoma; two others contained mature plus immature teratoma only. Embryonal carcinoma was present in 86 tumors, and teratomatous elements were a component of 79 (mature teratoma alone in 12, immature teratoma alone in 12, and both in 55).

Vessel invasion, i.e., tumor cells identified within an endothelial-lined space in the primary tumor, was identified in 34 patients (vascular in 7 tumors, lymphatic in 22, and both in 5) and noted to be absent in the remaining 66 patients. Vessel invasion was most common in the 22 tumors composed exclusively of either embryonal carcinoma, EST, or both (9 of 15, 60%) or of immature teratoma (no mature elements) and embryonal carcinoma with or without EST (4 of 7, 57%). In both categories, the added presence of seminoma, mature teratoma, or both decreased the proportion of tumors with vessel invasion.

Serum Markers

Either before or after orchiectomy, the level of serum AFP (alone) was elevated in 20 patients, of β-HCG (alone) in 9, and of both in 25, for a total of 54 patients; in 46 patients, no elevation of either biomarker was ever observed. The absence of an elevation before orchiectomy did not preclude one later if the patient relapsed; four patients who relapsed had normal biomarkers before orchiectomy, but in all 4, one or both biomarkers were elevated when they later relapsed.

Duration of Follow-up

Follow-up for the 69 patients who never suffered a relapse ranged from 9 months to 67 months (median 33 months). All but one patient—whose last follow-up examination was 9 months after orchiectomy but who committed suicide at 13 months—were observed for a minimum of 12 months. In fact, among those patients continuously free of disease, 62 were monitored for at least 18 months, 45 at least 24 months, and 29 for 36 or more months. One patient developed a second primary germ cell tumor (pure seminoma) 16 months after orchiectomy, for which he received no therapy. The second tumor is not considered to be a relapse; 61 months have passed since orchiectomy (45 months after his second tumor), and he is free of disease.

Relapse

Interval to Relapse

Metastatic tumor became apparent in 31 patients from 2 to 25 months (median, 4 months) after orchiectomy (Table 40–1). Metastasis occurred in 20 patients (65%) within 5 months of orchiectomy and in only 3 (10%) after 1 year (13, 23, and 25 months). Thus, among those patients who were destined to relapse, metastatic disease had appeared in about two thirds by the second follow-up visit and in all but 7% by their follow-up visit 12 months after entry.

Serum Biomarker Status

At the time of relapse only five patients had normal serum levels of AFP and β-HCG (the marker status of one patient was unknown). In the other 25 relapsing patients, one or both biomarkers were elevated: AFP only in 7, β-HCG only in 6, and both in 12.

Site of Relapse

Among the 31 patients who relapsed, 23 had radiographic or physical evidence of tumor in the lungs, retroperitoneum, supraclavicular lymph nodes, or some combination of these sites (Table 40–2). In 8 patients, the only evidence of tumor was elevated serum biomarkers, although 2 of these patients did manifest retroperitoneal tumor masses after chemotherapy was started. Nine other patients had tumor apparent in the retroperitoneum alone, for a total of 11 (35%); 14 patients (45%) had documented disease outside the retroperitoneum; and the 6 others (19%) who had only elevated biomarkers could potentially have tumor outside the retroperitoneum.

TABLE 40–1.

Time Postorchiectomy to Relapse

Interval (mo) (Median, 4 mo)	No. of Patients (n = 31)	Cumulative Proportion (%)
2	1	3
3	9	32
4	7	55
5	3	65
6	3	74
7	2	81
10	3	90
13	1	94
23	1	97
25	1	100

TABLE 40–2.
Site of Relapse

Site	Patients (n = 31)	
	No.	%
Lung only	9	29
Retroperitoneum only	9	29
Lung* + retroperitoneum	5	16
Biomarker ↑ only†	8	26

*Includes one patient with tumor in supradiaphragmatic lymph nodes + retroperitoneum.
†Two patients developed retroperitoneal tumor after chemotherapy.

Treatment

All but one patient who relapsed underwent delayed treatment (Table 40–3). The exception was a patient who had pure embryonal carcinoma and was discovered to have tiny nodules in the lungs and minimal elevations of serum AFP and β-HCG 23 months after orchiectomy. He "died in his sleep" at home less than 1 week later; no autopsy was performed. Twenty-eight patients received primary chemotherapy, 14 because of extraretroperitoneal tumor (stage III) and 14 because of retroperitoneal masses (stage II) or elevated biomarkers. We treated each patient until serum biomarkers were normal and all visible disease had disappeared or achieved maximum regression and then gave two more courses of chemotherapy. Nine patients had residual masses that were surgically excised, 6 by retroperitoneal lymphadenectomy and 3 by thoracotomy; histologically, all were only fibrosis or mature teratoma. Retroperitoneal lymphadenectomy was the primary therapy for 2 patients, 1 of whom showed extranodal extension of tumor and later needed chemotherapy because of rising biomarkers.

Present Status

Ninety-seven patients are alive today without evidence of disease, having completed any treatment they required. One patient, a chronically depressed 45-year-old man with juvenile diabetes, committed suicide 13 months after orchiectomy, still clinically disease-free, and one patient relapsed and died before ever receiving treatment for an apparently modest tumor burden. The third death was clearly secondary to tumor. The patient relapsed 5 months after orchiectomy in the retroperitoneum, at the site labeled "suspicious" on lymphangiogram. Although he initially responded to chemotherapy with apparent complete regression of the mass, it recurred there 7 months later and also in the lungs; the patient failed to respond to several salvage chemotherapy programs and died 31 months postorchiectomy.

TABLE 40–3.
Treatment Received by Relapsing Patients

Treatment	Patients (n = 31)
None	1
Primary lymphadenectomy	2
Only	1
Plus chemotherapy	1
Primary chemotherapy	28
Only	19
Plus lymphadenectomy	6
Plus thoracotomy	3

DISCUSSION

More accurate clinical staging and a better understanding of the natural history of testis cancer led investigators in the late 1970s to wonder whether some patients with low-stage NSGCTT could be spared routine lymphadenectomy. Only the development of consistently effective chemotherapy programs, however, made it safe to test this hypothesis. Preliminary reports of orchiectomy alone for patients with clinical stage I NSGCTT confirmed the feasibility of such an approach: relapse rates ranged between 16% and 20%, although these series included patients who had only short follow-up intervals after orchiectomy (Peckham et al. 1982; Johnson et al. 1984; Sogani et al. 1984).

The rationale behind orchiectomy alone, or surveillance, lies less with its morbidity than with the fact that retroperitoneal lymphadenectomy is unnecessary in about 80% of patients and insufficient in at least 10%. The operative mortality of staging lymphadenectomy is virtually zero, and postoperative morbidity is infrequent (7%–15%) and minor (Whitmore 1979; Babaian and Johnson 1980). However, a high percentage of patients suffer a decreased volume of ejaculate with its attendant compromise in fertility as well as other problems of sexual dysfunction when the lymphadenectomy is performed in the traditional manner (Schover and von Eschenbach 1985). Recent modifications of the surgical boundaries for patients who have no grossly positive lymph nodes have reduced the incidence of compromised ejaculation, but data are insufficient to determine the effect of these modifications on the accuracy of staging (Pizzocaro et al. 1985; Richie and Garnick 1985).

There is no doubt that a complete retroperitoneal lymphadenectomy provides the smallest staging error, but thorough clinical staging including AFP and β-HCG measurement, CT scans, and lymphangiography should be able to assess the retroperitoneum with 80% to 85% accuracy—perhaps a little less if the lymphangiogram is omitted. Among the 100 patients reported here, only 16 ever developed tumor in the retroperitoneum, and 5 of these also had metastases elsewhere. Thus, lymphadenectomy would have been unnecessary in 84% of the patients. Furthermore, despite its morbidity (even the lesser morbidity with modified boundaries), retroperitoneal lymphadenectomy may be insufficient to control most metastatic tumor. Tumor spreads hematogenously to the lungs or other viscera even if the retroperitoneal lymph nodes are removed. This occurs in about 10% of patients with pathologically negative nodes (Whitmore 1979) and in at least 20% of those who have microscopically positive lymph nodes determined on lymphadenectomy (and who would have had a negative clinical workup as did the patients in our surveillance series) (Donohue et al. 1979; Skinner and Scardino 1980).

Our data demonstrate that only 9 patients relapsed with tumor in the retroperitoneum alone and 5 others in the retroperitoneum plus lung or supraclavicular lymph nodes. Eight patients had serum biomarker elevations without radiographically apparent tumor. If we assume that no patient had clinically unrecognized disease in the lungs to account for the marker elevation, then the most pessimistic estimate would identify *no more* than 22 patients (all with retroperitoneal relapses plus biomarker elevations) whose disease was potentially resectable by initial lymphadenectomy, 5 of whom also had disease outside the retroperitoneum that may or may not have progressed stepwise from the retroperitoneum. Although most of our patients were treated with primary chemotherapy when they relapsed, 14 of these patients would, by today's treatment policies, get a retroperitoneal lymphadenectomy anyhow, but delayed and therapeutic as opposed to an immediate lymphadenectomy for staging (Logothetis et al. 1987).

Our highest relapse rate (6 of 9, 67%) occurred among patients with pure embryonal carcinoma, although 8 of the 15 patients (53%) with embryonal carcinoma and/or EST—

known to have a high rate of vessel invasion—also had a relapse. No patient without embryonal carcinoma present had a relapse, nor did any of the 5 patients with pure mature teratoma. Despite the apparent ameliorating influence of teratoma (especially mature), we were unable to show a significant difference between the relapse rate for patients with and without a teratomatous element independent of whether vessel invasion was present (Table 40–4). Clearly, if the primary tumor has invaded vessels, a patient is at higher risk for relapse (19 of 34, 56%) than if vessel invasion is absent (12 of 66, 18%), regardless of cell type. However, if the patient has no evidence of vessel invasion, he appears to be at a lesser risk of relapse if his primary tumor has teratomatous elements present, although this is still not statistically significant. A separate analysis of 93 patients also addresses this interrelationship (Dunphy et al. 1988).

The early reports that noted relapse rates of 20% or less clearly reflect the short follow-up time after orchiectomy for some patients. One should not be surprised that the rates of relapse being cited now are closer to 30% (Hoskin et al. 1986; Pizzocaro et al. 1986) if one considers the understaging error in the retroperitoneum to be 15% to 20% and the rate of relapse outside the retroperitoneum to be 10% to 15% (at least 10% for pathologically negative lymph nodes and at least 20% for microscopically positive lymph nodes). Theoretically, we should expect an ultimate relapse rate of 30% to 35% if all patients with clinical stage I NSGCTT are included. Our relapse rate of 31% overall is in excellent agreement, although we may still see additional relapses later since our minimum follow-up in this series is only 12 months. Our median interval to relapse of 4 months and the predominance of early relapses is also typical. However, a few late relapses have occurred: one each at 21 and 24 months (see Herr et al., Chapter 41), one each at 22 and 36 months (Pizzocaro et al. 1986), and one each at 25 and 30 months (Peckham 1985). Thus, although close to 90% of relapses become apparent within 1 year of orchiectomy, continued follow-up is important to diagnose the late relapses correctly and in a timely fashion.

Based on the published experience of many investigators, however, it is now obvious that there are certain prognostic indicators that can predict for high likelihood of subsequent "relapse," which is, of course, simply metastatic disease undiagnosed by clinical staging methods. These variables include, but are not necessarily limited to, locally advanced tumors ($>pT_1$), spermatic cord invasion, vascular or lymphatic invasion in the primary tumor, and possibly histologic type, although this may not be an independent factor (Moriyama et al. 1985; Hoskin et al. 1986; Pizzocaro et al. 1986; Rodriguez et al. 1986; Hoeltl et al. 1987; Packham and Brada 1987). The reported relapse rate in any series reflects the patient population studied; therefore, by limiting entry to a protocol based on these prognostic variables, the investigator might drop his "relapse" rate from around 30% to 20%, or even less. If we had excluded patients with vessel invasion, our relapse rate would be reported as 18% instead of 31%. We believe that orchiectomy alone and close surveillance is still appropriate for many of these higher-risk patients, however, because the data so far do not permit us to predict with sufficient accuracy where these patients will relapse (Table 40–5).

TABLE 40–4.
Relapses by Histologic Type and Vessel Invasion

Vessel Invasion	Relapse (Rate)		
	Teratoma* Present	Teratoma* Absent	Total
Absent	4/10 (40%)	8/56 (14%)	12/66 (18%)
Present	5/11 (46%)	14/23 (61%)	19/34 (56%)
Total	9/21 (43%)	22/79 (28%)	31/100 (31%)

*Mature, immature, or both.

TABLE 40–5.
Site of Relapse by Cell Type and Lymphatic Invasion of the Primary
Tumor

	Teratoma		Vessel Invasion	
Metastatic Site	No (21)	Yes (79)	No (66)	Yes (34)
Lung only	3	6	3	6
Retroperitoneum only	2	7	4	5
Lung* + retroperitoneum	3	2	2	3
Biomarker only	1	7	3	5
Total	9	22	12	19

*Includes one patient with both supradiaphragmatic lymph node and retroperitoneal
metastases.

We prefer to observe these patients closely, emphasizing to the patient the relatively high risk of relapse and possible need for subsequent therapy, and then to treat the disease appropriately when it appears. Some patients are thus spared a retroperitoneal lymphadenectomy when chemotherapy alone may cure them (Logothetis et al. 1986, 1987).

Of our 100 patients, 97 are currently alive and clinically disease free off all therapy; 3 have died, 1 of suicide clinically free of disease, 1 with apparent low-volume tumor never treated, and 1 secondary to tumor progression despite treatment. Other investigators have reported similar death rates. At Memorial Sloan-Kettering Cancer Center, 2 patients among the first 81 died of progressive tumor (see Herr et al., Chapter 41). In Milan, one patient—who refused therapy after relapse—among 59 died of cancer (Pizzocaro et al. 1986), and at the Royal Mardsen Hospital 1 of 126 patients died of cancer (Hoskin et al. 1986). Thus, in these four centers with the greatest reported experience with orchiectomy alone for clinical stage I NSGCTT, the mortality due to cancer has been 6 of 366, or 1.6%.

CONCLUSION

Our results with orchiectomy alone (surveillance) for 100 patients with clinical stage I NSGCTT monitored until relapse or for a minimum of 12 months confirm that this approach is safe, rational, and effective. Although 31 patients relapsed, only 2 died of cancer (1 untreated), because delayed therapy—usually chemotherapy or surgery, less commonly both—has been highly successful for late "recurrences." We believe it is rational because only 11 patients demonstrated disease in the retroperitoneum alone, and thus retroperitoneal lymphadenectomy would probably not have eradicated all disease in many patients. Finally, we believe this approach to the management of NSGCTT is effective because it spared many patients a lymphadenectomy that was either unnecessary (84 patients never had tumor in the retroperitoneum) or insufficient (disease outside the retroperitoneum was documented in 14 patients and potential in 8 more who had elevated serum biomarkers). Further experience, by investigators who must always remember that the highest possible survival rate is the top priority and achieving it with less treatment-related morbidity the second priority, should help define the prognostic indicators that identify the patients who will benefit most from this approach.

REFERENCES

1. Babaian RJ, Johnson DE. 1980. Management of stages I and II nonseminomatous germ cell tumors of the testis. *Cancer* 45:1775–1781.

2. Donohue JP, Perez JM, Einhorn LH. 1979. Improved management of nonseminomatous testis tumors. *J Urol* 121:425–428.

3. Dunphy CH, Ayala AG, Swanson DA, et al. 1988. Stage I nonseminomatous and mixed germ cell tumors of the testis: A clinicopathologic study of 93 cases. *Cancer* 62:1202–1206.

4. Hoeltl W, Kosak D, Pont J, et al. 1987. Testicular cancer: Prognostic implications of vascular invasion. *J Urol* 137:683–685.

5. Hoskin P, Dilly S, Easton D, et al. 1986. Prognostic factors in stage I nonseminomatous germ-cell testicular tumors managed by orchiectomy and surveillance: Implications for adjuvant therapy. *J Clin Oncol* 4:1031–1036.

6. Johnson DE, Lo RK, von Eschenbach AC, et al. 1984. Surveillance alone for patients with clinical stage I nonseminomatous germ cell tumors of the testis: Preliminary results. *J Urol* 131:491–493.

7. Logothetis CJ, Samuels ML, Selig DE, et al. 1986. Cyclic chemotherapy with cyclophosphamide, doxorubicin, and cisplatin plus vinblastine and bleomycin in advanced germinal tumors: Results with 100 patients. *Am J Med* 81:219–228.

8. Logothetis CJ, Swanson DA, Dexeus F, et al. 1987. Primary chemotherapy for clinical stage II nonseminomatous germ cell tumors of the testis: A follow-up of 50 patients. *J Clin Oncol* 5:906–911.

9. Moriyama N, Daly JJ, Keating MA, et al. 1985. Vascular invasion as a prognosticator of metastatic disease in nonseminomatous germ cell tumors of the testis: Importance in "surveillance only" protocols. *Cancer* 56:2492–2498.

10. Peckham MJ. 1985. Orchidectomy for clinical stage I testicular cancer: Progress report of the Royal Marsden Hospital study. *J R Soc Med* 78(suppl):41–42.

11. Peckham MJ, Brada M. 1987. Surveillance following orchidectomy for stage I testicular cancer. *Int J Androl* 10:247–254.

12. Peckham MJ, Husband JE, Barrett A, et al. 1982. Orchidectomy alone in testicular stage I nonseminomatous germ-cell tumours. *Lancet* 2:678–680.

13. Pizzocaro G, Salvioni R, Zanoni F. 1985. Unilateral lymphadenectomy in intraoperative stage I nonseminomatous germinal testis cancer. *J Urol* 134:485–489.

14. Pizzocaro G, Zanoni F, Milani A, et al. 1986. Orchiectomy alone in clinical stage I nonseminomatous testis cancer: A critical appraisal. *J Clin Oncol* 4:35–40.

15. Richie JP, Garnick MB. 1985. Limited retroperitoneal lymphadenectomy for patients with clinical stage I testicular tumor (abstract). *J Urol* 133:247A.

16. Rodriguez PN, Hafez GR, Messing EM. 1986. Nonseminomatous germ cell tumor of the testicle: Does extensive staging of the primary tumor predict the likelihood of metastatic disease? *J Urol* 136:604–608.

17. Schover LR, von Eschenbach AC. 1985. Sexual and marital relationships after treatment for nonseminomatous testicular cancer. *Urology* 25:251–255.

18. Skinner DG, Scardino PT. 1980. Relevance of biochemical tumor markers and lymphadenectomy in management of non-seminomatous testis tumors: Current perspective. *J Urol* 123:378–382.

19. Sogani PC, Whitmore WF Jr, Herr HW, et al. 1984. Orchiectomy alone in the treatment of clinical stage I nonseminomatous germ cell tumor of the testis. *J Clin Oncol* 2:267–270.

20. Whitmore WF Jr. 1979. Surgical treatment of adult germinal testis tumors. *Semin Oncol* 6:55–68.

Chapter 41

Germ Cell Tumors: Memorial Sloan-Kettering Cancer Center Experience With Surveillance for Clinical Stage I Disease*

Harry W. Herr, M.D.

Pramod C. Sogani, M.D.

Michael J. Morse, M.D.

George J. Bosl, M.D.

Robin C. Watson, M.D.

Victor Reuter, M.D.

Willet F. Whitmore, Jr., M.D.

Optimal management of stage I nonseminomatous germ cell tumor (NSGCT) following orchiectomy has been controversial for several decades. Radiotherapy and retroperitoneal lymphadenectomy each has its proponents, and recently chemotherapy has been advocated by some investigators. Comparison of the results of radiation therapy with those of surgery shows no significant difference between the cure rates achieved. In both instances, salvage chemotherapy is required in 5% to 20% of patients to achieve those results. A large-scale, prospective, randomized trial would be necessary to determine any superiority in disease control per se of one modality over the other. However, quite apart from the practical difficulties of implementing such a study, the question itself is of diminishing importance. In fact, it is probably more important to consider whether the end result of treatment could be improved by decreasing treatment toxicity. Given the increasing accuracy of clinical staging, the feasibility and accuracy of follow-up techniques, and the success of salvage

*This study was supported in part by grant 1 RO 1 CA28639-01 from the National Cancer Institute, National Institutes of Health, Bethesda, Md.

treatment, the more important question is whether any further treatment after orchiectomy is justified in patients with clinical stage I NSGCT.

Disease control, morbidity of treatment, quality of life after treatment, cost-effectiveness, treatment availability, and patient compliance must all be considered in evaluating the results of any management. Toward this end, several groups are currently investigating a surveillance policy in which patients are monitored closely after orchiectomy, and additional therapy is employed only in the event of relapse.

ORCHIECTOMY ALONE FOR STAGE I NONSEMINOMATOUS GERM CELL TUMOR

Since 1979, we have conducted a prospective clinical trial at Memorial Sloan-Kettering Cancer Center (MSKCC) (Sogani et al. 1984). Selected patients with clinical stage I NSGCT are offered the option of electing no treatment other than orchiectomy unless recurrent disease becomes clinically evident. The surveillance policy is based on the following considerations: (1) Clinical staging, using tumor markers, computerized tomographic (CT) scan, and pedal lymphangiography, has become more accurate. At MSKCC, clinical staging of consecutive patients with NSGCT has detected retroperitoneal lymph node deposits with an overall accuracy of 86% (Barzell and Whitmore 1979). Retroperitoneal lymph node dissection has shown that only 10% to 15% of patients with clinical stage I disease have microscopically involved nodes. (2) Close and meticulous follow-up can detect relapse early. (3) The probability is high that patients with small-volume relapses can be cured by modern multimodal therapy. (4) Unnecessary treatment (surgery, radiation therapy, or chemotherapy) can be avoided. (5) Ejaculatory function and the potential for fertility can be preserved.

Patient Selection

To be accepted for the observation protocol, patients must meet specific criteria. They must be between 15 and 40 years old, and their tumor must be designated clinical stage I after noninvasive staging (performed or confirmed at MSKCC). Furthermore, it must be a T_1 tumor, limited to the body of the testis and not extending to the rete testis, epididymis, spermatic cord, or scrotal wall. Circulating levels of α-fetoprotein (AFP), human chorionic gonadotropin (HCG), and lactic dehydrogenase (LDH) must either be normal or have fallen in accordance with normal half-life values after orchiectomy. Patients must have no history of scrotal violations, be cooperative and reliable, and be willing to attend regular follow-up visits.

Patients are excluded from the protocol who have pure choriocarcinoma or classic seminoma; T_2, T_3, or T_4 primary testis tumors; a history of scrotal incision, orchiectomy, or orchiopexy; and levels of AFP and HCG that remain persistently elevated after orchiectomy. Patients are also excluded if they are judged to be unreliable or logistically unavailable for frequent follow-up visits. Recently, the protocol was modified to exclude patients whose tumors show intratumoral vascular or lymphatic invasion, because of the possible adverse prognostic implications of these pathologic features (Stephenson et al. 1986).

Between September 1979 and April 1983, 73 patients with stage I NSGCT were evaluated by one of us (H.W.H.) for the surveillance protocol (Herr et al. 1986). Of these, 10 patients (14%) were deemed eligible. Three subsequently relapsed but were salvaged. Sixty-three patients (86%) were excluded for various reasons: 2 (3%) refused, 16 (25%) had a suspect or positive lymphangiogram, 22 (40%) had a positive CT scan, 6 (9%) had one or more elevated tumor markers, 3 (5%) were less than 15 or more than 40 years old, 8 (13%) had had a prior orchiopexy or scrotal violation, 4 (6%) had extension to the spermatic cord, and 2 (3%) were unavailable for monthly follow-up in our Center.

The complementary value of lymphangiography to the CT scan became apparent. Nine patients had abnormal lymphograms despite normal CT scans. Of these nine, seven had positive nodes. If these 9 had been included with the 10 entered in the observation study, the relapse rate would have been 63% (12 of 19), an unacceptably high number of failures. Another variable encountered was that in ten instances we believed the CT scans from the outside reports were inadequate and either repeated or reinterpreted them. The end result of such reevaluation often was to exclude these patients from the observation protocol. Moreover, of the 63 patients excluded, 36 (58%) had negative and 27 (43%) had positive nodes identified by retroperitoneal lymphadenectomy. Our data demonstrate that, in interpreting staging procedures, we tended to err more toward finding evidence of metastatic disease that excluded patients from study than toward adopting more lenient criteria favorable to enrolling more patients in the protocol.

Since April 1983, it has been our impression that more than 14% of patients meet the criteria for clinical stage I NSGCT and are eligible for surveillance only. This may be the result of a wider referral base as the protocol has become known or, more likely, the result of stage migration in which more patients are presenting with earlier-stage disease (G. J. Bosl, unpublished data, 1988), a larger proportion of which is clinical stage I. The fact that the relapse rate of around 20% and the predominant relapse site in the retroperitoneum have remained constant suggests that some of the patients included recently had unrecognized nodal micrometastases.

Surveillance Protocol

Patients with clinical stage I NSGCT are considered for entry into the study after orchiectomy. They undergo a careful history and physical examination and extensive staging investigations, including serial tumor marker determinations, chest x-ray, CT scan of the abdomen and pelvis, ipsilateral lymphangiogram, and routine hematologic and biochemical screening. Those who meet the eligibility criteria are admitted to the study after they give informed consent.

We evaluate patients monthly for the first 2 years by serum tumor marker measurement, chest x-ray, and abdominal x-ray until the lymphangiogram contrast material disappears; CT scans are performed every 3 months. During the third year of follow-up, the serum marker determinations and chest x-ray are repeated every 3 months and the CT scan every 6 months. Radiographic studies performed at outside facilities are submitted for review at MSKCC.

Results

One hundred seven patients have now been entered in the protocol. This report focuses on 81 patients entered between September 1979 and April 1985, which provides a minimum 2-year follow-up. Sixty-two of the 81 patients (76.5%) have been continuously free of disease for a median of 36 + months and are presumed cured by orchiectomy alone. Nineteen patients (23.5%) have relapsed. Relapses occurred at 3 to 7 months after orchiectomy in 17 of the 19 patients; one relapse occurred at 21 months and another at 24 months. Relapses occurred in the retroperitoneal lymph nodes alone in 13 patients and in the lungs alone in 4 patients. One patient's relapse occurred in both the retroperitoneal lymph nodes and the lungs; another had a serologic relapse: serum AFP levels were elevated, but there was no radiologic evidence of disease. A summary of results is shown in Table 41–1.

All 19 relapsing patients received further treatment, determined by the stage of disease. Two underwent retroperitoneal lymphadenectomy alone; seven had chemotherapy followed by surgery; six underwent lymph node dissection followed by adjuvant chemotherapy; three had chemotherapy alone. One patient with a stage III relapse underwent chemotherapy and thoracotomy; after a second relapse, he required salvage chemotherapy and had a second thoracotomy and retroperitoneal lymph node dissection, both with negative findings. He subsequently developed brain metastasis and required radiation therapy, but survived his tortuous clinical course.

Among the 19 patients who relapsed, 17 are alive and have been disease free for 12 to 63 months (median, 21 months) following salvage treatment with surgery, chemotherapy, or both. Two patients died with progressive disease. Thus, 79 of 81 patients (97.5%) are currently free of disease, and 62 of 81 (76.5%) have required no treatment other than orchiectomy (see Table 41–1).

The rapid growth of testis tumor metastasis is suggested by the relapses in the lymph nodes: in 11 of 13 patients, the metastatic tumors were stage IIB. Although these patients have been salvaged with further treatment, improvement in retroperitoneal lymph node surveillance procedures is clearly desirable. We now perform a CT scan of the abdomen at 6- to 8-week intervals during the first year, when the risk of relapse is high.

Risk of Relapse

To ascertain variables associated with a high risk of relapse, we have studied the cell type, size, and the presence or absence of vascular or lymphatic invasion of the primary tumor. The relapse rate was higher in patients with embryonal carcinoma (with or without seminoma) than in those with teratocarcinoma, although the difference was not statistically significant. Five of 16 patients with embryonal carcinoma (31%) relapsed, compared to 14 of 65 patients with teratocarcinoma (22%). The size of the tumor did not correlate with the risk of relapse. However, the presence of vascular or lymphatic space invasion in the primary tumor was associated with a significantly higher risk of relapse. Five of 11 patients (46%) who had vascular or lymphatic invasion relapsed, compared to 14 of 70 (20%) with no such invasion. Accordingly, we now believe that patients with vascular or lymphatic invasion within the primary tumor should not be included in the surveillance protocol.

Preorchiectomy serum levels of AFP and HCG were measured in 62 patients; in 39 (63%), levels of one or both markers were elevated. However, in this study, preorchiectomy

TABLE 41–1.
MSKCC Results of Surveillance for Stage I NSGCT*

Disease Status	Patients (n = 81)		Treatment	Follow-up (Mo)	
	No.	%		Median	Range
No relapse	62	76.5	Orchiectomy	36	25–84
Relapse	19	23.5	Orchiectomy, chemother-apy, and/or surgery	21	12–63
Dead of disease	2	2.5			
Overall survival	79	97.5			

*MSKCC = Memorial Sloan-Kettering Cancer Center; NSGCT = nonseminomatous germ cell tumors.

levels of serum tumor markers do not seem to have any prognostic significance. Of 39 patients with elevated markers, 9 (23%) relapsed, compared to 6 of 23 patients (26%) with normal tumor-marker levels.

Multivariate regression analysis of variables predictive of relapse after orchiectomy for stage I NSGCT has been performed by others (Hoskin et al. 1986) and is currently under study at MSKCC. Preliminary analysis indicates significant prognostic variables for relapse appear to be local T category, lymphatic tumor invasion within the primary tumor, and a pure embryonal carcinoma. The presence of yolk-sac elements within the primary tumor may confer a protective effect against relapse. None of these, nor any other factor, has correlated with a relapse in only extranodal sites, although definite blood-vessel invasion detected within the primary tumor may portend a higher incidence of hematogenous dissemination and subsequent failure in the lung.

Results From Other Centers

The surveillance policy is currently under evaluation in several other centers around the world (Table 41–2). Cumulative data show that, among 406 patients evaluated for periods ranging from 2 months to more than 7 years, the relapse rate is 25%. Of 103 patients who relapsed, 96 (93%) have been salvaged with delayed therapy. In general, when relapses occurred, they did so within 9 months of orchiectomy; they occurred most commonly in the retroperitoneal lymph nodes or the lungs, and most patients were salvaged with chemotherapy, surgery, or both. Seven patients (2%) have died from disease; the overall survival rate is 98% (399 of 406 patients).

COMMENTS

The data from over 400 patients suggest that a surveillance policy is a feasible option for patients with clinical stage I testicular NSGCT, although its safety remains to be established. This approach to treatment should be tested carefully and not be allowed merely to serve as an easy option for the patient or the physician. All patients must be selected appropriately and monitored closely by experienced physicians equipped with excellent diagnostic facilities. Because the meticulous follow-up required for therapeutic success is not as readily performed outside the specialty setting, this procedure may or may not translate well to the community-

TABLE 41–2.
International Results of Surveillance for Clinical Stage I NSGCT*

Center	No. of Patients	Relapses No.	Relapses %	No. Salvaged
MSKCC, New York	81	19	23	17
Royal Marsden Hospital, London	132	35	26.5	34
Princess Margaret Hospital, Toronto	24	10	42	10
UT M. D. Anderson Cancer Center, Houston	31	5	16	5
Royal Prince Alfred Hospital, Sydney	12	2	18	2
National Tumor Institute, Milan	59	18	30	15
University Hospital, Groningen	67	14	21	13
Total	406	103	25	96

*NSGCT = nonseminomatous germ cell tumors; MSKCC = Memorial Sloan-Kettering Cancer Center.

hospital level. Nonetheless, we have had recent success providing support to local urologists and medical oncologists who evaluated their patients regularly and sent them to our Center for periodic examinations and a review of blood studies and radiographs.

When the therapeutic procedure is feasible, the next concern is quality of life. Although the majority of patients (77%) on the surveillance protocol are apparently cured with orchiectomy alone (avoiding the morbidity of lymphadenectomy or radiation therapy), some patients with subsequent metastases are subjected to a greater therapeutic burden (usually both chemotherapy and surgery). This double therapy may or may not have been necessary had the patient been treated immediately and not observed first. On the other hand, an unnecessary, albeit safe, retroperitoneal lymphadenectomy does not benefit the patient medically (although knowing the nodes are negative may be psychologically beneficial for some) and carries a low but definite morbidity. Our continuing experience suggests that most patients are willing to accept the risk of relapse to avoid a major operation.

Another primary concern is fertility. Retroperitoneal lymphadenectomy may interfere with this function, and facing the potential loss of childbearing is often deeply disturbing to the young married man and his partner in a childless marriage. This factor then becomes the predominant motivation behind considering and accepting surveillance. Some physicians dismiss this concern, assuming that patients who have testicular tumors are subfertile compared with otherwise healthy young men. Although this may be true for some, for many patients it is not true. Among 22 men oligospermic or azospermic shortly after orchiectomy, serial semen analyses returned to normal during the observation period in 11, usually within 6 to 12 months (Carroll et al. in press). Moreover, we have witnessed spouses' pregnancies during the surveillance of our patients, including several who subsequently relapsed. The fact that fertility has been proved renders rather meaningless data concerning its overall frequency within the testis tumor population when an individual patient with stage I disease is facing therapeutic options. The potential for fertility is a tremendous incentive to accept an observation regimen, and for many is equal in importance to survival.

The best method of follow-up has not yet been determined. We need to discover how often and for how long surveillance studies (including CT scan) should be performed, evaluate newer imaging modalities such as magnetic resonance imaging, and identify at what point the patient may be considered cured. Although 90% of relapses have occurred within the first 9 months after orchiectomy, some have been as late as 2 years; this mandates caution in follow-up, which should continue for a minimum of 5 years. Furthermore, the cost-effectiveness of a protocol that requires intensive and repeated expensive investigations will need to be documented. Nonetheless, expectant therapy for patients with clinical stage I NSGCT is predicted to increase, since it seems that 75% of the patients observed for more than 2 years probably are cured by orchiectomy. Patient awareness (and even demand) of this option has increased accordingly, a fact that will continue to compel physicians to evaluate properly and to educate patients (and other physicians) regarding the value, safety, and benefit of surveillance.

REFERENCES

1. Barzell WE, Whitmore WF Jr. 1979. Clinical significance of biological markers: Memorial Hospital experience. *Semin Oncol* 6:48–52.
2. Carroll PR, Herr HW, Morse MJ, et al. In press. Fertility status of patients with clinical stage I testis tumors on a surveillance protocol. *J Urol.*
3. Herr HW, Whitmore WF Jr, Sogani PC, et al. 1986. Selection of testicular tumor patients for omission

of retroperitoneal lymph node dissection. *J Urol* 135:500–503.

4. Hoskin P, Dilly S, Easton D, et al. 1986. Prognostic factors in stage I non-seminomatous germ-cell testicular tumors managed by orchiectomy and surveillance: Implications for adjuvant chemotherapy. *J Clin Oncol* 4:1031–1036.

5. Sogani PC, Whitmore WF Jr, Herr HW, et al. 1984. Orchiectomy alone in the treatment of clinical stage I nonseminomatous germ cell tumor of the testis. *J Clin Oncol* 2:267–270.

6. Stephenson RA, Reuter V, James BC, et al. 1986. Surveillance for patients with stage I NSGCT: Variables associated with relapse. *J Urol* 135:142A.

Chapter 42

Adjuvant Chemotherapy After Retroperitoneal Lymphadenectomy (Pathologic Stage II)

William D. DeWys, M.D.,

for the Testicular Cancer Intergroup Study*

Between May 1979 and October 1984, the collaborating investigators of the Testicular Cancer Intergroup Study (DeWys et al. 1984) entered 195 evaluable patients who had pathologic stage II testicular cancer into a randomized, controlled clinical trial comparing two strategies of management. One strategy involved monthly examination plus chemotherapy if there was evidence of recurrent disease (referred to as the control group) (DeWys 1979). The other strategy involved administering two cycles of multiagent chemotherapy beginning 2 to 4 weeks after completion of surgery (referred to as the adjuvant therapy group) (Vugrin et al. 1981, 1983; Pizzocaro and Manfardini 1984). The patients have been monitored for a minimum of $2^{1}/_{2}$ years, and the data collected form the basis for this chapter.

STUDY POPULATION AND PROTOCOL

All patients had testicular cancer other than pure seminoma or pure choriocarcinoma. Patients had an orchiectomy to establish the histologic diagnosis. Studies were performed to exclude patients who had disease beyond the scope of retroperitoneal lymphadenectomy or who had medical conditions that would interfere with administration of chemotherapy. Staging studies included a bipedal lymphangiogram or a computed tomography (CT) scan, or both, followed by a retroperitoneal lymph node dissection. A bilateral lymphadenectomy was performed if serum markers were elevated after orchiectomy, if lymphangiogram or CT scan were positive, or if clinically suspect nodes were found at the time of lymphadenectomy. If the aforementioned conditions were not present, a more limited dissection (modified bilateral) was permitted (Williams et al. 1987b). Criteria for inclusion in the protocol included removal of all grossly visible metastatic disease and postoperative normalization of serum levels of α-fetoprotein (AFP) and β-human chorionic gonadotropin (β-HCG).

*Including the Southeastern Cancer Study Group, Eastern Cooperative Oncology Group, Southwestern Oncology Group, Northern California Oncology Group, Walter Reed Army Medical Center, and others.

Patients were stratified based on the stage of the primary tumor and the number and size of involved retroperitoneal lymph nodes and were randomly assigned to the control or the adjuvant chemotherapy group. The patients in the control group were monitored with a history, physical examination, chest x-ray, and serum marker determinations at monthly intervals for 1 year and at 2-month intervals for the second year. The patients in the adjuvant therapy group received two cycles of combination chemotherapy followed by periodic monitoring as in the control group. Investigators prospectively chose one of the chemotherapy protocols shown in Table 42–1 (Einhorn et al. 1981; Reynolds et al. 1981; Bosl et al. 1986). Patients in the control group whose disease relapsed usually received four cycles of one of the chemotherapy programs shown in Table 42–1 or as modified by the investigator.

Categorical variables were compared using the chi square and Fisher's exact tests. Standard parametric and nonparametric univariate analyses were performed. Relapse-free intervals were evaluated with the log-rank statistic. Reported P values are two-tailed unless otherwise specified.

RESULTS

Two hundred thirteen patients were entered into the study, and 18 were excluded from analyses (7 control and 11 adjuvant therapy), leaving 195 evaluable patients (98 control and 97 adjuvant therapy). Reasons for exclusion included elevated markers at the time of entry (9 patients), failure to ascertain markers prior to entry (7), and delayed entry (2). The randomized groups were generally comparable as to surgical treatment, extent of disease, pathologic data, and marker status at entry into the study (Table 42–2). Choriocarcinoma elements ($P = .09$) and yolk sac elements ($P = .02$) were seen more frequently in the adjuvant therapy group, but these features occurred infrequently and so this imbalance is not likely to bias the results.

Tumor recurred in 48 of 98 control patients, and 5 have died, 3 from tumor, 1 from an automobile accident, and 1 by suicide. One of the 3 who died from tumor had refused chemotherapy after one cycle. A second developed an elevated level of serum β-HCG but did not receive chemotherapy until $3^{1}/_{2}$ months later after retrocrural node involvement was discovered; he received chemotherapy with modest delays and dose reductions, responded, but subsequently relapsed and died. The third patient developed an elevated level

TABLE 42–1.
Adjuvant Chemotherapy Drugs, Dose, and Schedule

Drug	Dose	Schedule
VBP		
Vinblastine	0.15 mg/kg	days 1 and 2
Bleomycin	30 units	days 2, 9, 16, and 23
Cisplatin	20 mg/m²	days 1, 2, 3, 4, and 5
Repeat cycle		day 29
VAB		
Vinblastine	4 mg/m²	day 1
Dactinomycin (Actinomycin D)	1 mg/m²	day 1
Bleomycin	30 mg	day 1
	and 15 mg/m²/day	days 1–6, continuous infusion
Cisplatin	120 mg/m²	day 7
Cyclophosphamide	600 mg/m²	day 1
Repeat cycle		day 29

TABLE 42–2.
Characteristics of the Study Population

Characteristic*	Randomized Group	
	Control (%)	Adjuvant Therapy (%)
Orchiectomy		
Inguinal	92	90
Scrotal	2	1
Combined	6	9
Node dissection		
Full bilateral	62	51
Modified	38	48
Less than above	0	1
Tumor extent		
Limited to testes	64	61
Involved cord	15	13
Involved scrotum†	19	26
Unknown	1	0
Nodal stage		
Microscopic only	31	33
Grossly pos, <2 cm	20	23
Grossly pos, >2 cm	44	36
Extranodal	5	8
Pathology		
Pure embryonal	38	32
Teratoma elements	44	47
Choriocarcinoma elements	8	19
Yolk sac elements	3	12
Vascular invasion	17	24
Marker status‡		
β-HCG>10 IU/L	35	36
AFP<25 ng/ml	35	46

*pos = positive; β-HCG = beta human chorionic gonadotropin; AFP = α-fetoprotein.
†Tumor extending to scrotum, scrotal orchiectomy or biopsy, or previous scrotal surgery.
‡Marker status prior to lymphadenectomy.

of serum lactic dehydrogenase (LDH) but did not receive chemotherapy until a recurrence was discovered in the retroperitoneal and supraclavicular areas; he had delays in chemotherapy, responded poorly, and died.

Tumor recurred in 6 of 97 patients assigned to the adjuvant therapy group. Five of those six patients, however, had not received adjuvant therapy, either because of refusal (1) or because disease relapsed between assignment and the initiation of therapy (4). Thus only 1 patient who actually received adjuvant therapy has had a relapse. In this patient, tumor had extended along the spermatic cord and involved 17 nodes; the involved nodes were large (3.5 cm). This patient had received a unilateral node dissection instead of the bilateral dissection specified in the protocol, and an 8-week delay had occurred between node dissection and the initiation of chemotherapy. He relapsed several months later, developed drug-resistant tumor, and died. Two other patients in the adjuvant therapy group died, 1 from an automobile accident and 1 from metastases from a primary cutaneous melanoma. The 5 patients whose tumor recurred before they received chemotherapy subsequently received chemotherapy and survived.

The disease-free survival rates for the two groups are shown in Figure 42–1. The difference between the disease-free survival rates is highly significant ($P < .001$), but the difference between overall survival rates (5 deaths vs. 3 deaths) is not. Similarly the difference in deaths from testicular cancer (3 vs. 1) is not significant; a difference of this degree or larger could be expected to occur by chance 31% of the time (one-tailed test).

Three patients have developed a second primary testis tumor, 2 of them after chemotherapy (1 after adjuvant therapy and 1 after therapy for recurrent disease). As noted above, 1 patient in the adjuvant therapy group developed a primary cutaneous melanoma. Second primary tumors can be expected to develop, based on the known excess of second testicular tumors in patients with a testicular cancer (Hainsworth and Greco 1983).

The sites of tumor recurrence in patients in the control group were predominantly lung and lymph nodes (Table 42–3). In 22 patients, an elevated serum marker was the first evidence of recurrence before disease could be detected anatomically. Many patients had more than one indicator of recurrence, such as a lung tumor plus an elevated marker. Only one patient had initial recurrence in bone, and none had the first recurrence in liver or brain. The pattern observed confirms the validity of the follow-up examinations specified in the protocol— physical examination, chest x-ray, and serum marker determinations.

Analysis of the relationship between pretreatment characteristics and recurrence in the 95 control patients who did not receive adjuvant therapy (3 patients assigned to the control group who demanded and received adjuvant therapy are excluded) disclosed several borderline predictive factors (Table 42–4). The risk of recurrence was higher when tumor extended along the spermatic cord (when this group was compared to all patients not having this extension, $P = .09$, chi square, one-tail). The risk of recurrence was also higher with higher nodal stage (microscopic nodal involvement vs. gross nodal involvement, $P = .08$, chi square, one-tail). Additional variables that were analyzed and found not to be predictive for recurrence include age of the patient, history of undescended testicle, size of the primary tumor, weight of the primary tumor, type of orchiectomy, type of node dissection, pathologic categories shown in Table 42–4, other histologic subgroupings not shown, vascular invasion, and marker status prior to lymphadenectomy.

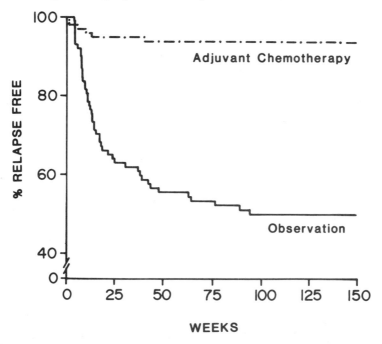

FIG 42–1.
Disease-free survival rate of all eligible patients.

TABLE 42–3.
Sites of Recurrence in the Control Group (n = 98)

Site	No. of Recurrences (Total = 48)
Elevated marker	34 (22 elevated marker only)
Lung	18 (8 lung only)
Lymph nodes	9 (2 lymph nodes only)
Bone	1

TABLE 42–4.
Prognostic Factors in the Control Group (n = 95)

Prognostic Factor*	Recurred/Total	%
Node dissection		
Full bilateral	29/60	48
Modified	19/35	54
Tumor extent		
Limited to testes	27/61	44
Involved cord	10/15	67
Involved scrotum†	10/18	56
Nodal stage		
Microscopic only	12/30	40
Grossly pos, <2 cm	9/17	53
Grossly pos, >2 cm	26/43	60
Extranodal	1/5	20
Tumor type		
Pure embryonal	10/36	56
Teratoma elements	17/42	40
Chorior elements	4/8	50
Yolk sac elements	1/3	33
Vascular invasion		
Yes	8/17	47
No	36/72	50
Unknown	4/6	67
Marker status‡		
β-HCG >10 IU/L	18/33	55
AFP >25 ng/ml	12/34	56
Both elevated	13/22	59

*pos = positive; β-HCG = β-human chorionic gonadotropin; AFP = α-fetoprotein.
†Tumor extending to scrotum, scrotal orchiectomy or biopsy, or previous scrotal surgery.
‡Marker status prior to lymphadenectomy.

The toxic effects of adjuvant chemotherapy were compared to the toxic effects of chemotherapy for recurrent cancer (Table 42–5) (Weiss et al. 1986). When chemotherapy was for recurrent cancer, the toxicity was more severe in the pulmonary, renal, allergic, and fevers/infection categories. This difference suggests that the presence of recurrent tumor affects the ability of normal tissues to withstand or repair the toxic effects of chemotherapy (DeWys and Mansky 1973). This difference in toxicity must be balanced by the observation that only 48 of 98 (49%) of the control group required chemotherapy for recurrent cancer.

TABLE 42–5.
Toxic Effects of Adjuvant Chemotherapy Compared to Toxic
Effects of Chemotherapy for Recurrent Cancer*

Toxicity Category	Adjuvant Chemotherapy		Chemotherapy for Recurrence (%)*	
	No.	(%)*	No.	(%)
Pulmonary	2	(2)	25	(20)
Renal	6	(0)	23	(5)
Fever	30	(0)	45	(25)
Dermatologic	24	(6)	38	(13)
Hematologic	78	(22)	85	(34)

*Percent having toxic reactions (% serious toxic reactions).

DISCUSSION

This study has documented the high degree of effectiveness of node dissection plus chemotherapy for patients with pathologic stage II testicular cancer (2% mortality from cancer). Two cycles of adjuvant chemotherapy prevented recurrence of cancer in nearly 100% of patients so treated, confirming previous studies (Vugrin et al. 1981, 1983; Pizzocaro and Manfardini 1984). The success of brief chemotherapy appears to be dependent on total removal of all retroperitoneal disease. The only patient who had a recurrence and who died in this group had had a unilateral node dissection, but the observation of grossly enlarged nodes indicates a high likelihood that contralateral nodal metastases were present and remained in situ (Donohue et al. 1981).

The alternate management strategy—frequent monitoring and chemotherapy for recurrence—yielded a similar cure rate while avoiding chemotherapy in approximately 50% of patients. The success of this strategy depends on close follow-up and optimum chemotherapy for recurrence. The three patients in this group who died from cancer had delays in therapy or deviations from protocol dose or schedule.

The analysis of prognostic factors has shown that patients with tumor extension along the spermatic cord and more extensive nodal involvement have a higher risk of relapse. Patients whose tumor does not extend along the spermatic cord and whose nodal involvement is only microscopic have a risk of recurrence of only 9 of 26, or 35%, and may be considered for the management strategy of frequent monitoring and chemotherapy for recurrence. In contrast, patients with tumor extending along the cord or with grossly visible nodal involvement have a risk of recurrence of 39 of 69, or 57%, and may be candidates for adjuvant chemotherapy. For the latter patients, we would suggest the recently reported more effective and less toxic etoposide (VP-16-213), cisplatin, and bleomycin chemotherapy (Williams et al. 1987a) and could consider omitting node dissection.

The incidence of new primary tumors in the contralateral testis (3/213, 1.4%) is consistent with previous reports (Hainsworth and Greco 1983). It is noteworthy that two of these patients had received prior chemotherapy, suggesting that chemotherapy may not be able to eradicate premalignant lesions as has been suggested by other investigators (von der Masse et al. 1985). Patients who have been cured of a testicular tumor should perform testicular self-examination and receive periodic medical examination.

CONCLUSION

A cure rate of nearly 100% can be achieved for patients with pathologic stage II testicular cancer treated with retroperitoneal node removal plus adjuvant chemotherapy or chemotherapy for recurrent tumor. Analysis of failures emphasizes the necessity of adhering to protocol specifications regarding completeness of node dissection, frequency of follow-up, and dose and schedule of chemotherapy.

REFERENCES

1. Bosl GJ, Glickman R, Geller NL, et al. 1986. An effective chemotherapy regimen for patients with germ cell tumors. *J Clin Oncol* 4:1493–1499.
2. DeWys WD. 1979. Basis for adjuvant chemotherapy for stage II testicular cancer. *Cancer Treat Rep* 63:1693–1695.
3. DeWys WD, Green SB, Einhorn LH, et al. 1984. Adjuvant chemotherapy for testicular cancer, in Jones SE, Salmon SE (eds): *Adjuvant Therapy of Cancer IV*. Orlando, Fla, Grune & Stratton, pp 529–537.
4. DeWys WD, Mansky J. 1973. Delayed hematologic recovery after cyclophosphamide in the presence of an advanced cancer. *Cancer Res* 33:2662–2667.
5. Donohue JP, Zachary JM, Maynard BR. 1981. Distribution of nodal metastases in nonseminomatous testis cancer. *J Urol* 128:315–320.
6. Einhorn LH, Williams SD, Troner M, et al. 1981. The role of maintenance therapy in disseminated testicular cancer. *N Engl J Med* 305:727–731.
7. Hainsworth JD, Greco F. 1983. Testicular germ cell neoplasms. *Am J Med* 75:817–832.
8. Pizzocaro G, Monfardini S. 1984. Adjuvant chemotherapy in selected patients with pathologic stage II nonseminomatous germ cell tumors of the testis. *J Urol* 131:677–680.
9. Reynolds TF, Vugrin D, Cvitkovic E, et al. 1981. VAB-3 combination chemotherapy of metastatic testicular cancer. *Cancer* 48:888–898.
10. von der Maase H, Berthelsen JG, Jacobsen GK, et al. 1985. Carcinoma-in-situ of testis eradicated by chemotherapy (letter). *Lancet* 1:98.
11. Vugrin D, Whitmore W, Cvitkovic E, et al. 1981. Adjuvant chemotherapy with VAB-3 of stage II-B testicular cancer. *Cancer* 48:233–237.
12. Vugrin D, Whitmore WF Jr, Herr HW, et al. 1983. VAB-6 combination chemotherapy in resected stage II-B testis cancer. *Cancer* 51:5–8.
13. Weiss RB, Stablein DM, Muggia FM, et al. 1986. Toxicity of chemotherapy as adjuvant or salvage treatment in early stage non-seminomatous testicular cancer (NSTC) (abstract). *Proc Am Soc Clin Oncol* 5:99.
14. Williams SD, Birch R, Einhorn LH, et al. 1987a. Disseminated germ cell tumors: Chemotherapy with cisplatin plus bleomycin plus either vinblastine or etoposide. *N Engl J Med* 316:1435–1440.
15. Williams SD, Stablein DM, Einhorn LH, et al. 1987b. Pathologic stage II testis cancer: Immediate adjuvant chemotherapy versus observation with treatment at relapse. A report from the Testicular Cancer Intergroup Study. *N Engl J Med* 317:1433.

Chapter 43

Primary Chemotherapy for Retroperitoneal Nodal Disease (Clinical Stage II)

Christopher J. Logothetis, M.D.

David A. Swanson, M.D.

Sheryl Ogden, R.N.

Appropriate therapeutic options for stages II and III nonseminomatous germ cell tumors of the testis (NSGCTT) are significantly different from each other. Patients with stage III disease depend completely on chemotherapy for long-term disease-free survival, but those with stage II may derive therapeutic benefit from radiation or surgery as well. In the United Kingdom, radiation is employed for stage II disease, and in North America retroperitoneal lymph node dissections have been popular.

Before chemotherapy was introduced as treatment of stage II nonseminomatous testicular tumors, long-term survival was determined by the volume of retroperitoneal disease and secondarily by the histologic type of the tumor. Those patients with gross retroperitoneal metastases (>2 cm in diameter) had a survival rate of approximately 50%. Those whose retroperitoneal metastases were <2 cm in diameter or were only microscopically present at lymphadenectomy had the highest cure rate (≥70%) (Staubitz et al. 1973; Whitmore 1979).

Today, the long-term disease-free survival rate is high as a result of the current active chemotherapy regimens. Survival is nearly universal and minimally influenced by volume of disease, but the likelihood of postchemotherapy surgery is related to both the volume of retroperitoneal disease and the histologic type of the tumor. The treatment of retroperitoneal germ cell tumors currently accepted by most physicians in North America includes a retroperitoneal lymph node dissection followed by adjuvant chemotherapy or close observation. Adequate data have been accumulated so one may, with a high degree of reliability, predict the likelihood of postsurgery relapse. A retroperitoneal lymph node dissection plus postoperative chemotherapy results in a survival rate in excess of 95% (Samuels and Johnson 1980; DeWys et al. 1984).

THE UNIVERSITY OF TEXAS M. D. ANDERSON CANCER CENTER EXPERIENCE

In view of this excellent survival rate and our ability to predict the likelihood of relapse, we initiated in 1982 a prospective trial of primary chemotherapy for clinical stage II NSGCTT at The University of Texas M. D. Anderson Cancer Center. The purpose of this trial was to administer primary chemotherapy to those patients who have a very high likelihood of achieving a complete remission with chemotherapy alone and who would probably require chemotherapy after a retroperitoneal lymph node dissection. The benefit derived should be a reduction in unnecessary lymph node dissections.

Between 1982 and 1985, all patients who had metastasis involving the retroperitoneum only received primary chemotherapy. Chemotherapy regimens included cisplatin, cyclophosphamide, and doxorubicin (Adriamycin II) with vinblastine and bleomycin IV (CISCA$_{II}$/VB$_{IV}$) and, in a small group of patients, alternative chemotherapy regimens because of contraindications to intensive myelosuppressive therapy. Chemotherapy was delivered with a flexible number of courses, as determined by individual patient response. Patients received two courses of chemotherapy after achieving either a complete remission (defined as normal serum biomarker levels and a radiographically negative abdomen) or stable radiographic mass and normal serum biomarkers. These latter patients then underwent retroperitoneal lymphadenectomy.

Patients were divided into four clinical categories (Table 43–1). The study population consisted of 50 patients, of whom 43 received CISCA$_{II}$/VB$_{IV}$. The clinical characteristics and the type of therapy for each are listed in Table 43–2. The majority had elevated serum biomarker levels, and many had both a positive lymphangiogram and a positive computed tomography (CT) scan. The histologic distribution of the tumors was typical of the nonseminomatous germ cell tumor population seen at UT M. D. Anderson Cancer Center during this study period. Of importance is a conspicuous absence of tumors with choriocarcinomatous elements throughout this study population.

Ninety-six percent of the patients studied achieved long-term disease-free survivals. Seventy-eight percent were spared a retroperitoneal lymph node dissection, despite the fact that some of them were in clinical categories considered advanced disease in other series.

Histologic tumor type was the most important predictor of postchemotherapy node dissection. Thirty-six percent of patients with embryonal plus teratomatous elements (Dixon-Moore category IV) required a retroperitoneal lymph node dissection (Table 43–3), whereas only two patients with Dixon-Moore category II (embryonal ± seminoma) required retroperitoneal lymphadenectomy. This difference was highly significant ($P = .014$). The results of postchemotherapy surgery were very similar to those we have found after CISCA$_{II}$/VB$_{IV}$

TABLE 43–1.
UT M. D. Anderson Cancer Center Classification of Clinical Stage II
Nonseminomatous Germ Cell Testicular Tumors

Clinical Stage	Criteria*
II$_A$	Rising levels of serum biomarkers (AFP and β-HCG) after orchiectomy
II$_B$	Retroperitoneal mass <2 cm maximum diameter
II$_C$	Retroperitoneal mass ≥2 cm and <5 cm in maximum diameter
II$_D$	Retroperitoneal mass ≥5 cm and <10 cm in maximum diameter

*AFP = α-fetoprotein; β-HCG = β-human chorionic gonadotropin.

TABLE 43–2.
The Influence of Clinical Presentation on Therapy

| Clinical Presentation | Therapy | | | |
| | Chemotherapy Alone | Chemotherapy + Surgery | | Total |
		No.	%	
Tumor ≥5–<10 cm	6	3	33	9
Tumor >2–<5 cm	15	4	21	19
Positive lymphangiogram only	10	1	9	11
Elevated AFP, β-HCG, or both only	8	3	27	11
Total	39	11	22	50

*AFP = alpha-fetoprotein; β-HCG = beta-human chorionic gonadotropin.

TABLE 43–3.
Influence of Dixon-Moore Classification on Treatment

| Primary Testicular Tumor | Therapy | | | | |
| | Chemotherapy Alone | | Chemotherapy and Surgery | | Total No. |
	No.	%	No.	%	
Dixon-Moore IV	14	64	8	36	22 ⎱
Dixon-Moore II	24	92	2	8	26 ⎰ *P* = .014
Seminoma + elevated AFP*	0	0	1	100	1
Total	38	78	11	22	49

*AFP = alpha-fetoprotein.

among patients with stage III disease (Table 43–4). Two patients had foci of yolk-sac tumor, both of whom remain alive and disease free after adequate resection. The finding of mature teratoma in the postchemotherapy surgical specimen was highest among patients with initial Dixon-Moore IV tumors and occurred in only 1 of the 26 with embryonal elements plus seminoma.

We conclude from this experience that aggressive primary chemotherapy delivered to patients with clinical stage II NSGCTT can achieve a very high complete-remission rate (Fig 43–1). This complete-remission rate is equivalent to that of patients with pathologically defined stage II disease. The majority of patients in the study have been spared a retroperitoneal lymph node dissection and remain alive and disease free. We believe that these patients had high volumes of disease and, if treated first with lymphadenectomy, would probably not have been spared chemotherapy. Patients with teratomatous elements in the primary tumor were least likely to benefit from this approach. These patients nearly universally survived, but 36% of them required double therapy (surgery after chemotherapy).

Primary chemotherapy for stage II NSGCTT has also been used at the Royal Marsden Hospital, as reported by Peckham and Hendry (1985). Their experience has been similar to ours. Although the long-term disease-free survival rate for patients who had masses in the retroperitoneum of greater than 5 cm in diameter was 74%, their cure rate was uniformly high when disease was less than 5 cm in diameter.

DISCUSSION

When treating patients with clinical stage II NSGCTT, our current purpose is to maintain

TABLE 43–4.
Pathologic Findings at Retroperitoneal Lymphadenectomy

Primary Tumor Type	No.	Fibrosis	Teratoma	Yolk-Sac
Embryonal ± teratoma (Dixon-Moore IV)	22	1	6	1
Embryonal ± seminoma (Dixon-Moore II)	26	1	1	0
Seminoma + elevated AFP	1			1
Total	49	2	7	2

*AFP = alpha-fetoprotein.

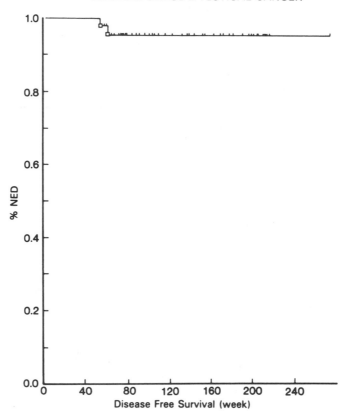

FIG 43–1.
Disease-free survival of 50 patients with primary clinical stage II nonseminomatous germ cell tumors of the testis. (*NED* = no evidence of disease).

the present high cure rate and simultaneously to reduce the frequency of unnecessary therapy. Previous reports have suggested that patients whose primary tumor contains teratomatous elements and those with elevated α-fetoprotein serum levels are less likely to develop distant metastases (Freedman et al. 1987), whereas those with pure embryonal carcinoma have a high likelihood of metastases. With these differences in mind, we are presently engaged in a prospective trial in which patients with clinical stage II pure embryonal carcinoma of the testis receive primary chemotherapy and those with teratomatous elements in the testicular tumor are treated by primary retroperitoneal lymphadenectomy and postoperative observation. Our hope is that the latter patients, who are unlikely to be able to avoid a retroperitoneal lymphadenectomy, will nevertheless be able to omit the adjuvant chemotherapy with its potentially morbid side effects. In contrast, the group with pure embryonal carcinoma may well be able to omit a lymphadenectomy, since primary chemotherapy can totally eradicate their retroperitoneal disease.

Recently some authors, attempting to spare patients the adverse side effects of retroperitoneal lymphadenectomy—impotence and infertility—have advocated limiting the scope of this surgical procedure. Infertility, a result of sympathetic nerve interruption, is indeed reduced in patients who have limited node dissections. Unfortunately, however, patients with clinical stage II NSGCTT are not appropriate candidates for this procedure, because their retroperitoneal lymph nodes are grossly involved with disease. If the extent of retroperitoneal lymphadenectomy were to be limited in patients with clinical stage II disease, its therapeutic benefit would be reduced. A more appropriate role for limited retroperitoneal lymph node dissection in these patients would be as a diagnostic procedure, where its findings could be compared with those of CT scan and lymphangiography.

Patients who have clinical stage II NSGCTT compose a category of patients who are likely to present to the oncologist with increasing frequency—this because of the routine availability of biomarker analysis and CT and a better understanding of the role of chemotherapy. Therapeutic decisions for these patients should be based not only on cure rates, which, in the hands of experienced oncologists using contemporary combination chemotherapies, are high, but also on morbidity rates. It should be understood that patients with clinical stage II NSGCTT are likely to have a higher volume of disease than their counterparts with pathologic stage II disease. Therefore, reductions in systemic chemotherapy should only be made cautiously. Individualizing therapy for this select group of patients is likely to maintain their high cure rate while reducing the overall morbidity of their treatment.

REFERENCES

1. DeWys WD, Green SB, Einhorn LH, et al. 1984. Adjuvant chemotherapy of testicular cancer, in Jones SE, Salmon SE (eds): *Adjuvant Therapy of Cancer IV. Proceedings of the Fourth International Conference on the Adjuvant Therapy of Cancer.* Orlando, Fla, Grune & Stratton, pp 529–537.
2. Freedman LS, Jones WG, Peckham MJ, et al. 1987. Histopathology in the prediction of relapse of patients with stage I testicular teratoma treated by orchiectomy alone. *Lancet* 2:294–298.
3. Peckham MJ, Hendry WF. 1985. Clinical stage II non-seminomatous germ cell tumours: Results of management by primary chemotherapy. *Br J Urol* 57:763–768.
4. Samuels ML, Johnson DE. 1980. Adjuvant therapy of testis cancer: The role of vinblastine and bleomycin. *J Urol* 124:369–371.
5. Staubitz WJ, Early KS, Magoss IV, et al. 1973. Surgical treatment of non-seminomatous germinal testis tumors. *Cancer* 32:1206–1212.
6. Whitmore WF. 1979. Surgical treatment of adult germinal testis tumors. *Semin Oncol* 6:55–68.

Chapter 44

The Management of Advanced Nonseminomatous Germ Cell Tumors at Memorial Sloan-Kettering Cancer Center*

George J. Bosl, M.D.

Nancy L. Geller, Ph.D.

Germ cell tumors are the most curable solid neoplasms treated by the oncologist. Advances in their management came quickly after high doses of cisplatin were introduced as therapy in the mid-1970s. In this chapter we summarize our experience with these tumors at Memorial Sloan-Kettering Cancer Center (MSKCC).

BACKGROUND

In the 1960s, dactinomycin (actinomycin D) was identified as an active single agent that produced rare but definite long-term complete responses (CR) (Mackenzie 1966). Vinblastine and bleomycin were also found to be active, both as single agents and in combination (Samuels and Howe 1970; Blum et al. 1973; Samuels et al. 1976). These agents were combined in the first VAB regimen (VAB-1) (Table 44–1). In 1974, cisplatin (60 mg/m²) was added (VAB-2). Although the proportions of patients achieving CR and cure were both higher than previously reported, they were not higher than those for patients treated with vinblastine and continuous-infusion bleomycin (Samuels et al. 1976).

In an attempt to abrogate the nephrotoxicity of cisplatin, Hayes et al. (1977) conducted a phase I trial of cisplatin ($\geq$120 mg/m²) with mannitol diuresis. Five of 9 patients with refractory germ cell tumors responded to the higher doses of cisplatin. As a result, two cycles of high-dose cisplatin at 120 mg/m² were then added into the VAB regimen (VAB-3), as was doxorubicin (Adriamycin) (Monfardini et al. 1972). The proportions of both CRs and cures increased (Reynolds et al. 1981). At subsequent operation, some patients with a residual mass

*This research was supported in part by grant CA-05826 and contract CM-07337 from the National Cancer Institute, National Institutes of Health, Bethesda, Md.

TABLE 44–1.
Summary of Treatment Programs at Memorial Sloan-Kettering Cancer Center

Regimen*	No. of Patients	% CR[†]	% Relapse	Reference
VAB-1	47	15	28	Wittes et al. 1976
VAB-2	50	50	56	Cheng et al. 1978
VAB-3	74	61	31	Reynolds et al. 1981
VAB-4	41	80	12	Vugrin et al. 1981
VAB-5	38	47	22	Vugrin et al. 1983
VAB-6	161	78	12	Bosl et al. 1986a

*See text for explanation of regimen.
[†]CR = complete response.

were found to have only mature teratoma, implying that adjunctive surgery would be necessary to define the completeness of response (Hong et al. 1977). A 31% relapse rate was observed, perhaps because of the 5- to 6-month interval between the cisplatin-containing induction cycles.

A third induction cycle of high-dose cisplatin was incorporated into VAB-4 (Vugrin et al. 1981). The proportion of patients achieving CR increased, and the proportion relapsing decreased. Pretreatment elevated serum tumor marker levels and extensive metastases were correlated with a lesser chance of achieving a CR, and for this condition a more intensive program (VAB-5) was introduced (Vugrin et al. 1983). Unfortunately, the proportion of CRs was not higher than that expected for poor-prognosis patients.

We learned several lessons from these studies: (1) Durable CR could be achieved with high doses of cisplatin, and the relapse rate could be minimized by three induction cycles. (2) Surgery after chemotherapy was important, since residual masses in the presence of normal marker values often meant necrotic debris or mature teratoma rather than viable residual cancer; not only would such operations determine whether viable tumor was present, but also they would be therapeutic for those patients in whom viable tumor was totally resected (Brenner et al. 1982). (3) The duration of therapy might be too long; since cisplatin was not a part of the maintenance regimen, perhaps maintenance chemotherapy could be decreased in duration or eliminated altogether. (4) Similarly high CR rates had been reported with the three-drug regimen of cisplatin, bleomycin, and vinblastine (PVB) (Einhorn and Donahue 1977); therefore, perhaps the number of agents could be decreased.

VAB-6 TRIAL

The trial of VAB-6 (cisplatin, bleomycin, actinomycin D, cyclophosphamide, and vinblastine [Table 44–2]) ran from January 1979 through November 1982 (Bosl et al. 1986a). One hundred and sixty-six patients with advanced germ cell tumors (161 evaluable) of testicular or extragonadal origin were treated (Table 44–3). It is noteworthy that the proportion of patients with elevated serum tumor marker values decreased during this study (Bosl et al. 1983b).

Response and Survival

One hundred and twelve of 142 evaluable patients (79%) with primary testicular tumors and 14 of 19 patients (74%) with extragonadal tumors achieved a CR. Eighteen patients

TABLE 44–2.

The VAB-6 Treatment Program

Vinblastine, 4.0 mg/m² day 1, IV
Cyclophosphamide, 600 mg/m² day 1, IV
Dactinomycin, 1.0 mg/m² day 1, IV
Bleomycin, 30 units day 1, IV push
Bleomycin, 20 units/m² days 1–3, continuous IV infusion
Cisplatin, 120 mg/m² day 4, IV, with mannitol diuresis
    Repeat every 4 weeks × 3 cycles
    No bleomycin in the third cycle
    Consider surgery after three cycles

TABLE 44–3.

VAB-5: Patient Characteristics and Results

	Origin of Tumor	
Variable	Testicular	Extragonadal
Patients		
Total	147	19
Evaluable	142	19
Median age (yr)	28	33
Histologic type* (%)		
Seminoma	15	43
EC ± S ± YS	27	26
T ± EC ± S ± YS	31	5
C ± others	27	21
"Anaplastic carcinoma"	0	5
Sites (%)		
None (marker only)	11	0
1–2	73	63
>3	16	37
Marker status (%)		
Elevated LDH	43	90
Elevated HCG	38	28
Elevated AFP	38	39
Response (% evaluable)		
Complete	79	74
Incomplete	21	26
Relapse from CR	11	21

*EC = embryonal carcinoma; S = seminoma; YS = yolk-sac; T = teratoma;
C = choriocarcinoma; LDH = lactic dehydrogenase; HCG = human chorionic gonadotropin; AFP = α-fetoprotein; CR = complete response.

achieving CR required resection of viable residual cancer. Histologic tumor type played some role in determining which patients would respond completely. All 8 patients with extragonadal seminoma achieved a durable CR, whereas only 3 of 11 with extragonadal nonseminomatous germ cell tumors (NSGCT) achieved a durable CR. However, the survival distributions for seminoma and NSGCT of testicular origin were similar. Maintenance chemotherapy did not alter survival or relapse patterns.

Of the 126 patients who achieved a CR, 15 (12%) relapsed. The proportion of relapses was greater in patients with extragonadal tumors (3/14, 21%) than in patients with testicular tumors (12/112, 11%) (Bosl et al. 1986a).

Toxicity

The acute toxicity of VAB-6 was predictable. All patients experienced nausea, vomiting, and alopecia. The median white blood count nadir in the third cycle of therapy was 2,700/ml, the platelet count nadir 132,000/ml, and the hemoglobin nadir 9.9 g/dl. Neither Raynaud's phenomenon nor treatment-induced death occurred as a consequence of treatment.

Because the major end-organ toxicity of cisplatin-based chemotherapy is renal, late renal toxicity was evaluated in 24 normotensive patients. Seventy-four percent had increased plasma renin activity (Bosl et al. 1986b). Increased urinary excretion and serum levels of aldosterone were also documented. A statistically significant decrease in serum phosphorous and increase in serum blood urea nitrogen and creatinine were also found when values after chemotherapy were compared to pretreatment values. The median nadir of serum magnesium was 1.3 mEq/L, implying that the majority of treated patients had a serum magnesium level that was below the lower limits of normal (1.4 mEq/L). The lowest observed serum magnesium level was 0.5 mEq/L, despite the fact the patient's last treatment was more than 2 years prior to the evaluation. Hypomagnesemia and vascular toxicity have been linked in patients treated with vinblastine plus bleomycin and PVB (Vogelzang et al. 1981, 1985; Vogelzang 1984).

Gonadal function was also studied. We compared treated patients to previously untreated patients to discover differences in the levels of serum luteinizing hormone (LH), follicle-stimulating hormone (FSH), and testosterone. To detect possible pituitary defects, we performed provocative testing with gonadotropin-releasing hormone (GnRH). Previously untreated patients had high normal levels of LH, comparable to those of previously treated patients, indicating an antecedent state of Leydig cell dysfunction. Follicle stimulating hormone levels in untreated patients were normal. After GnRH administration, peak levels of LH and FSH were significantly higher in treated patients than in untreated patients (Leitner et al. 1986). Testosterone levels were normal in both previously treated and untreated patients. These data indicate that untreated patients have some degree of Leydig cell insensitivity, that the pituitary is normal in its response to GnRH, that the Leydig cell suffers additional damage after chemotherapy, and that all treated patients have a compensated state of hypogonadism. The abnormalities tended to be less severe in patients younger than 25 years at the time of treatment and to normalize over time.

GOOD- AND POOR-RISK STUDIES

Selection Criteria

During these years of VAB development, it became clear that a proportion of patients would fail to achieve a CR; these patients generally died of their disease. In patients likely to achieve a CR ("good-risk" patients), the consequences of late toxicity from chemotherapy are important considerations; maintaining a high CR rate while minimizing toxicity is the goal for these patients. However, for patients unlikely to achieve CR ("poor-risk" patients), toxicity is important but efficacy takes precedence. Thus, we identified a need to distinguish between good- and poor-risk patients. The VAB experience (Israel et al. 1985; Bosl et al. 1986a) identified patients with extragonadal NSGCT as poor-risk, a conclusion similar to that of others (Garnick et al. 1983; Logothetis et al. 1985), and those with seminoma as good-risk. However, the patients with testicular NSGCT had varying outcomes.

Therefore we performed a multivariate analysis of prognostic variables in an attempt to identify those clinical characteristics that would independently predict a patient's outcome. In a study of 171 patients treated with high-dose cisplatin regimens, a patient's actual pretreatment serum values of lactate dehydrogenase (LDH) and human chorionic gonadotropin

(HCG) and the total number of sites of metastasis were the only independent variables contributing to a mathematical model that predicted CR (Bosl et al. 1983a). This model was validated on an independent data set from the University of Minnesota in which PVB was used to treat patients who had germ cell tumors. Beginning in December 1982, we used this model prospectively to allocate patients to either good- or poor-risk studies. The good-risk group encompassed all patients with seminoma and all patients with testicular NSGCT whose calculated probability of CR was greater than 0.5. The poor-risk category included all patients with extragonadal NSGCT and those with testicular NSGCT whose calculated probability of CR was less than 0.5.

Good-Risk Studies

Based on the ability of etoposide-and-cisplatin-based chemotherapy to cure some patients with resistant germ cell tumors (Bosl et al. 1985), 164 evaluable good-risk patients were randomly allocated to receive either VAB-6 or etoposide plus cisplatin (EP). Of 82 patients receiving VAB-6, 96% achieved CR, and of 82 patients receiving EP, 93% achieved CR. The relapse rate in both arms was 12%. The relapse-free, event-free, and total survival distributions for the two arms were not significantly different. Of interest, 31 of the 164 patients (19%) were found to be in the Einhorn "advanced disease" category (Birch et al. 1986), including 6 with hepatic metastases, 2 with bone metastases, and the remainder with either bulky pulmonary or bulky abdominal and pulmonary disease. Of these 31 patients, 27 (87%) remain in durable CR.

The toxicities of VAB-6 and EP differed. Quantitative emesis ($P = .05$), median white blood cell nadir ($P = .06$), platelet nadir ($P = .01$), and serum magnesium nadir ($P = .0001$) were less severe with EP than with VAB-6 (Bosl et al. 1988b). Bleomycin was discontinued in 16% of the patients receiving VAB-6 because of a more than 20% decrease in vital capacity, carbon monoxide diffusion capacity, or both. No treatment-related deaths occurred. Thus, among nearly 250 patients receiving VAB-6 and over 80 patients receiving EP in successive trials, none died as a result of treatment.

Poor-Risk Studies

The first poor-risk study used six cycles—three of VAB-6 and three of EP in alternate months. Of 41 patients treated, 21 (51%) achieved CR (Bosl et al. 1987b). Unfortunately, 7 of 21 patients (33%) relapsed from CR, leaving only 14 of 41 (34%) with a durable CR. This proportion of durable CRs in patients with poor-risk germ cell tumors is lower than that in other series. However, all patients with seminoma have been excluded, and those with bone or hepatic metastases or with a palpable abdominal mass with or without pulmonary metastases have not been categorized as poor-risk unless the calculated probability of their achieving CR was less than 0.5. The poor-risk criteria of MSKCC, the National Cancer Institute (NCI), the European Organization on Research and Treatment of Cancer (EORTC), and Indiana University differ considerably (Bosl et al. 1987a). Of 118 patients examined for assignment to good- and poor-risk groups, 31% were ascribed poor-risk status by MSKCC criteria, 49% by NCI criteria, 51% by the criteria of Indiana University, and 62% by EORTC criteria. Thus, some patients considered good-risk by one institution are included in poor-risk studies at another.

Current Studies

At MSKCC, patients continue to be allocated to good- and poor-risk programs based on pretreatment marker values and the number of sites of metastases.

In May 1985, we initiated a prospective phase II trial of etoposide plus carboplatin plus bleomycin for poor-risk patients. Carboplatin had been reported to be at least partially non–cross-resistant with cisplatin in animal studies and had a low but definable level of activity in a phase II study (Motzer et al. 1987). Thus, the possibility existed that an etoposide, bleomycin, carboplatin regimen might be more active than an etoposide, bleomycin, cisplatin regimen. Of the first 15 patients, 7 achieved CR, but in only 4 was the CR durable (Motzer et al. 1987). These results closely resemble the outcome of poor-risk patients treated on the initial VAB-6 trial (Bosl et al. 1988a).

The current good-risk study, which opened in December 1986, is a randomized comparison of EP vs. etoposide plus carboplatin. Carboplatin can be administered as outpatient therapy, has diminished nephrotoxicity, and causes less neurotoxicity and ototoxicity. Outpatient delivery would allow a reduction not only in drug-induced host toxicity but also in the financial burden of repeated hospitalization. Obviously, efficacy is the ultimate end result, and lessened toxicity is useful only if the regimens are equally active.

Acknowledgments

Prospective phase II and phase III trials evaluating treatment of patients with germ cell tumors at MSKCC have now included more than 800 patients. The contributions of the many investigators over the years who have participated in these trials cannot be overestimated. In particular, the contributions and insights of Drs. Robert Golbey and Willet F. Whitmore, Jr., have been present ever since the first report of "triple therapy" (Li et al. 1961). To the patients who participated in these trials we owe a debt of gratitude, for without them the studies summarized above could not have been accomplished.

REFERENCES

1. Birch R, Williams S, Long A, et al. 1986. Prognostic factors for favorable outcome in disseminated germ cell tumors. *J Clin Oncol* 4:400–407.
2. Blum RH, Carter SK, Agre K. 1973. A clinical review of bleomycin: A new antineoplastic agent. *Cancer* 31:903–914.
3. Bosl GJ, Bajorin D, Geller NL. 1987a. An analysis of poor risk assignment in patients with germ cell tumors. *Int J Androl* 10:285–289.
4. Bosl GJ, Geller NL, Bajorin D. 1988a. Identification and management of poor risk patients with germ cell tumors: The Memorial Sloan-Kettering Cancer Center experience. *Semin Oncol* In press.
5. Bosl GJ, Geller NL, Bajorin D, et al. 1988b. A randomized trial of etoposide + cisplatin versus vinblastine + bleomycin + cisplatin + cyclophosphamide + actinomycin D (VAB-6) in patients with good prognosis germ cell tumors. *J Clin Oncol* 6:1231–1238.
6. Bosl GJ, Geller NL, Cirrincione C, et al. 1983a. Multivariate analysis of prognostic variables in patients with metastatic testicular cancer. *Cancer Res* 43:3403–3407.
7. Bosl GJ, Geller NL, Cirrincione C, et al. 1983b. Serum tumor markers in patients with metastatic germ cell tumors of the testis. *Am J Med* 75:29–35.
8. Bosl GJ, Geller NL, Vogelzang NJ, et al. 1987b. Alternating cycles of etoposide + cisplatin and VAB-6 in the treatment of poor risk patients with germ cell tumors. *J Clin Oncol* 5:436–440.
9. Bosl GJ, Gluckman R, Geller NL, et al. 1986a. VAB-6: An effective chemotherapy regimen for patients with germ cell tumor. *J Clin Oncol* 4:1493–1499.

10. Bosl GJ, Leitner SP, Altas SA, et al. 1986b. Increased plasma renin and aldosterone in patients treated with cisplatin-based chemotherapy for metastatic germ cell tumors. *J Clin Oncol* 4:1684–1689.

11. Bosl GJ, Yagoda A, Golbey RB, et al. 1985. Role of etoposide-based chemotherapy in the treatment of patients with refractory or relapsing germ cell tumor. *Am J Med* 78:423–428.

12. Brenner J, Vugrin D, Whitmore W. 1982. Cytoreductive surgery for advanced nonseminomatous germ cell tumors of the testis. *Urology* 19:571–575.

13. Cheng E, Cvitkovic E, Wittes R, et al. 1978. Germ cell tumors: VAB II in metastatic testicular cancer. *Cancer* 42:2162–2168.

14. Einhorn LH, Donahue J. 1977. Cis-diamminedichloroplatinum, vinblastine, and bleomycin combination chemotherapy in disseminated testicular cancer. *Ann Intern Med* 87:293–298.

15. Garnick MB, Canellos GP, Richie JP. 1983. Treatment and surgical staging of testicular and primary extragonadal germ cell tumors. *JAMA* 250:1733–1741.

16. Hayes DM, Cvitkovic E, Golbey RB, et al. 1977. High dose cis-platinum diammine dichloride: Amelioration of renal toxicity by mannitol diuresis. *Cancer* 39:1372–1381.

17. Hong WK, Wittes RE, Hajdu ST, et al. 1977. The evolution of mature teratoma from malignant testicular tumors. *Cancer* 40:2987.

18. Israel A, Bosl GJ, Golbey RB, et al. 1985. The results of chemotherapy for extragonadal germ-cell tumors in the cisplatin era: The Memorial Sloan-Kettering Cancer Center experience (1975 to 1982). *J Clin Oncol* 3:1073–1078.

19. Leitner DP, Bosl GJ, Bajorunas D. 1986. Gonadal dysfunction in patients treated for metastatic germ cell tumors. *J Clin Oncol* 4:1500–1505.

20. Li MC, Whitmore WF, Golbey R, et al. 1961. Effects of combination drug therapy on metastatic cancer of the testis. *JAMA* 174:145–150.

21. Logothetis CJ, Samuels ML, Selig DE, et al. 1985. Chemotherapy of extragonadal germ cell tumors. *J Clin Oncol* 3:316–325.

22. Mackenzie AR. 1966. Chemotherapy of metastatic testis cancer: Results in 154 patients. *Cancer* 19:1369–1376.

23. Monfardini S, Bassetta E, Musumeli R, et al. 1972. Clinical use of adriamycin in advanced testicular cancer. *J Urol* 108:293.

24. Motzer RJ, Tauer K, Bosl GJ, et al. 1987. Phase II trial of carboplatin in patients with advanced germ cell tumors refractory to cisplatin. *Cancer Treat Rep* 71:197–198.

25. Reynolds TF, Vugrin D, Cvitkovic E, et al. 1981. VAB-3 combination chemotherapy of metastatic testicular cancer. *Cancer* 48:888–898.

26. Samuels ML, Howe CD. 1970. Vinblastine in the management of testicular cancer. *Cancer* 25:1009–1017.

27. Samuels ML, Lanzotti VJ, Holoye PY, et al. 1976. Combination chemotherapy in germinal cell tumors. *Cancer Treat Rev* 3:185–204.

28. Vugrin D, Cvitkovic E, Whitmore W, et al. 1981. VAB-4 combination chemotherapy in the treatment of metastatic testis tumor. *Cancer* 47:833–839.

29. Vugrin C, Whitmore W, Golbey R. 1983. VAB-6 combination chemotherapy in prognostically poor risk patients with germ cell tumors. *Cancer* 51:1072–1075.

30. Vogelzang NJ. 1984. Vascular and other complications of chemotherapy for testicular cancer. *World J Urol* 2:32–37.

31. Vogelzang NJ, Bosl GJ, Johnson K, et al. 1981. Raynaud's phenomenon: A common toxicity after combination chemotherapy for testicular cancer. *Ann Intern Med* 95:288–292.

32. Vogelzang NJ, Torkelson J, Kennedy BJ. 1985. Hypomagnesemia, renal function, and Raynaud's phenomenon in patients treated with cisplatin, vinblastine and bleomycin. *Cancer* 56:2765–2770.

33. Wittes RE, Yagoda A, Silvay O. 1976. Chemotherapy of germ cell tumors of the testis. *Cancer* 37:637–645.

Chemotherapy for Advanced Germ Cell Tumors of the Testis: The Stanford Experience

Richard K. Lo, M.D.

Fuad S. Freiha, M.D.

Frank M. Torti, M.D.

With the introduction of cisplatin-based combination chemotherapy and surgical resection of residual masses, most patients with advanced nonseminomatous germ cell tumors of the testis (NSGCTT) can expect a favorable clinical outcome (Vugrin et al. 1981; Donohue et al. 1982; Bracken et al. 1983). At Stanford University and the Northern California Oncology Group (NCOG), we have employed a flexible chemotherapy regimen, tailored to the responses of the patients during treatment. Our experience has indicated that, despite differences in chemotherapeutic agents, dosages, and schedules compared to other cancer centers, this tailored approach to therapy may have some advantage in complete responses and survivals of patients over other similar regimens that use a fixed number of chemotherapy cycles.

CHEMOTHERAPY PROTOCOL

At Stanford University, we have used, consistently, the same schedules of cisplatin, vinblastine, and bleomycin (PVB) combination chemotherapy in treating advanced metastatic NSGCTT. Patients were given cisplatin, 100 mg/m^2 (continuous intravenous infusion over 24 hours), after heavy hydration. Bleomycin was given at 15 units/m^2 at weekly intervals, to a maximum of 255 units/m^2. Vinblastine was administered at a dose between 0.13 and 0.18 mg/kg intravenously on days 1 and 2, with the exact dose gauged to patient age, prior exposure to chemotherapy, and the Karnofsky performance status. Treatment cycles were repeated every 3 weeks, until the tumor markers α-fetoprotein (AFP) and the β-subunit of human chorionic gonadotropin (HCG) returned to normal on two consecutive cycles and radiographic abnormalities had either reverted to normal or stabilized on two successive cycles.

RESULTS

Of 105 patients with stages IIC (bulky abdominal disease) and III NSGCTT, 92 (88%) remained continuously free of disease at 1 year and 89 (85%) at 2 years; the minimum follow-up period was 2 years. These responders were not maintained on any chemotherapy regimens.

Our experience with residual masses after PVB chemotherapy (Freiha et al. 1984) should be highlighted here. We evaluated 35 patients who were found to have residual masses that required surgical resection. In all, 40 procedures were performed. Preoperatively, all patients had had normal tumor marker levels and stable masses for two consecutive cycles. After resection, all patients were monitored without further maintenance chemotherapy. The histopathologic status of the resected specimens is summarized in Table 45–1.

Only one patient in the entire group had residual carcinoma (99% mature teratoma and 1% endodermal sinus tumor). He has remained free of disease more than 3 years postoperatively. Twenty-two sites in 18 patients contained teratoma only. The other 16 patients had fibrosis or necrosis in the surgical specimens. These figures appear to be superior to those from other testicular cancer series (Table 45–2).

Three of these 35 patients subsequently relapsed with embryonal carcinoma. All three had previously had complete resections, two of mature teratoma and one of predominantly mature teratoma with one focus of immaturity. They were successfully salvaged with additional chemotherapy. No patients with fibrosis or necrosis in the surgical specimens relapsed.

TABLE 45–1.
Surgical Resection of Residual Masses After
Chemotherapy: Histopathology and Clinical Outcome

| Pathologic Finding | Patients | | | |
| | Resected | | Relapsed | |
	No.	%	No.	%
Residual carcinoma	1	3	0	0
Teratoma	18	51	3	17
Fibrosis/necrosis	16	46	0	0
Total	35	100	3	9

TABLE 45–2.
Residual Masses After Chemotherapy: Comparison
of Chemotherapy Results

| Histopathologic Finding | Patients per Category (%) | | |
	Stanford	Indiana	Memorial
Carcinoma	3	44	43
Teratoma	51	32	19
Fibrosis/necrosis	46	24	38

COMMENTS

Early (and probably premature) surgical resection of residual masses was associated with a larger percentage of patients with viable tumors (Vugrin et al. 1981; Donohue et al. 1982; Bracken et al. 1983), and, probably, more relapses. Others have observed a rapid progression of disease after surgically removing residual cancer (Lange et al. 1980), a phenomenon that does not occur in patients with scar or fibrosis. These observations, coupled with our own data, imply that early, aggressive chemotherapy continued until tumor markers normalize and masses are stable radiographically has the best chance of sterilizing viable tumor cells and, by extrapolation, since patients whose residual masses contain cancer do poorly, offers a better prognosis.

Decay of the serum tumor marker level is usually an accurate predictor of response to PVB chemotherapy. Failure of tumor marker levels to return to the normal range after therapy is complete indicates the persistence of tumor. The converse, however, is not necessarily true. Up to 30% of patients with normalized tumor marker levels after chemotherapy were found to have residual tumors in the resected masses.

In an attempt to devise a "rule" for predicting therapeutic outcome using serum tumor markers, we reviewed a group of 106 consecutive patients with stage III NSGCTT evaluated by Stanford University and the NCOG (Picozzi et al. 1984). Forty-two had an elevated level of HCG before beginning chemotherapy, and 40 of these were evaluable. As per the treatment protocol, tumor marker levels were determined at the beginning of each cycle (days 1, 22, 43, etc.) to measure response to chemotherapy. We then compared our predictions, based on declining HCG levels, with the actual clinical courses of the patients.

Using the day 1 and day 22 HCG levels, we developed an empirically derived rule and tested it for its predictive value. If the ratio of the day 22 HCG level to the day 1 level was more than 1:200 (0.005), and the level on day 22 was elevated, an incomplete response was predicted (Fig 45–1). Of 19 patients who had an incomplete response, 17 belonged in this category, for a sensitivity of 90% and a predictive value of 94%. Conversely, a favorable therapeutic outcome could be predicted, with a sensitivity of 95%, if the HCG level fell to or below the 1:200 rule. The overall, long-term accuracy of this rule was confirmed in 37 of 40 patients ($P < .001$).

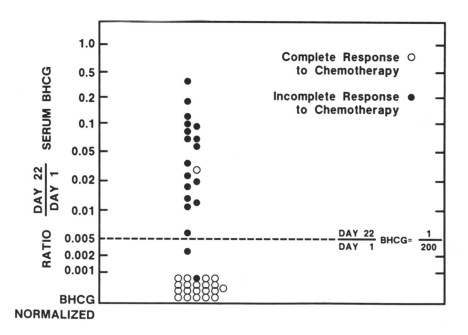

FIG 45–1.
Response to chemotherapy according to level of β-human chorionic gonadotropin (*BHCG*) at day 1 and day 22.

CONCLUSION

We have presented our data on the treatment of advanced NSGCTT, and they are superior or comparable to those of other institutions. Given these impressive survival statistics, the next step is to identify those who may ultimately fail and to change the chemotherapeutic agents early, before these patients become too pancytopenic to undergo salvage chemotherapy. We, like other institutions, have substituted etoposide (VP-16-213) for vinblastine to minimize marrow toxicity. The preliminary results indicate equal efficacy with slightly less toxicity for this regimen.

Treatment with flexible chemotherapy programs such as ours will minimize the number of patients with residual tumors and maximize the percentage of durable responders.

REFERENCES

1. Bracken RB, Johnson DE, Frazier OH, et al. 1983. The role of surgery following chemotherapy for stage III germ cell neoplasms. *J Urol* 129:39–43.
2. Donohue JP, Roth LM, Zachary JM, et al. 1982. Cytoreductive surgery for metastatic testis cancer: Tissue analysis of retroperitoneal masses after chemotherapy. *J Urol* 127:1111–1114.
3. Freiha FS, Shortliffe LD, Rouse RV, et al. 1984. The extent of surgery after chemotherapy for advanced germ cell tumors. *J Urol* 132:915–917.
4. Lange PH, Hekmat K, Bosl G, et al. 1980. Accelerated growth of testicular cancer after cytoreductive surgery. *Cancer* 45:1498–1506.
5. Picozzi VJ, Freiha FS, Hannigan JF, et al. 1984. Prognostic significance of a decline in serum human chorionic gonadotropin levels after initial chemotherapy for advanced germ-cell carcinoma. *Ann Intern Med* 100:183–186.
6. Vugrin D, Whitmore WF, Sogani PC, et al. 1981. Combined chemotherapy and surgery in treatment of advanced germ cell tumors. *Cancer* 47:2228–2231.

Chapter 46 _____

Chemotherapy of Advanced Germ Cell Tumors: Overview of Australasian Germ Cell Tumor Group Studies

Derek Raghavan, M.B.B.S., Ph.D., F.R.A.C.P.

John Levi, M.B.B.S., F.R.A.C.P.

Damien Thomson, M.B.B.S., F.R.A.C.P.

Michael Byrne, M.B.B.S., F.R.A.C.P.

Vernon Harvey, M.D., M.R.C.P.

Martin H. N. Tattersall, M.D., F.R.C.P.,
F.R.A.C.P.

Richard Fox, M.B.B.S., Ph.D., F.R.A.C.P.

Richard Abbott, M.B.B.S., F.R.A.C.P.

Ivon Burns, M.B.B.S., F.R.A.C.P.

James Bishop, M.B.B.S., F.R.A.C.P., F.R.C.P.A.

Thomas Sandeman, M.D., Ch.B., D.M.R.T.
F.R.C.R., F.R.A.C.R.

Zoltan Kerestes, Ph.D.

Members of the Australasian
Germ Cell Trial Group

The introduction of cisplatin into chemotherapy regimens has revolutionized the management of metastatic germ cell tumors, improving cure rates from less than 20% to more than 60% to 90%, depending on the stage and volume of disease. The Australasian Germ Cell Trial (AGCT) Group has carried out a series of trials with the aim of further rationalizing the use of chemotherapy in the treatment of this disease by reducing toxicity and improving the cost-effectiveness of schedules of delivery. In this chapter, we review the design and application of the trials conducted since 1979.

PATIENTS AND METHODS

Patients with biopsy-proved germ cell tumors were entered into three sequential trials outlined in Table 46–1. Each patient had inoperable stage II or III tumors, classified according to the system developed at The University of Texas M. D. Anderson Cancer Center (Samuels et al. 1976). In the initial study, all patients were treated according to a common protocol (Levi et al. 1988). Prognostic factors for survival were determined from the results of this trial and were validated by comparison with other large clinical studies (Einhorn 1981; Peckham et al. 1981; Bosl et al. 1983). These factors formed the basis of two subsequent trials for patients with "poor-prognosis" and "good-prognosis" tumors (see Table 46–1). Although reported in detail elsewhere (Levi et al. 1988), these prognostic groups were classified on the basis of tumor mass and sites of involvement. The characteristics of the patients are summarized in Table 46–2.

Before the commencement of chemotherapy, patients underwent detailed clinical staging, including a complete history and physical examination, chest x-ray, full blood count, biochemical profile including renal and liver function, and measurement of serum α-fetoprotein (AFP) and β-subunit human chorionic gonadotropin (β-HCG). Tumor mass was assessed clinically and by computed tomography, plain x-rays, lymphography, and radionuclide scans, as appropriate. Serial audiography and pulmonary function tests were performed for most patients.

The details of the treatment programs have been reported elsewhere (Levi et al. 1986, 1988; Raghavan, Thomson, Levi, and Bishop unpublished data) and are summarized in Table

TABLE 46–1.
Trial Design*

Study	Drug	Dose	Schedule	Accrual	Status	Comments
1	cDDP	100 mg/m²	IV, day 1 3 × weekly	1979–1983	Closed	If CR, randomized to ± VBX maintenance. See text for total dosage.
	VBX	6 mg/m²	IV, days 1 + 2 3 × weekly			
	Bleo	30 units	IM/IV weekly			
2†	cDDP	70 mg/m²	IV, days 1 + 2	1984–1985	Closed	Failures retreated with PVB or POMBACE
	VP-16	120 mg/m²	IV, days 1–3			
3†	cDDP	100 mg/m²	IV, day 1 3 × weekly	1985–present	Ongoing	—
	VBX	6 mg/m²	IV, days 1 + 2 3 × weekly			
	± Bleo	30 units	IM/IV weekly			See text for total dosage.

*cDDP = cisplatin; VBX = vinblastine; Bleo = bleomycin; IV = intravenous; IM = intramuscular; CR = complete remission; VP-16 = etoposide; PVB = cisplatin, vinblastine, and bleomycin; POMBACE = Charing Cross regimen, with cisplatin, vincristine, methotrexate, bleomycin, actinomycin D, cyclophosphamide, and etoposide.
†Note: Study 2 for patients with "poor-prognosis" tumors and Study 3 for patients with "good-risk" disease (see text).

TABLE 46–2.
Characteristics of Patients*

Characteristic	Trial		
	AGCT1	AGCT2	AGCT3
No.			
Entered into study	260	29	184
Assessed	253	28	152
Age			
Median	29	30	29
Range	15–65	16–59	14–67
ECOG status			
0–1	215	22	143
2–3	32	6	41
4	6	0	0
Sites of primary tumor			
Testis	223	23	152
Extragonadal	23	5	0
Ovary	7	0	0
β-HCG>1,000 IU/L	53	12	21
AFP>1,000 ng/ml	47	7	13
Prior radiotherapy	33	4	10
Prior chemotherapy	3	5	0
Prognostic groups	All	"Poor-risk"	"Good-risk"

*AGCT = Australasian Germ Cell Trial; ECOG = European Co-operative Oncology Group; β-HCG = β-human chorionic gonadotropin; AFP = α-fetoprotein.

46–1. The number of courses of induction chemotherapy was determined by clinical and tumor-marker response without an empirical upper limit. Patients were reassessed clinically, and tumor markers were measured after each course of chemotherapy; the other investigations noted above were repeated after every two courses. If complete remission (CR) were achieved, two additional courses of induction treatment were administered. In the first trial (see Table 46–1), patients achieving CR were randomized to receive maintenance vinblastine or no further treatment. In the second and third trials, maintenance chemotherapy was not given.

Patients with residual masses after induction chemotherapy underwent surgical resection whenever possible (provided that circulating tumor-marker levels were normal). If the resected specimen were composed of necrotic tissue, fibrosis, or differentiated teratoma, patients were then considered to be in CR. If viable cancer were found in the specimen but had been completely removed, the patients were classified as having no residual evidence of disease (NED), received two further courses of induction chemotherapy (first trial) or alternative chemotherapy (second and third trials), and were subsequently monitored.

Patients in whom surgical resection was incomplete, those who had persistently raised levels of tumor markers, and those with obvious clinical tumor progression during or after chemotherapy were classified as treatment failures. Most of these patients were treated according to salvage protocols at the discretion of the investigator.

The durations of response and of survival were calculated from the date chemotherapy began until the time of relapse, death, or last follow-up.

RESULTS

The response rates achieved in the first and second trials are summarized in Table 46–3. Interim response data for the two arms in the third trial are also documented in this table, although it is emphasized that these are *preliminary* data, as the study is not yet complete.

The major side effects of chemotherapy were myelosuppression, nausea and vomiting, alopecia, and pulmonary toxicity. In the first trial, neutropenia was the major hematologic side effect: 23% of patients developed nadir white blood cell counts lower than $1,000/\mu l$. Thrombocytopenia (platelet nadir $<100,000/\mu l$) occurred in 32% of patients, but no significant hemorrhagic episodes resulted. These hematologic problems were more severe in patients who had received prior radiotherapy than in those who had only undergone surgery ($P<.01$). Severe (grade 3–4) renal dysfunction occurred in only 3% of patients, in all instances in conjunction with septicemia.

Bleomycin-related pulmonary toxicity was documented in 46% of patients, was severe in 4%, and was the direct cause of death in eight. Seven of these deaths occurred among the first 100 patients treated in the trial. By contrast, in the latter 153 cases, the administration of bleomycin was terminated when serial pulmonary function studies showed a fall in diffusing lung capacity of carbon dioxide (DLCO) of greater than 25%, and only one death occurred.

A similar pattern of toxicity was noted in the PVB (cisplatin, vinblastine, bleomycin) arm of the third trial, also reflecting the experience reported in other studies (Einhorn 1981; Peckham et al. 1981; Stoter et al. 1986). By contrast, in the third trial, the two-drug combination (cisplatin-etoposide) induced a significantly lower rate of acute toxicity ($P<.01$), with fewer episodes of leukopenia, thrombocytopenia, and renal dysfunction. Of particular importance, no episodes of pulmonary toxicity occurred after the two-drug combination, as compared with 30% after PVB in this randomized trial.

Analogous to treatment with vinblastine and cisplatin, the use of etoposide and 140 mg/m² cisplatin was associated with modest toxicity. Only 11% of patients had white blood cell counts less than $1,000/\mu l$, although 40% had grade 4 thrombocytopenia. Although nausea and vomiting were severe in 53%, there were no severe cases of pulmonary or auditory toxicity, or neurotoxicity, and only three cases of grade 3 renal dysfunction. No treatment-related deaths resulted from this regimen.

In the first AGCT, a 5-year actuarial disease-free survival rate of 81% was demonstrated for patients achieving CR/NED; for the total series, the rate was 61% (Levi et al. 1988). The total long-term survival rate of all treated patients was 68% (84% for those achieving CR/NED status). In the second trial, patients with "poor-prognosis" tumors had a long-term survival rate of 54%. In the third AGCT, preliminary analysis has shown 3-year actuarial survival

TABLE 46–3.
Objective Response*

Study	Regimen	Total No. of Patients	CR/NED No.	CR/NED %	Comments
1	PVB	253	191	76	All tumors
2	PE	28	12	43	"Poor risk" tumors
3[†]	PVB	75	67	89	"Good risk"
	PV	77	68	88	tumors

*P = cisplatin; V = vinblastine; B = bleomycin; E = etoposide; CR = complete remission; NED = no evidence of residual disease after surgery.
†Ongoing.

figures of greater than 90% for both the two-drug i.e., PV, and PVB combinations. Again, it is emphasized that this study is ongoing and the data are preliminary.

DISCUSSION

Cisplatin-containing chemotherapy regimens now have a proven role in the management of advanced germ cell tumors (Einhorn 1981; Peckham et al. 1981; Bosl et al. 1986a), and most patients with this disease will be cured. However, analogous to the situation in advanced Hodgkin's disease, concern is increasing regarding the possibility of late toxicity or of treatment-related deaths from the use of these complicated combination chemotherapy regimens (Vogelzang 1984; Levi et al. 1986). In addition to well-documented acute toxicity (Einhorn 1981; Peckham et al. 1981; Bosl et al. 1986a), chronic side effects have been documented, including pulmonary damage (Weiss and Muggia 1980), vascular complications (Rothberg 1978; Sundstrup 1978; Edwards et al. 1979; Vogelzang et al. 1980, 1984; Bosl et al. 1986b), and occasional second malignancies (Mead et al. 1983). As a result, emphasis has increasingly been placed on attempts to ameliorate the toxicity of the treatment regimens (Bosl et al. 1980; Wettlaufer et al. 1984; Stoter et al. 1986) without losing the high cure rates achieved with conventional therapy.

The initial Australasian Germ Cell Trial demonstrated the comparable efficacy of a regimen of vinblastine, bleomycin, and a 1-day schedule of administration of 100 mg/m^2 cisplatin and that reported for the conventional 5-day schedule (Einhorn 1981; Peckham et al. 1981; Stoter et al. 1986), although this was not a randomized trial. This study also confirmed the earlier report (Einhorn 1981) that the use of adjuvant vinblastine did not improve outcome.

The toxicity of treatment also was similar to that reported for the conventional 5-day regimen. Of importance, myelosuppression was significantly greater in patients who had previously received radiotherapy. The introduction of more sophisticated indices of pulmonary function into routine practice during the latter period of the first trial, with appropriate modification of bleomycin dosage, resulted in a reduced prevalence of severe pulmonary toxicity. Nevertheless, this side effect was somewhat unpredictable, despite the monitoring of DLCO.

In this large, nonrandomized trial, univariate analysis yielded the following adverse prognostic factors: extent of disease, poor performance status, an extragonadal origin for the primary tumor, and circulating levels of AFP or β-HCG greater than 1,000 ng/ml or 1,000 IU/L, respectively. However, multivariate regression analysis showed only extent of disease and pretreatment elevated blood level of β-HCG as independent adverse prognostic factors (Levi et al. 1988). These factors are similar to those reported by others (Einhorn 1981; Bosl et al. 1983; Birch et al. 1986), although lactate dehydrogenase (LDH) was not routinely measured in our study. On the basis of these data, it was possible to divide the patient population for subsequent studies into those with "good-prognosis" and "poor-prognosis" disease, and to attempt to define different strategies of treatment for each group.

In view of the activity of high-dose cisplatin (200 mg/m^2) in the management of "poor-prognosis" germ cell tumors (Ozols et al. 1983), the second AGCT was initiated in which a moderate dose escalation of cisplatin was effected (140 mg/m^2, divided into two doses) for patients with "poor-risk" tumors. This dose was chosen to avoid the severe toxicity associated with higher doses. Although the response rate was comparable to that achieved with the PVB regimen, there was no obvious benefit to this approach apart from a possible reduction in acute toxicity. Further evaluation of this regimen has not been pursued pending a judgment of the duration of response. Since the patients who achieved CR have remained in CR, this approach may be incorporated into future studies. Of particular interest, there was no obvious increase in nephrotoxicity or ototoxicity with the increased dose of cisplatin, despite the fact that hypertonic saline was not used in the schedule of delivery.

The current AGCT, which is not yet complete, is assessing the safety and efficacy of omitting bleomycin from the conventional three-drug PVB regimen for patients who have good-risk metastatic testicular cancer (Levi et al. 1986). This study is still accruing patients, and a minimum follow-up period of 3 years for all patients will be required before a definitive statement can be made. To date, there is no significant difference in response rate or overall duration of survival, although a statistically significant difference in acute toxicity has been shown. This is true particularly for pulmonary toxicity and treatment-related deaths. Nevertheless, a slightly higher relapse rate after the two-drug regimen *at present* must be monitored closely.

Future trials in Australia and New Zealand will explore the utility of carboplatin, a less toxic analogue of cisplatin, in combination regimens for the routine management of germ cell tumors. In addition, the policy of active surveillance only for patients with stage I germ cell tumors has been assessed prospectively (Raghavan et al. 1984, in press; Dewar et al. 1987). The cautious application of well-structured, innovative trials and the development of less toxic chemotherapeutic agents and improved diagnostic tests will allow investigators to maintain the high cure rates achieved for this disease while reducing the morbidity suffered by the patient. In this fashion, the treatment of germ cell tumors will serve as a model for the development of therapeutic strategies against other cancers.

Acknowledgments

We gratefully acknowledge the collaboration and active participation of our colleagues in the Australasian Germ Cell Trial Group: Alan Coates, Royal Prince Alfred Hospital, Sydney, NSW; David Dalley, St. Vincent's Hospital, Sydney, NSW; Albert Freedman, Prince of Wales Hospital, Sydney, NSW; Grantley Gill, Royal Adelaide Hospital, Adelaide, South Australia; Alan Gray, Wellington Hospital, Wellington, New Zealand; Geoff Hawson, Prince Charles Hospital, Brisbane, Queensland; Richard Kefford, Westmead Hospital, Sydney, NSW; Ray Lowenthal, Royal Hobart Hospital, Hobart, Tasmania; Ken MacMillan, Peter MacCallum Clinic, Hobart, Tasmania; Max Schwarz, Alfred Hospital, Melbourne, Victoria; Keiran Phadke, St. George Hospital, Sydney, NSW; Raymond Snyder, St. Vincent's Hospital, Melbourne, Victoria; Bert Sundstrup, Peter MacCallum Clinic, Launceston, Tasmania; Robert Woods, Repatriation General Hospital, Sydney, NSW.

REFERENCES

1. Birch R, Williams S, Cone A, et al. 1986. Prognostic factors for favorable outcome in disseminated germ cell tumors. *J Clin Oncol* 4:400–407.
2. Bosl GJ, Geller N, Cirrincione C, et al. 1983. Multivariate analysis of prognostic variables in patients with metastatic testicular cancer. *Cancer Res* 43:3403–3407.
3. Bosl GJ, Gluckman R, Geller NL, et al. 1986a. VAB-6: An effective chemotherapy regimen for patients with germ cell tumors. *J Clin Oncol* 4:1493–1499.
4. Bosl GJ, Kwong R, Lange PH, et al. 1980. Vinblastine, intermittent bleomycin, and single-dose cis-dichlorodiammineplatinum(II) in the management of stage III testicular cancer. *Cancer Treat Rep* 64:331–334.
5. Bosl GJ, Leitner SP, Atlas SA, et al. 1986b. Increased plasma renin and aldosterone in patients treated with cisplatin-based chemotherapy for metastatic germ-cell tumors. *J Clin Oncol* 4:1684–1689.
6. Dewar JM, Spagnolo DV, Jamrozik KD, et al. 1987. Predicting relapse in stage I non-seminomatous germ cell tumours of the testis (letter). *Lancet* 1:454.

7. Edwards GS, Lane M, Smith FE. 1979. Long-term treatment with cis-dichlorodiamminoplatinum (II)-vinblastine-bleomycin: Possible association with severe coronary artery disease (letter). *Cancer Treat Rep* 63:551–552.
8. Einhorn LH. 1981. Testicular cancer as a model for a curable neoplasm. The Richard and Hinda Rosenthal Foundation Award Lecture. *Cancer Res* 41:3275–3280.
9. Levi J, Raghavan D, Harvey V, et al. 1986. Deletion of bleomycin from therapy for good prognosis advanced testicular cancer: A prospective randomized study (abstract). *Proc Am Soc Clin Oncol* 5:97.
10. Levi JA, Thomson D, Sandeman T, et al. 1988. A prospective study of cisplatin based combination chemotherapy in advanced germ cell malignancy: Role of maintenance and long term follow-up. *J Clin Oncol* 6:1154–1160.
11. Mead GM, Green JA, Macbeth FR, et al. 1983. Second malignancy after cisplatin, vinblastine, and bleomycin (PVB) chemotherapy: A case report (letter). *Cancer Treat Rep* 67:410.
12. Ozols RF, Deisseroth AB, Javadpour N, et al. 1983. Treatment of poor prognosis nonseminomatous testicular cancer with "high dose" platinum combination chemotherapy regimen. *Cancer* 51:1803–1807.
13. Peckham MJ, Barret A, McElwain TJ, et al. 1981. Non-seminoma germ cell tumours (malignant teratoma) of the testis: Results of treatment and an analysis of prognostic factors. *Br J Urol* 53:162–172.
14. Raghavan D. 1984. Expectant therapy for clinical stage A nonseminomatous germ-cell cancers of the testis? A qualified "yes." *World J Urol* 2:59–63.
15. Raghavan D, Colls B, Levi J, et al. 1988. Surveillance for stage I nonseminoma germ cell tumours of the testis (NSGCT): The optimal protocol has not yet been defined. *Br J Urol* 61:522–526.
16. Raghavan D, Thomson D, Levi J, et al. (submitted for publication). Etoposide and 140 mg/m² cisplatin as induction treatment for "bad-risk" advanced germ cell tumours.
17. Rothberg H. 1978. Raynaud's phenomenon after vinblastine-bleomycin chemotherapy. *Cancer Treat Rep* 62:569–570.
18. Samuels ML, Lanzotti VJ, Holoye PY, et al. 1976. Combination chemotherapy in germinal cell tumors. *Cancer Treat Rev* 3:185–204.
19. Stoter G, Sleyfer DT, Ten Bokkel Huinink WW, et al. 1986. High-dose versus low-dose vinblastine in cisplatin-vinblastine-bleomycin combination chemotherapy of non-seminomatous testicular cancer: A randomized study of the EORTC Genitourinary Tract Cancer Cooperative Group. *J Clin Oncol* 4:1199–1206.
20. Sundstrup B. 1978. Raynaud's phenomenon after bleomycin treatment (letter). *Med J Aust* 2:266.
21. Vogelzang NJ. 1984. Vascular and other complications of chemotherapy for testicular cancer. *World J Urol* 2:32–37.
22. Vogelzang NJ, Frenning DH, Kennedy BJ. 1980. Coronary artery disease after treatment with bleomycin and vinblastine. *Cancer Treat Rep* 64:1159–1160.
23. Weiss RB, Muggia FM. 1980. Cytotoxic drug-induced pulmonary disease: Update 1980. *Am J Med* 68:259–266.
24. Wettlaufer JN, Feiner AS, Robinson WA. 1984. Vincristine, cisplatin, and bleomycin with surgery in the management of advanced metastatic nonseminomatous testis tumors. *Cancer* 53:203–209.

Long-Term Follow-up of Patients Treated with Cyclic CISCA$_{II}$/VB$_{IV}$ at The University of Texas M. D. Anderson Cancer Center

Christopher J. Logothetis, M.D.

Clayton D.K. Chong, M.D.

Sheryl Ogden, R.N.

A regimen of cyclophosphamide, cisplatin, and doxorubicin (Adriamycin) alternating with vinblastine and bleomycin (CISCA$_{II}$/VB$_{IV}$) (Table 47–1) has been used to treat patients with germ cell tumors at The University of Texas M. D. Anderson Cancer Center since 1981. The original report of that experience (Logothetis et al. 1985) suggested that treatment induced a high complete-remission (CR) rate accompanied by near-universal sterilization of retroperitoneal metastasis and a virtual absence of late relapses. In a subsequent update of CISCA$_{II}$/VB$_{IV}$, we analyzed the results of treatment of 100 patients with metastatic germ cell tumors (Logothetis et al. 1986).

In that report, we concluded that the morbidity of CISCA$_{II}$/VB$_{IV}$ was significant, although its mortality was low (1%). The side effects encountered were severe, but also acutely reversible. Because the initial results were encouraging and toxicity acceptable, we have expanded the study to now include 167 patients. Thirteen of the original patients had extragonadal tumors, and all others had testicular primary tumors. In this review, we analyze our experience with all 167 patients placed on the protocol.

STUDY POPULATION

The 167 patients evaluable for response and survival had histologically confirmed germ cell tumors treated with CISCA$_{II}$/VB$_{IV}$ at UT M. D. Anderson Cancer Center. All patients who began the protocol were eligible for analysis, including those who required treatment adjustment because of toxicity.

TABLE 47–1.
CISCA$_{II}$/VB$_{IV}$ Dose Schema

Drug	Dosage
CISCA$_{II}$	
Cyclophosphamide	500 mg/m^2 BSA* on day 1, day 2
Adriamycin	45 mg/m^2 BSA on day 1, day 2
Cisplatin	100–120 mg/m^2 BSA on day 13
VB$_{IV}$	
Vinblastine	3 mg/m^2 BSA × 5 (continuous infusion)
Bleomycin	30 mg/m^2 × 5 (continuous infusion)

*BSA = body surface area.

RESULTS

Survival

The term "survival," as used in this study, indicates disease-free survival. In this analysis, all patients who are alive with evidence of recurrent disease or have died of complications attributed to chemotherapy have been tabulated as dead of disease. Only patients who have died of clearly unrelated causes have been included in the group tabulated as alive and disease free at their most recent visit. All patients were either clinically evaluated at UT M. D. Anderson Cancer Center or the records of their most recent physical examination and laboratory data from their private physicians were obtained. In addition, all patients were contacted by telephone.

Survival rates were tabulated according to M. D. Anderson stage (Table 47–2), histologic type (Table 47–3), and Indiana stage (Table 47–4). Histologic type did not significantly influence long-term disease-free survival, although patients with choriocarcinoma had the lowest survival rate (56%). In our earlier experience, a multivariate analysis showed that only those patients with pure choriocarcinoma and serum biomarkers elevated above 50,000 mU/ml were associated with a poor survival rate; this relationship continues. Stage and site of origin were influential only in that those patients with extragonadal primary tumors had a poor survival rate. Overall, patients with minimal disease (clinical stage II, Samuels clinical stage III-B$_3$) achieved a nearly 100% long-term disease-free survival rate; only those with stages IIIB$_4$ and IIIB$_5$ disease appeared to have lower survival rates. The survival rate of patients with truly extragonadal germ cell tumors was significantly inferior to that of patients with testicular primary tumors.

According to the staging system employed by the Indiana University Hospital, patients with moderate and minimal disease nearly universally survived: the rates exceeded 90%. Disease-free survival rates were not significantly different for these two categories, and the anticipated outcome was excellent. The disease-free survival rate for patients with advanced disease was 69%.

Our follow-up has ranged from 5 to 394 weeks (median, 185 weeks). All patients considered disease free have been monitored sequentially for 18 months.

Toxicity

Only the first 100 patients have been meticulously analyzed for toxicity. The results, which were reported previously, were tabulated into two broad groups, acute toxicity (Table 47–5) and long-term toxicity (Table 47–6). Acute toxicity was severe and frequent. Morbidity

TABLE 47–2.
CISCA$_{II}$/VB$_{IV}$: Influence of Clinical Stage on Subsequent Disease-Free Survival

	Patients		
		Disease-Free	
Stage	Total	No.	%
Testicular			
Clinical II	59	55	93
IIIA	3	3	100
IIIB$_1$	3	3	100
IIIB$_2$	23	21	91
IIIB$_3$	16	14	88
IIIB$_4$	28	22	79
IIIB$_5$	22	16	73
Extragonadal	13	8	62
Total	167	142	85

TABLE 47–3.
CISCA$_{II}$/VB$_{IV}$: Influence of Histologic Type on Subsequent Survival Rate

	Patients		
		Disease-Free	
Cell Type	Total	No.	%
Seminoma (Dixon-Moore I)	5	5	100
Embryonal carcinoma (Dixon-Moore II)	59	53	90
Mature teratoma (Dixon-Moore III)	0	0	—
Teratocarcinoma (Dixon-Moore IV)	85	74	87
Choriocarcinoma (Dixon-Moore V)	9	5	56
Pure endodermal sinus tumor	6	4	67
No histologic analysis	3	1	33
Total	167	142	85

TABLE 47–4.
CISCA$_{II}$/VB$_{IV}$: Relationship Between Indiana Stage and Subsequent Disease-Free Survival Rate

	Patients		
		Disease-Free	
Indiana Stage	Total	No.	%
Minimal	87	81	93
Moderate	29	26	90
Advanced	51	35	69
Total	167	142	85

TABLE 47–5.
Incidence of Acute Toxicity

Type	CISCA$_{II}$ Courses		VB$_{IV}$ Courses	
	No.	%	No.	%
Stomatitis				
Grade 1	52	19.0	98	45.0
Grade 2	11	4.0	39	18.0
Grade 3	2	0.7	7	3.0
Intestinal toxicity				
Obstipation			62	29.0
Paralytic ileus			7	3.0
Pericarditis			6	3.0
Hypertension	2	0.7	9	4.0
Leukopenic fever				
Culture-negative	98	36.0	95	44.0
Culture-positive	15	5.0	17	8.0
Soft-tissue infection	10	4.0	5	2.0
Urinary-tract infection	5	2.0	9	4.0
Pneumonia	5	2.0	2	0.9
Drug-induced hepatitis	6	2.0	4	2.0
Pancreatitis				
Rectal abscess	1	0.4		
Inappropriate secretion of antidiuretic hormone	7	3.0	1	0.5
Anaphylactic reaction	1	0.4		
Clinical systemic candidiasis			1	0.5
Rhabdomyolyis			1	0.5
Viral myocarditis	1	0.4		
Granulomatous disease of unknown origin			1	0.5

TABLE 47–6.
Incidence of Chronic Toxicity

Type	Patients	
	No.	%
Bleomycin lung toxicity		
Positive results on gallium scanning	7	7
Positive results on gallium scanning plus drop in forced vital capacity of more than 10%	1	1
Renal toxicity	3	3
Hearing loss		
Documented hearing loss	3	3
Tinnitus	2	2
Peripheral neuropathy	10	10
Raynaud's phenomenon	1	1
Cardiac toxicity	1	1

was very high, but the mortality was very low (2/167 patients; only 1 in the first 100). By its nature, acute toxicity was reversible, but the chronic toxicity persisted and became a significant factor affecting these patients' future lives.

Long-term toxicity occurred at a low frequency; cisplatin neuropathy and nephrotoxicity were the most frequent. A single patient suffered cardiomyopathy and had a transient drop in ejection fraction but recovered fully. Although attributed to Adriamycin, we believe that this reaction in reality represented a viral myocarditis. No histologic proof of Adriamycin cardiotoxicity was obtained.

Bleomycin pulmonary toxicity is evaluated at UT M. D. Anderson Cancer Center with a combination of a 48-hour gallium scan and spirometry. If a previously negative gallium scan converts to a positive one, bleomycin is deleted. A 10% drop in forced vital capacity is considered to be significant, and bleomycin is deleted if this occurs, also. Only a single patient had both a drop in the forced vital capacity and a converted gallium scan, although the gallium scans of 7 additional patients among the first 100 treated converted to positive. No patient has suffered fatal or clinically significant bleomycin pulmonary toxicity that restricted pulmonary function.

The late deaths occurred in one patient who died suddenly from unknown causes at 100 weeks after therapy, one who died in an automobile accident, one who died of a colon carcinoma, and three who died with the acquired immune deficiency syndrome (AIDS). Two of the three patients who developed AIDS had recognized risk factors associated with this condition.

Late Relapses

Only three patients had a late recurrence of their tumor (defined as >100 weeks disease-free survival). All three patients had late regrowth of teratoma. The mass in one patient could not be excised; the patient refused further therapy and died of growing teratoma in the mediastinum. One patient had a single site of teratoma excised and remains disease free. A third patient's disease has also been controlled with chemotherapy and excision of the remaining teratoma. Late death related to tumor occurred in only one patient. All late relapses were associated with persistent teratomatous elements radiographically visible at the time chemotherapy was completed. Two patients had unrecognized persistent teratoma. In each case the radiographs were misinterpreted: the mass was either considered to reveal the presence of a lymphocele or simply was not seen (one patient each). One patient had an unresectable mediastinal teratoma that was observed and showed evidence of late regrowth.

DISCUSSION

Our experience with CISCA$_{II}$/VB$_{IV}$ continues to demonstrate the effectiveness of this regimen. The 93% disease-free survival rate compares favorably with the rate reported from other intense regimens. The very intense regimen of cisplatin, vincristine, dactinomycin (actinomycin D), methotrexate, chlorambucil, bleomycin, and etoposide (VP-16-23) (POM-BACE) reported by Newlands et al. (1983) also achieves a high CR rate. The one subcategory of patients with a relatively low CR rate is that of patients with a high serum level of β-human chorionic gonadotropin (β-HCG), defined as 50 mIu/ml at our institution. Similar poor prognostic groups of patients have been identified by other investigators (Bosl et al. 1983; Stoter et al. 1984). These patients remain a therapeutic challenge: they have an overall relatively low cure rate and require an intensive therapeutic approach to achieve a CR. Nevertheless, we are convinced that CISCA$_{II}$/VB$_{IV}$ achieves results superior to those achieved with standard cisplatin, vinblastine, and bleomycin (PVB) combination chemotherapy regimens. Our conviction is based on the higher CR rate achieved when our patients with very far advanced disease by the Indiana staging system are compared to PVB-treated patients similarly staged.

The toxicity of $CISCA_{II}/VB_{IV}$ is substantial. Severe myelosuppression is routine. Stomatitis occurs frequently, and other acute side effects involving the gastrointestinal tract, emesis, and infections due to myelosuppression are nearly universal. Despite this, mortality is low. In the hands of experienced oncologists, the toxicity of $CISCA_{II}/VB_{IV}$ is very manageable. However, this regimen should always be delivered cautiously by experienced oncologists and with adequate support facilities available to avoid life-threatening complications.

Toxicity is currently measured in many institutions by the frequency and degree of myelosuppression, the frequency of infections, and the severity of gastrointestinal side effects (mucositis and emesis). These side effects are significant and require meticulous management, but the more important toxicity in a patient population expected to achieve durable CRs is that which is associated with long-term side effects. Such side effects after $CISCA_{II}/VB_{IV}$ therapy include cisplatin neuropathy, bleomycin pulmonary toxicity, Adriamycin cardiotoxicity, and cisplatin nephrotoxicity. These side effects are likely to inhibit significantly the patient's return to a normal existence after chemotherapy.

In our patients, bleomycin pulmonary toxicity, which results in significant morbidity and occasional mortality from the use of intermittent bleomycin, is very rare. Clinically significant restrictive lung disease has not occurred in any patient we have treated with $CISCA_{II}/VB_{IV}$. Nor has any patient developed significant persistent Adriamycin cardiac toxicity, and the reported vascular complications of PVB chemotherapy (Raynaud's phenomenon, myocardial infarction) have not represented a significant problem. These differences in toxicity between $CISCA_{II}/VB_{IV}$ and PVB can perhaps be attributed to the low total cumulative dose of each individual drug delivered by alternating two high-dose chemotherapy regimens. Although acute toxicity is determined by the dose of each individual drug delivered, long-term toxicity is more related to the total dose of each of the individual drugs. Cisplatin neuropathy and cisplatin nephrotoxicity appear to occur at a lower frequency in patients receiving $CISCA_{II}/VB_{IV}$ than in those receiving standard and repeated doses of cisplatin, although no comparative trial has been performed.

For patients in the advanced categories on the Indiana staging system, Williams et al. (1987) report a 38% CR rate after PVB therapy compared to a 63% CR rate after treatment with bleomycin, etoposide, and cisplatin (BEP). When we use the Indiana system to stage patients who were treated with $CISCA_{II}/VB_{IV}$, we note that the patients with truly advanced disease have a 69% disease-free survival rate. The long-term disease-free survival rate of the patients with advanced disease who were treated with $CISCA_{II}/VB_{IV}$ at UT M. D. Anderson Cancer Center is higher than the overall CR rate achieved with either PVB or BEP for patients with equally advanced disease.

Other differences in outcome also point to the superior results of $CISCA_{II}/VB_{IV}$. Although a significant portion of patients treated with PVB are found to have viable carcinoma at surgical exploration, this finding is extremely unusual for patients treated with $CISCA_{II}/VB_{IV}$. Patients with teratomatous elements treated with PVB have a relapse rate that approaches 33% of those whose mature teratoma is resected. Also encountered is the presence of unusual sarcomatoid teratomatous elements at surgery following PVB chemotherapy. In contrast, the frequency of relapse from teratoma of patients treated with $CISCA_{II}/VB_{IV}$ is extremely low. Only three patients who had unresectable or unrecognized persistent teratoma have shown evidence of regrowth. In addition, we have not encountered sarcomatoid elements at surgery after chemotherapy in any of the patients treated with $CISCA_{II}/VB_{IV}$.

CONCLUSION

From the long-term follow-up of 167 patients treated with CISCA$_{II}$/VB$_{IV}$, we conclude that cure is nearly universal for patients with minimal disease. Patients with very far-advanced disease also have a very high cure rate except in the presence of a β-HCG level elevated to above 50,000 mIu/ml. When the β-HCG level is very high, however, the overall cure rate remains low. Our current approach is to reduce the intensity of therapy for those patients with minimal disease and to increase the intensity of chemotherapy for those with a very high serum β-HCG level, who have an overall poor prognosis.

REFERENCES

1. Bosl GJ, Geller N, Cirrincione C, et al. 1983. A multivariate analysis of prognostic variables in patients (pts) with metastatic germ cell tumors of the testis (GCT). *Cancer Res* 43:3403–3406.
2. Logothetis CJ, Samuels ML, Selig D, et al. 1986. Cyclic chemotherapy with cyclophosphamide, doxorubicin, and cisplatin plus vinblastine and bleomycin in advanced germinal tumors: Results with 100 patients. *Am J Med* 81:219–228.
3. Logothetis CJ, Samuels ML, Selig D, et al. 1985. Improved survival with cyclic chemotherapy for nonseminomatous germ cell tumors of the testis. *J Clin Oncol* 3:326–335.
4. Newlands ES, Rustin GJS, Begent RHJ, et al. 1983. Further advances in the management of malignant teratomas of the testis and other sites. *Lancet* 1:948–951.
5. Stoter G, Vendrik CPJ, Struyvenberg A, et al. 1984. Five-year survival of patients with disseminated nonseminomatous testicular cancer treated with cisplatin, vinblastine, and bleomycin. *Cancer* 54:1521–1524.
6. Williams SD, Stablein DM, Einhorn LH, et al. 1987. Immediate adjuvant chemotherapy versus observation with treatment at relapse in pathological stage II testicular cancer. *N Engl J Med* 317:1433–1438.

_____

Chapter 48

High-Dose Chemotherapy Regimens for the Treatment of Poor-Prognosis Nonseminomatous Germ Cell Tumors

Robert F. Ozols, M.D.

Daniel C. Ihde, M.D.

W. Marston Linehan, M.D.

Robert C. Young, M.D.

For patients with germ cell cancer who present with features predictive for a favorable outcome, the major clinical issues today revolve around the development of less toxic therapies, since greater than 90% of these patients can be cured with standard cisplatin-based combination chemotherapy. In contrast, the goal in treating patients with poor-prognosis nonseminomatous germ cell tumors is to develop a more effective treatment. To that end, several aggressive chemotherapy regimens intended primarily for patients with poor prognostic features have been investigated.

A number of different classification systems have been proposed to identify patients at high risk who would be suitable candidates for such innovative and aggressive therapeutic approaches (Birch et al. 1986; Vogelzang 1987). In addition, multivariate analysis techniques have been applied to data from patients with metastatic germ cell cancer in an effort to determine which factors are capable of prospectively identifying patients who have an unfavorable prognosis (Bosl et al. 1983; Stoter et al. 1987). However, disagreements remain as to the specific clinical and laboratory criteria used to define high-risk patients. It appears that both the serum levels of human chorionic gonadotropin (HCG) and the volume of metastases are the most important factors predicting for a poor prognosis (Vogelzang 1987).

The characteristics that have been used to identify those patients with an unfavorable prognosis have been derived from retrospective analysis of treatment results in the last decade. During this time period, the results of standard therapy have improved without an apparent change in the drug regimens or in the intensity of the treatment (Einhorn 1986). The specific reasons for this improvement in therapeutic results are not clear but are probably due to the more effective use of standard chemotherapy regimens. In particular, it is probable that cisplatin has been administered at a more effective dose and schedule as physicians have become more aware of the patterns of its toxicity and ways to decrease it.

We initially demonstrated that double-dose cisplatin could be administered without significant nephrotoxicity (Ozols et al. 1984a). In addition, a new drug combination termed PVeBV, consisting of double-dose cisplatin, vinblastine, bleomycin, and etoposide (VP-16-213), produced complete responses in 6 of 6 patients who had poor prognostic features (Ozols et al. 1983). Since that initial report, high-dose platinum regimens (Schmoll et al. 1984; Daugaard and Rorth 1986) have been evaluated in several noncontrolled phase II trials. These studies, plus those using other aggressive chemotherapy regimens in which high-dose cisplatin was not employed (Logothetis et al. 1985), have produced an apparent improvement in complete-response rates in high-risk patients over those in previous reports.

Because the studies were not controlled, their results must be viewed with caution. Clearly, before a new drug regimen can be judged an improvement over standard therapy for patients at high risk for germ cell cancer, it must be prospectively compared in a randomized fashion to a standard regimen that is also administered in an optimal manner.

PVeBV CHEMOTHERAPY FOR PATIENTS WITH GERM CELL TUMORS

We initially reported our pilot experience with PVeBV chemotherapy (Table 48–1) for 10 patients with poor-prognosis germ cell tumors, 4 previously treated and 6 untreated, in 1983. PVeBV represents a major modification of the standard cisplatin, etoposide, and bleomycin (PVeB) regimen (cisplatin, 20 mg/m² daily for 5 days; vinblastine, 0.3 mg/kg on day 1; and bleomycin, 30 units/week for 12 weeks). The rationale for this new drug combination was as follows: (1) Cisplatin has been shown to have an important dose-response relationship in patients with germ cell cancers (Samson et al. 1984). The renal toxicity of the cisplatin had previously limited the dose to 100-120 mg/m² per cycle, but experimental studies in murine tumors had demonstrated that hypertonic saline can protect against the nephrotoxicity of cisplatin (Litterst 1981). Consequently, we administered high-dose cisplatin in 250 ml of 3% saline with concomitant aggressive hydration consisting of 6 L/day of normal saline, each liter containing 20 mEq KCl. (2) Bleomycin and vinblastine were retained because of their demonstrated clinical synergy. The dose of vinblastine, however, was decreased from the standard 0.3 mg/kg of PVeB to 0.2 mg/kg. (3) Etoposide was added because of its demonstrated effectiveness in patients previously treated for testicular cancer (Williams et al. 1980). PVeBV chemotherapy was administered on a 21-day cycle without dose modifications for hematologic toxicity.

TABLE 48–1.
PVeBV Chemotherapy (21-Day Cycles)

Drug	Dosage
Cisplatin	40 mg/m² IV daily × 5*
Vinblastine	0.2 mg/kg IV day 1
Bleomycin	30 units IV weekly × 9–12
VP-16-23 (etoposide)	100 mg/m² IV daily × 5

*Cisplatin administered in 250 ml 3% normal saline over 30 minutes. Hydration consists of 250 ml/hour of normal saline with 20 mEq KCl per liter. Hydration continues for the 5 days of cisplatin treatment.

All six previously untreated patients with poor-prognosis germ cell cancer achieved a complete remission (Ozols et al. 1983), and all remain alive and free of disease. In addition, all four previously treated patients with refractory germ cell cancer who were treated with PVeBV as salvage chemotherapy responded to therapy (2 partial remissions and 2 complete remissions). It is of note that nephrotoxicity was no longer dose limiting and that high-dose cisplatin could be administered safely to this group of patients. Approximately half the patients had obstructive uropathy, which frequently led to decreased renal function. Even in this group of patients, high-dose cisplatin was not associated with any significant increase in serum creatinine or decrease in creatinine clearance rate (Ozols et al. 1984a). However, PVeBV in the pilot study was associated with severe hematologic toxicity. White blood cell counts fell below 1,000/μl in all patients sometime during their course of therapy; platelet transfusions were administered to all patients with platelet counts below 20,000/μl.

PVeB VS. PVeBV IN GERM CELL CANCER PATIENTS

A randomized trial of PVeBV vs. PVeB has been completed at the Medicine Branch of the National Cancer Institute, and the preliminary results have recently been reported (Ozols et al. 1984b, 1987). The trial was initiated in 1981 and completed for patient entry in January 1986. The protocol design is shown in Figure 48–1, and eligibility criteria are listed in Table 48–2. Fifty-two consecutive patients with poor-prognosis germ cell cancer were included, 34 randomized to PVeBV and 18 to PVeB. There have been no exclusions from analysis; that is, all patients are evaluable for response, toxicity, and survival. Median follow-up in this study is 36 months (range, 6–48 months).

All patients who were randomized to PVeBV received three cycles of therapy. If after three cycles their serum tumor markers (AFP or HCG) were elevated, they received an additional cycle of PVcBV. When tumor markers were normal after either three or four cycles, the patients were restaged. If computed tomography (CT) scans of the abdomen or lungs were normal, the patients were considered to be in a complete remission. Those patients who had residual masses following chemotherapy underwent surgery, and attempts were made to resect completely any residual disease. After surgery, if the resected mass contained

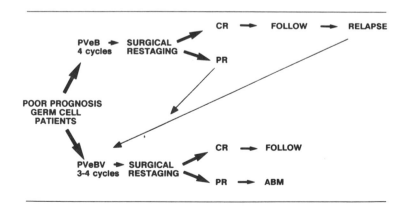

FIG 48–1.
Protocol design for a randomized trial of PVeB (cisplatin, etoposide, bleomycin) vs. PVeBV (double-dose cisplatin, etoposide, bleomycin, vinblastine) for patients who have poor-risk germ cell cancer. *CR* = complete response; *PR* = partial response; *ABM* = autologous bone marrow.

TABLE 48–2.
Eligibility Criteria for PVeBV vs. PVeB Trial
_____

Bulky metastases
　Advanced abdominal disease
　　Palpable mass
　　10 cm if not palpable
　　Liver metastases
　Advanced lung disease
　　Mediastinal mass or pulmonary nodule >5.0 cm
　　Multiple nodules (>5) with at least one >2.0 cm
　　>5 metastases per lung if each lesion is >1.0 cm
　　Pleural effusion
　　Tumor-associated hypoxia (partial pressure of oxygen
　　　[PO_2] <75 mm Hg)
　Other visceral metastases
　Central nervous system metastases
Histologic type
　Pure choriocarcinoma
　Extragonadal primary tumors
Serum tumor markers*
　AFP >1,000
　HCG >10,000

*AFP = alpha-fetoprotein; HCG = human chorionic
　gonadotropin.
_____

only fibrosis, necrotic tissue, or immature or mature teratoma, patients were also considered to have achieved a complete remission and received no further therapy. If the resected mass contained viable residual embryonal carcinoma or if the serum tumor markers were elevated after four cycles of PVeBV chemotherapy, the patients were then treated with high-dose therapy consisting of etoposide (200 mg/m² IV on days 1–5) together with high-dose cisplatin, as described above, followed by reinfusion of stored autologous bone marrow.

All patients randomized to the standard PVeB regimen received four cycles of therapy unless they had evidence of disease progression. After completing PVeB chemotherapy, they were restaged as described above for patients who had normal markers after PVeBV chemotherapy. Those patients with PVeB whose disease progressed while on therapy or who had residual embryonal cancer after four cycles of PVeB were crossed over to receive salvage therapy with high-dose cisplatin plus etoposide.

Patients who achieved a complete remission with PVeB induction therapy and then relapsed were treated with three cycles of high-dose cisplatin plus etoposide. Any patients whose mass was regrowing at a time when their tumor markers were normal underwent surgical exploration to define the disease status. If the resected mass did not contain any embryonal carcinoma and, instead, consisted only of teratoma, fibrosis, or both, the patients received no further therapy.

Figure 48–2 depicts the preliminary results for the 34 patients randomized to receive PVeBV. Thirty (88%) achieved a complete response. Of these 30, 67% required only three cycles of therapy and 30% required four cycles. Only one patient required autologous bone marrow infusion. Twenty-seven of the 34 patients (79%) remain alive. Twenty-five patients are continually disease-free, 1 is alive after relapsing with embryonal cancer and undergoing salvage therapy, and 3 are alive who had recurrent teratoma only. Seven patients randomized to receive PVeBV have died. Four of these, including 2 who presented in pulmonary failure, did not achieve a complete response. Two patients achieved a complete remission but died from bleomycin lung toxicity, and 1 patient relapsed after a complete response to induction

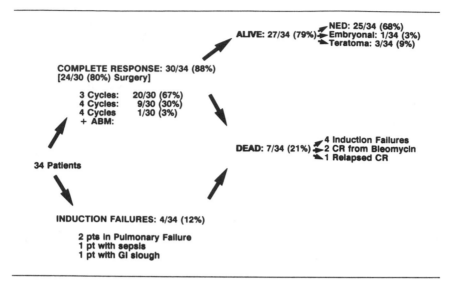

FIG 48–2.
Clinical course and preliminary results of patients with poor-prognosis germ cell cancer randomized to receive PVeBV (double-dose cisplatin, etoposide, bleomycin, vinblastine). *ABM* = autologous bone marrow; *NED* = no evident disease; *CR* = complete response; *GI* = gastrointestinal.

therapy with PVeBV and had only a transient response to salvage therapy.

Figure 48–3 summarizes the preliminary results for those patients randomized to receive PVeB. Of 18 patients entered in the study, 12 (67%) achieved a complete response. However, only 9 of the 18 (50%) are alive, and only 33% remain without evidence of disease. Three patients relapsed after achieving a complete response, only 1 of whom is alive. Two patients have relapsed with teratoma. All patients who did not achieve a complete remission with PVeB have died of progressive disease.

DISCUSSION

The selection criteria used in this trial identified a high-risk group of patients with germ cell cancer. Standard PVeB therapy produced only a 50% overall survival rate, whereas the overall survival rate for patients randomized to receive PVeBV was 78%. PVeBV therapy, however, was more toxic. The number of patients treated with PVeBV who developed white blood cell counts below 1,000/μl, who became febrile, or who required prophylactic platelet administration for thrombocytopenia was signficantly greater than that of those who received PVeB (*P*<.05). However, since the majority of patients randomized to receive PVeBV required only three cycles of therapy, the hematologic toxicity was manageable. The major toxicity in this study was due to bleomycin. Three patients, two randomized to PVeBV and one to PVeB, died of pulmonary fibrosis at a time when they had no evidence of embryonal cancer. Bleomycin lung toxicity occurred even with careful monitoring, which included physical examinations, chest x-rays, and pulmonary function tests. Widespread pulmonary metastases may increase the incidence of bleomycin lung toxicity in this group of patients.

This study also demonstrates that patients cannot be treated initially with less toxic chemotherapy and then crossed over to an aggressive arm if they do not achieve a complete remission. In this study, none of the six patients who did not achieve a complete remission with PVeB was salvageable by crossing over to high-dose platinum plus etoposide. Patients who achieved complete remission with PVeB and then relapsed were able to achieve a second complete remission with high-dose platinum plus etoposide, although only one of these second complete remissions was durable.

The greater effectiveness of PVeBV in this patient population may be due to the double dose of platinum, the addition of etoposide, or a synergistic effect of this combination. On the basis of recently performed prospective randomized trials comparing bleomycin, etoposide, and platinum (BEP) with PVeB, it is clear that etoposide should be included for all patients with germ cell cancer who receive chemotherapy (Williams et al. 1987). Studies are currently in progress to determine if the double dose of platinum is a critical factor. At Indiana University, patients are being randomized to receive either BEP in standard doses or double-dose platinum plus etoposide and bleomycin. This should answer the question of the relative importance of high-dose platinum vs. etoposide to patients with high-risk germ cell cancer.

It is likely that other innovative approaches may be useful in treating patients with germ cell cancer who present with poor prognostic features. Studies are in progress using ifosfamide-containing regimens, and it appears that this agent is very active against germ cell cancer. Another study at Indiana University is investigating carboplatin plus etoposide at accelerated doses together with autologous bone marrow transplantation for patients whose disease is refractory to standard chemotherapeutic regimens. If it can be demonstrated that the dose-response relationship to these agents is important, then this approach will need to be examined in previously untreated patients who have poor prognostic features. On the basis of the encouraging preliminary results of these aggressive regimens, it appears that the outlook has improved and will continue to improve for patients who present with high-risk germ cell cancers.

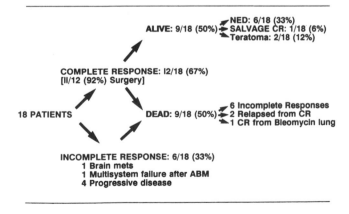

FIG 48–3.
Clinical course and preliminary results of patients with poor-prognosis germ cell cancer randomized to PVeB (cisplatin, etoposide, bleomycin). *NED* = no evident disease; *CR* = complete response; *mets* = metastases; *ABM* = autologous bone marrow.

REFERENCES

1. Birch R, Williams S, Cone A, et al. 1986. Prognostic factors for favorable outcome in disseminated germ cell tumors. *J Clin Oncol* 4:400–407.
2. Bosl GJ, Geller NL, Cirrincione C, et al. 1983. Multivariate analysis of prognostic variables in patients with metastatic testicular cancer. *Cancer Res* 43:3403–3407.
3. Daugaard G, Rorth M. 1986. High-dose cisplatin and VP-16 with bleomycin in the management of advanced metastatic germ cell tumors. *Eur J Cancer Clin Oncol* 22:477–485.
4. Einhorn LH. 1986. Have new aggressive chemotherapy regimens improved results in advanced germ cell tumors? *Eur J Cancer Clin Oncol* 22:1289–1293.
5. Litterst CL. 1981. Alterations in the toxicity of cis-dichlorodiammineplatinum-II and in tissue localization of platinum as a function of NaCl concentration in the vehicle of administration. *Toxicol Appl Pharm* 61:99–108.
6. Logothetis CJ, Samuels ML, Selig D, et al. 1985. Improved survival with cyclic chemotherapy for nonseminomatous germ cell tumors of the testis. *J Clin Oncol* 3:326–335.
7. Ozols RF, Corden BJ, Jacob J, et al. 1984a. High-dose cisplatin in hypertonic saline. *Ann Intern Med* 100:19–24.
8. Ozols RF, Deisseroth AB, Javadpour N, et al. 1983. Treatment of poor prognosis nonseminomatous testicular cancer with "high-dose" platinum combination chemotherapy regimen. *Cancer* 51:1803–1807.
9. Ozols RF, Ihde D, Jacob J, et al. 1987. Poor prognosis nonseminomatous testicular cancer: Mature results of a randomized trial of PVeBV vs. PVeB (abstract). *Proc Am Soc Clin Oncol* 6:107.
10. Ozols RF, Ihde D, Jacob J, et al. 1984b. Randomized trial of PVeBV vs. PVeB in poor prognosis nonseminomatous testicular cancer (abstract). *Proc Am Soc Clin Oncol* 3:155.
11. Samson MK, Rivkin SE, Jones SE, et al. 1984. Dose-response and dose-survival advantage for high versus low-dose cisplatin combined with vinblastine and bleomycin in disseminated testicular cancer. *Cancer* 53:1029–1035.
12. Schmoll HJ, Arnold H, Mayr T, et al. 1984. Platinum-ultra high dose etoposide-bleomycin (DDP-HD/VP16/BLM): An effective regimen for testicular cancer with poor prognosis (abstract). *Proc Am Soc Clin Oncol* 3:639.
13. Stoter G, Sylvester R, Sleijfer DT, et al. 1987. Multivariate analysis of prognostic factors in patients with disseminated nonseminomatous testicular cancer: Results from a European Organization for Research on Treatment of Cancer multiinstitutional phase III Study. *Cancer Res* 47:2714–2718.
14. Vogelzang NJ. 1987. Prognostic factors in metastatic testicular cancer. *Int J Androl* 10:225–237.
15. Williams SD, Birch R, Einhorn LH, et al. 1987. Treatment of disseminated germ-cell tumors with cisplatin, bleomycin, and either vinblastine or etoposide. *N Engl J Med* 316:1435–1440.
16. Williams SD, Einhorn LH, Greco FA, et al. 1980. VP-16-213 salvage therapy for refractory germinal neoplasms. *Cancer* 46:2154–2158.

Chapter 49

Chemotherapy for Extragonadal Germ Cell Tumors: The M. D. Anderson Experience

Clayton D.K. Chong, M.D.

Christopher J. Logothetis, M.D.

The mechanism by which germ cell tumors arise in extragonadal sites is unknown. They are usually midline tumors and can be found in multiple locations (pineal gland, anterior mediastinum, retroperitoneum, presacral area, and other unusual sites). The anterior mediastinum and the retroperitoneum are the most common sites for the disease. Separating germ cell tumors that are truly of extragonadal origin from those that actually represent occult testicular carcinomas poses a major clinical dilemma. Classification of the tumors and care for the patients are complicated by the fact that tumors that develop in many young men (atypical teratoma syndrome) are poorly differentiated and mimic extragonadal germ cell tumors (Fox et al. 1979). Some of these poorly differentiated tumors also secrete serum biomarkers, further complicating their subclassification.

Postmortem studies have revealed that testicular cancer has a characteristic mode of spread. Retroperitoneal lymph nodes are involved most frequently, followed by lungs, liver, brain, and then bone (Johnson et al. 1973). For anterior mediastinal metastases to develop without prior involvement of the retroperitoneal nodes is extremely unlikely (Garnick et al. 1983). Therefore, when a tumor in the anterior mediastinum has pathologic features diagnostic of germ cell tumors, it is unlikely to represent an occult primary testicular tumor.

Apparent primary retroperitoneal tumors, in contrast, can actually be metastases from an occult primary testicular carcinoma. Patients with this presentation show, on a subsequent orchiectomy, regression of the primary testicular tumor and persistent "scars" or viable tumor. In other patients, frequently an occult primary testicular carcinoma is diagnosed later. Because of the concern that many patients diagnosed as having extragonadal primary tumors in reality have occult primary testicular tumors, Azzopardi and Hoffbrand (1965) established specific pathologic criteria for a regressed gonadal primary tumor. Some investigators consider only upper primary retroperitoneal tumors as truly extragonadal. Abell et al. (1965) also adopted rigid criteria for primary retroperitoneal germ cell tumors: the tumor must arise in the "upper abdomen," must be "encapsulated," and pelvic nodal involvement must be absent. In all instances, a careful search for a testicular primary tumor is necessary.

Nevertheless, anterior mediastinal germ cell tumors can indeed be true extragonadal tumors. As further supporting evidence, investigators have documented that extragonadal tumors have a different histologic distribution than retroperitoneal metastases and are uniquely associated with Klinefelter's syndrome, a congenital abnormality (Friedman 1951; Chaussain et al. 1980; Logothetis et al. 1985; Dexeus et al. 1986).

TREATMENT

In the prechemotherapy era, chances of survival after surgical resection of primary anterior mediastinal germ cell tumors were dismal (Martini et al. 1964; Oberman and Libcke 1964; Utz and Buscemi 1971; Raghavan et al. 1982). All patients who had nonseminomatous germ cell tumors (NSGCT) in the anterior mediastinum showed subsequent regrowth after resection. A few patients with anterior mediastinal pure seminomas, however, were cured with the combination of surgery and radiation, or with radiation therapy only. Table 49–1 summarizes previous experiences using surgery with or without radiation therapy.

Since the introduction of chemotherapy, results for patients with testicular germ cell tumors have improved significantly (Samuels et al. 1976; Einhorn 1981). However, despite chemotherapy, those with extragonadal germ cell tumors continued to have poor results. Table 49–2 summarizes the recent experience using chemotherapy for extragonadal tumors. In the Southwest Oncology Group study, cisplatin, vinblastine, and bleomycin (PVB) produced very poor results in patients with anterior mediastinal germ cell tumors; only a rare patient survived (Feun et al. 1980). Similar results were reported by Kuzur et al. (1982), who identified only a rare survivor among patients with pure endodermal sinus tumors in the anterior mediastinum treated with PVB. It is clear, therefore, that the true extragonadal germ cell tumor in the anterior mediastinum is unlikely to be cured with conventional PVB chemotherapy.

At The University of Texas M. D. Anderson Cancer Center, our experience has spanned the era of vinblastine/bleomycin to our most recent, most intense chemotherapy regimen $CISCA_{II}/VB_{IV}$ (cisplatin, cyclophosphamide, doxorubicin [Adriamycin] alternating with vinblastine and bleomycin) (Logothetis et al. 1985). In Table 49–3, the UT M. D. Anderson Cancer Center experience with extragonadal tumors is summarized. Using $CISCA_{II}/VB_{IV}$, patients with pure yolk-sac tumors of the anterior mediastinum have a high likelihood of remaining disease free (Chong et al. 1986) (Table 49–4), whereas patients with choriocarcinoma have the poorest prognosis (Table 49–5). The patients with high-volume choriocarcinoma typically present in a catastrophic clinical state with hemoptysis, pulmonary hemorrhage, respiratory failure, and an unstable cardiovascular status. Such patients have a

TABLE 49–1.
Treatment of Extragonadal Germ Cell Tumors: Radiation ± Surgery

| | Tumor Location* | | | | |
| | Mediastinum | | Abdomen | | |
Investigator	NSGCT[†]	Seminoma	NSGCT[†]	Seminoma	Pineal
Utz and Buscemi (1971)	6 (2)	6 (4)	5 (1)	—	1 (1)
Raghavan et al. (1982)	—	6 (4)	—	—	—
Martini et al. (1964)	20 (1)	10 (5)	—	—	—
Oberman and Libcke (1964)	7 (0)	1 (1)	—	—	—
Abell et al. (1965)	—	—	—	10 (6)	—

*Number in parentheses indicates patients alive and disease free.
[†]NSGCT = nonseminomatous germ cell tumor.

TABLE 49–2.
Chemotherapy for Extragonadal Germ Cell Tumors*

		Patients			Clinical Presentation					
			Alive		Chest			Retroperitoneum		
						Disease-Free			Disease-Free	
Study	Treatment	Total[†]	No.	%	Total	No.	%	Total	No.	%
Vanderbilt + Indiana (Hainsworth 1982)	PVB ± surgery	31	18	58	10	7	70	18	11	61
Dana-Farber (Garnick 1983)	PVB ± surgery; consolidation with cyclophosphamide + doxorubicin (Adriamycin)	15	4	27	8	0	0	7	4	57
SWOG[‡] (Feun 1980)	PVB ± surgery	19	0	0	10	0	0	9	0	0
Madrid[§] (Funes 1981)	PVB ± surgery	14	6	43	14	6	43	—	—	—

*PVB = cisplatin, vinblastine, bleomycin; SWOG = Southwest Oncology Group.
[†]Results exclude endodermal sinus tumor for analysis.
[‡]Complete remissions only among patients with abdominal presentations.
[§]Shows follow-up of complete remissions (6–22 months); endodermal sinus tumor excluded from study.

TABLE 49–3.
Chemotherapy for Extragonadal Germ Cell Tumors: UT M. D. Anderson Cancer Center

| Clinical Presentation | No. of Patients | Chemotherapy*[†] | | | Total No. Disease-Free[†] |
		VB	CISCA_{II}	CTX + Cisplatin	
Seminoma					
Abdomen	15[‡]	1 (0%)	1 (100%)	13 (92%)	13[§]
Chest	4	0	1 (100%)	3 (100%)	4
Total	19	0/1 (0%)	2/2 (100%)	15[§]/16 (94%)	17/19 (89.5%)

		VB	VB_{III} + P	CISCA	CISCA_{II}/VB_{IV}	Total No. Disease-Free
Nonseminomatous germinal tumors						
Abdomen	15	6 (33%)	3 (66%)	3 (33%)	3 (100%)	15 (53%)
Chest	15	4 (0%)	0	6 (17%)	5 (60%)	15 (27%)
Total	30	10 (20%)	3 (66%)	9 (22%)	8 (75%)	12 (40%)

*VB = vinblastine, bleomycin; CISCA = cisplatin, cyclophosphamide, Adriamycin; CTX = cyclophosphamide; P = cisplatin; $CISCA_{II}/VB_{IV}$ = subscript numbers designate degree of dosage.
[†]Number in parentheses represents percent disease-free.
[‡]Four patients had failed chemotherapy elsewhere.
[§]One patient alive with disease.

TABLE 49–4.
Mediastinal Endodermal Sinus Tumor: UT M. D. Anderson Cancer Center*

| Patient | SVC[†] | Serum Biomarkers | | Chemotherapy | Survival (wk)[‡] |
		AFP	β-HCG		
1	(+)	2,603	(−)	CISCA/VB	72+
2	(+)	32,000	(−)	CISCA/VB	20
3	(+)	280	(−)	CISCA/VB	149
4	(−)	4,095	(−)	CISCA/VB	27.5
5	(+)	262	(−)	CISCA	46.5

*SVC = superior vena cava syndrome; AFP = α-fetoprotein; β-HCG = beta-human chorionic gonadotropin; CISCA = cisplatin, cyclophosphamide, Adriamycin; VB = vinblastine, bleomycin.
[†]Patients received post-thoracotomy radiation therapy.
[‡]All surviving patients are disease-free.

TABLE 49–5.
UT M. D. Anderson Cancer Center: Extragonadal Choriocarcinoma*[†]

Patient	Clinical Presentation	Chemotherapy	Biomarkers		Survival (wk)
			AFP	β-HCG	
1	Pulmonary metastases, hemoptysis	VB + P-CISCA$_{II}$	4.6	782,000	296.0+
2	Respiratory failure, hemoptysis requiring ventilatory support[‡]	CISCA$_{II}$	<1.0	1,326,200	4.5
3	Abdominal mass, hemoperitoneum, high-volume pulmonary metastasis	CISCA$_{II}$/VB	779.9	211,425	42.5+
4	Hemoptysis/respiratory failure	CISCA$_{II}$	45.7	476,400	21
5	Abdominal mass, hemoperitoneum	CISCA$_{II}$	3.6	146,000	18
6	Abdomen + abdominal wall invasion + chest	VB$_{III}$	NA	NA	579.5+
7	Abdomen + chest, hemoptysis	VB$_{III}$	NA	NA	32

*AFP = α-fetoprotein; β-HCG = beta-human chorionic gonadotropin; VB = vinblastine, bleomycin; P = cisplatin; CISCA = cisplatin, cyclophosphamide, Adriamycin. Subscript numerals designate degree of dosage.

[†]Five patients had a pure choriocarcinoma, 2 patients choriocarcinoma + embryonal carcinoma (Dixon-Moore class V).

[‡]Patient initially presented with high-volume pulmonary metastasis and pulmonary purpura; he continued to respond but died with progressive pulmonary fibrosis.

high response rate, but because of initial acuteness of their problems (respiratory failure), meticulous and intensive clinical care is required to achieve a cure.

The patients with poorly differentiated tumor mimicking an extragonadal germ cell tumor (atypical teratoma syndrome) are of great interest (Table 49–6). Some of these patients have a true germ cell tumor and are highly responsive to and potentially curable with chemotherapy. Other patients have poorly differentiated tumors of unknown origin; these also appear to be highly responsive to therapy but are only rarely curable. Subsequent autopsies revealed that their tumors frequently are not germ cell. Two recent studies by Greco et al. (1986) and Hainsworth et al. (1987) document that such patients have not benefitted from further pathologic subclassification but do have a high response rate to platinum-based chemotherapy. We used CISCA$_{II}$/VB$_{IV}$ to treat seven who had poorly differentiated tumors. Only transient responses were achieved, and all seven patients died with progressing disease after an initial response to therapy.

In the vinblastine/bleomycin era, patients with seminoma were unlikely to be cured (Samuels et al. 1980), but primary seminomatous tumors have a high cure rate with platinum-based chemotherapy. Treatment with CISCA$_{II}$ or cyclophosphamide, or both, and sequential cisplatin has cured the majority of these patients. Seminoma appears to be such a sensitive tumor that, regardless of volume and regardless of its origin (testicular vs. extragonadal), high cure rates can be achieved with intensive cisplatin-based therapy (see Table 49–3) (Israel et al. 1985; Logothetis et al. 1985).

Our experience in treating extragonadal germ cell tumors at UT M. D. Anderson Cancer Center reflects the unique behavior of this tumor. Our currently recommended therapy is

TABLE 49–6.
Atypical Teratoma Syndrome*

Study	No. of Patients	Elevated Biomarkers β-HCG ± AFP	Sites of Origin Chest	Abd.	Other	Treatment[†]	Disease-Free No.	%
Fox et al (1979)	5	1	5			VB (1), VB + P (4)	1	20
Richardson et al (1981)	12	6/10[‡]	8	1	2[§]	VB + P (12)	4	33
Logothetis et al (1985)	7	7	5	2		CISCA$_{II}$/VB$_{IV}$ (5) VB + P (2)	0	
Greco et al (1986)	67	10/3	21	28		PVB ± A (62) CISCA (2) Other (3)	9	13

*β-HCG = beta-human chorionic gonadotropin; AFP = alpha-fetoprotein; Abd. = abdomen; VB = vinblastine, bleomycin; P = cisplatin; CISCA = cisplatin, cyclophosphamide, doxorubicin (Adriamycin), PVB = cisplatin, vinblastine, bleomycin; A = Adriamycin. Subscript numerals designate degree of dosage.
[†]Number in parentheses indicates number treated in each category.
[‡]Serum biomarkers not evaluated in 2 patients.
[§]Pulmonary nodule without clear mediastinal origin.

CISCA$_{II}$/VB$_{IV}$. This therapy has significantly improved the survival rate of patients with endodermal sinus tumors, but patients with high-volume choriocarcinoma continue to have a poor prognosis. Choriocarcinoma remains a clinical problem that requires further developments in therapy. Treatment of extragonadal seminoma has been improved greatly by the introduction of cisplatin-based therapy.

In our experience, patients who have primary retroperitoneal tumors should be treated cautiously. These tumors may represent occult testicular primary tumors, and therefore a careful search for a testicular primary should be made. A delayed orchiectomy is recommended if the physician suspects a testicular tumor may exist. Patients with poorly differentiated tumors mimicking germinal tumors may benefit from cisplatin-based therapy, but unfortunately they are rarely cured.

CONCLUSION

It is our belief that adequate evidence exists that extragonadal germ cell tumors are a unique form of germ cell tumor. This belief is based on differences in histologic distribution, clinical response to therapy, and associated congenital anomalies between patients with these tumors and those with testicular carcinoma. Extragonadal germ cell tumors can be cured when treated appropriately. Conventional (PVB) chemotherapy results in an unacceptably low cure rate, but CISCA$_{II}$/VB$_{IV}$ achieves a higher rate of complete response and is our treatment of choice for extragonadal mixed germinal tumors, whereas cyclophosphamide and sequential cisplatin therapy is our choice for extragonadal seminoma (Table 49–7).

Because extragonadal germinal tumors are rare, it is unlikely that physicians seeing them at infrequent intervals will become experienced in treating them. Patients who have these tumors should be referred to a major treatment center experienced in caring for them to maximize the cure rate.

TABLE 49–7.
Extragonadal Germ Cell Tumors: Treatment at UT M. D. Anderson Cancer
Center, 1987

Tumor Type	Chemotherapy*
Seminoma	
Mediastinum[†]	Cyclophosphamide + sequential cisplatin
Abdomen[†]	Cyclophosphamide + sequential cisplatin
Nonseminoma[‡]	$CISCA_{II}/VB_{IV}$
Anterior mediastinum	$CISCA_{II}/VB_{IV}$
Abdomen[§]	$CISCA_{II}/VB_{IV}$

*$CISCA_{II}/VB_{IV}$ = cisplatin, cyclophosphamide, Adriamycin plus vinblastine, bleomycin.
Subscript numerals designate degree of dosage.
[†]Patients with a seminoma and elevated serum alpha-fetoprotein level are treated as if they
had mixed germ tumors.
[‡]Surgery for a persistent and stable biomarker-negative mass, after 2 courses of chemotherapy
past complete remission.
[§]Orchiectomy performed on patient with a palpable testis mass or an atrophic testis on the
side of dominant intra-abdominal tumor mass.

REFERENCES

1. Abell MR, Fayos JV, Lampe I. 1965. Retroperitoneal germinomas (seminomas) without evidence of testicular involvement. *Cancer* 18:273–290.
2. Azzopardi JG, Hoffbrand AV. 1965. Retrogression in testicular seminoma with viable metastases. *J Clin Pathol* 188:135–141.
3. Chaussain JL, Lemerle J, Roger M, et al. 1980. Klinefelter syndrome, tumor, and sexual precocity. *J Pediatr* 97:607–609.
4. Chong C, Logothetis C, Samuels ML, et al. 1986. The successful management of pure endodermal sinus tumors (EST) of adult males (abstract). *Proc Am Soc Clin Oncol* 5:379.
5. Dexeus F, Logothetis C, Samuels M, et al. 1986. Chromosomal and constitutional abnormalities in male patients (pts) with germ cell tumors (GCT) (abstract). *Proc Am Soc Clin Oncol* 5:98.
6. Einhorn L. 1981. Testicular cancer as a model for a curable neoplasm: The Richard and Hinda Rosenthal Foundation Award lecture. *Cancer Res* 41:3275–3280.
7. Feun LG, Samson MK, Stephens RL. 1980. Vinblastine (VCB), bleomycin (Bleo), cis-diamminedichloroplatinum (DDP) in disseminated extragonadal germ cell tumors. *Cancer* 45:2543–2549.
8. Fox RM, Woods RL, Tattersall MHN. 1979. Undifferentiated carcinoma in young men: The atypical teratoma syndrome. *Lancet* 1:1316–1318.
9. Friedman NB. 1951. The comparative morphogenesis of extra genital and gonadal teratoid tumors. *Cancer* 4:265–276.
10. Funes HC, Mendez M, Alonso E, et al. 1981. Mediastinal germ cell tumors treated with cisplatin, bleomycin, and vinblastine (abstract). *Proc Am Soc Clin Oncol* C–553.
11. Garnick MD, Canellos GP, Richie JP. 1983. Treatment and surgical staging of testicular and primary extragonadal germ cell cancer. *JAMA* 150:1773–1741.
12. Greco FA, Vaughn WK, Hainsworth JD. 1986. Advanced poorly differentiated carcinoma of unknown primary site: Recognition of a treatable syndrome. *Ann Intern Med* 104:547–554.
13. Hainsworth JD, Einhorn LH, Williams SD, et al. 1982. Advanced extragonadal germ cell tumors: Successful treatment with combination chemotherapy. *Ann Intern Med* 97:7–11.
14. Hainsworth JD, Wright ED, Gray GF, et al. 1987. Poorly differentiated carcinoma of unknown primary site: Correlation of light microscopic findings with response to cisplatin-based combination chemotherapy. *J Clin Oncol* 5:1275–1280.
15. Israel A, Bosl G, Golbey RB, et al. 1985. The results of chemotherapy for extragonadal germ-cell tumors in the cisplatin era: The Memorial Sloan-Kettering Cancer Center experience (1975–1982). *J Clin Oncol* 3:1073–1078.
16. Johnson DE, Laneri JD, Mountain CF, et al. 1973. Extragonadal germ cell tumors. *Surgery* 73:85–90.

17. Kuzur ME, Cobleigh M, Greco FA, et al. 1982. Endodermal sinus tumor of the mediastinum. *Cancer* 50:766–774.
18. Logothetis CJ, Samuels ML, Selig DE, et al. 1985. Chemotherapy of extragonadal germ cell tumors. *J Clin Oncol* 3:316–325.
19. Martini N, Golbey RB, Hajdo SI, et al. 1964. Primary mediastinal germ cell tumors. *Cancer* 33:763–769.
20. Oberman HA, Libcke JH. 1964. Malignant germinal neoplasms of the mediastinum. *Cancer* 17:498–507.
21. Raghavan D, Sullivan MJ, Peckham MJ, et al. 1982. Elevated serum alpha fetoprotein and seminoma: Clinical evidence for a histologic continuum. *Cancer* 50:982–989.
22. Richardson RL, Schoumacher RA, Fer MF, et al. 1981. The unrecognized extragonadal germ cell syndrome. *Ann Intern Med* 94:181–186.
23. Samuels ML, Lanzotti VJ, Holoye PY, et al. 1976. Combination chemotherapy in germinal tumors. *Cancer Treat Rep* 3:185–204.
24. Samuels ML, Logothetis CJ, Trindade A. 1980. Sequential weekly pulse dose cisplatin for far advanced seminoma (abstract). *Proc Am Soc Clin Oncol* 21:423.
25. Utz DC, Buscemi MF. 1971. Extragonadal testicular tumors. *J Urol* 105:271–274.

Chapter 50

Chemotherapy for Extragonadal and Poor-Prognosis Germ Cell Cancers: The Dana-Farber Cancer Institute Approach

Carlo Tondini, M.D.

Marc B. Garnick, M.D.

About 1% to 2% of all germ cell cancers have an extragonadal origin. These tumors present a spectrum of pathologic types similar to that of their primary testicular counterparts and include all types of seminomas and nonseminomas. The most common sites of extragonadal germ cell cancer (EGGCC) are the anterior mediastinum and retroperitoneum. In the mediastinum, EGGCC accounts for approximately 1% of all tumors. Symptoms are similar to symptoms of other malignancies in the same location, most often chest pain, dyspnea, hoarseness, cough, hemoptysis (especially with embryonal carcinoma or choriocarcinoma), gynecomastia (with choriocarcinoma), a chest-wall mass, or supraclavicular adenopathy. Superior vena cava syndrome has been reported in about a fifth of the patients. Occasionally, these tumors are asymptomatic and are discovered from a routine chest x-ray. Retroperitoneal tumors, because of their location, usually grow to large proportions before they are detected and may be accompanied by back and flank pain, abdominal fullness, nonspecific gastrointestinal complaints such as nausea, vomiting, constipation, fever, sweats, and weight loss.

Most series indicate that these tumors develop when the patient is in the middle of the third decade of life. They show a strong male predominance, occurring rarely in women. Seminomas are the most common, accounting for 40% to 50% of all EGGCCs. Embryonal carcinoma and teratocarcinoma account for approximately two thirds of the nonseminomas, and choriocarcinoma, endodermal sinus tumors, and mixed tumors make up the remaining third.

EGGCCs of the mediastinum and retroperitoneum exhibit clinical behaviors that distinguish them from primary testicular malignancies. Their differences in metastatic patterns and clinical syndromes may contribute to the poorer prognosis associated with them; for example, patients with EGGCC, especially seminomas, have a high incidence of bone metastases. Tumor bulk at presentation can also affect their clinical behavior. Testicular tumors are more easily detected and are therefore discovered in earlier stages. In addition, EGGCCs have no anatomic confining structures to limit growth; therefore most of them invade surrounding tissues and become very large before symptoms develop and a diagnosis is made.

Successful treatment programs for germinal cell cancer have achieved a cure in about 80% of patients (Einhorn 1981; Garnick et al. 1983). Chemotherapeutic regimens containing cisplatin and followed by tumor-reductive surgery have recently evolved from carefully designed studies focusing on the management of this virulent and once-fatal disease (Einhorn and Donohue 1977). Nonetheless, despite these great improvements, for a fraction of patients with advanced testicular tumors the prognosis is still unacceptably poor: a low complete-remission (CR) rate, high probability of relapse, and ultimately a low cure rate (Einhorn et al. 1981). Based on our original experience (Garnick et al. 1983), we believe that it is possible to include patients with EGGCC in this poor-prognosis group along with patients who have primary testicular nonseminomatous germ cell tumors (NSGCT) and negative prognostic features, such as bone metastases, central nervous system metastases, a human chorionic gonadotropin (HCG) serum titer greater than 2,000 ng/ml (10,000 IU/L), and liver metastases accompanied by an HCG titer greater than 2,000 ng/ml.

The combination of cisplatin, vinblastine, and bleomycin (PVB) is a standard regimen that has clearly proved its curative efficacy in most patients with germ cell tumors. However, using four cycles of PVB followed by surgery, we obtained a cure in only about 20% of the patients with EGGCC. Therefore, in 1982, we started a prospective trial designed to evaluate the feasibility and the therapeutic results of alternating two chemotherapeutic regimens as remission induction, followed by surgically removing residual radiographic abnormalities, to maximize the opportunity to achieve and to maintain a CR in both of these groups of patients with a poor prognosis.

PATIENTS AND TREATMENT PROGRAM

In the recent years, patients with EGGCC seen at the Dana-Farber Cancer Institute in Boston have been treated according to two consecutive programs that consisted of a remission-induction phase using chemotherapy followed by tumor-reductive surgery if patients had resectable residual abnormalities and if tumor markers had become normal.

The first study, conducted between 1979 and 1983 (Garnick et al. 1983), included 15 patients with EGGCC. The remission-induction chemotherapeutic phase for these patients was four consecutive cycles of PVB (cisplatin, 20 mg/m^2 intravenously [I.V.] on days 1 through 5; bleomycin, 30 units IV bolus days 1, 8, and 15; vinblastine sulfate, 0.15 to 0.2 mg/kg IV bolus on days 1 and 2; cycles repeated every 21 days). The original strategy called for tumor-reductive surgery for all patients who obtained either a CR or a partial response (PR) at the end of the remission-induction phase, followed by additional postoperative chemotherapy with cyclophosphamide and doxorubicin (Adriamycin). Midway through the study, however, we modified this approach. There was no evidence, in fact, that patients who had achieved a CR with chemotherapy needed to undergo pathologic confirmation and suffer the operative risks. Postchemotherapy surgery was retained for those patients who had resectable residual disease and whose previously abnormal levels of tumor markers had dropped to normal. Postoperative chemotherapy was eliminated for patients who had achieved a CR after the remission-induction phase and for those patients who, at surgery, were found to have only fibrosis or completely resectable teratoma. Patients found to have viable cancer at the surgical exploration were given further chemotherapy as originally planned.

The second study was conducted between 1982 and 1986. It included 30 patients, 13 with a diagnosis of primary EGGCC, 12 with a diagnosis of poor-prognosis primary testicular NSGCT (including patients with bone metastases, central nervous system metastases, an HCG titer >2,000 ng/ml, or liver metastases and an HCG titer >2,000 ng/ml), and 5 with a diagnosis of undifferentiated cancer but a clinical syndrome compatible with metastatic NSGCT (mediastinal undifferentiated cancer). The remission-induction phase, a total of six cycles of alternating chemotherapy, was administered over a period of 18 weeks. PVB was alternated every 3 weeks with a combination of cisplatin (same schedule as in PVB regimen), etoposide (100 mg/m² IV over 45 minutes, days 1 through 5), and bleomycin (same schedule as in PVB regimen) (PEB), alone or with Adriamycin (40 mg/m² IV bolus, on day 1) (PEBA). Because the therapeutic total of 360 units of bleomycin was reached after the first four cycles, this drug was not included in the fifth and sixth cycles.

Adriamycin was originally scheduled for all patients, but we noted that its use added significantly to myelosuppression and often interfered with the dose and the schedule of administration. Therefore, in 1983 we deleted it from the treatment protocol in an effort to diminish myelosuppression. In 1985, however, reviewing our experience about the possible benefit of using Adriamycin against refractory germ cell cancers, we found that its inclusion may have improved the response rate in this subset of patients (Lederman and Garnick 1986). Following this observation, we again added doxorubicin to the PVB/PEB treatment protocol. We administered the PVB regimen on cycles 1, 3, and 5 and the PEB or PEBA regimen on cycles 2, 4, and 6.

Tumor-reductive surgery was attempted in those patients who had achieved a clinical PR after the chemotherapeutic phase and who had normal marker levels and resectable residual abnormalities. The intent was to document the histologic nature of the residue and, if possible, to render the patient disease free after completely removing these residual abnormalities. If viable tumor was found, we administered further chemotherapy, adding cyclophosphamide to the other agents used in the initial induction regimen. The number of cycles was decided according to the amount of residual disease found and the patient's ability to tolerate the treatment.

The 13 patients with EGGCC in this study had a median age of 28 years (range, 18 months–38 years). Eight of these patients were treated with the PVB/PEB alternating regimen and 5 with the PVB/PEBA regimen. The median age of the 12 patients with primary testicular poor-prognosis NSGCT was 29.5 years (range, 15–51 years). Eight were treated with PVB/PEB and 4 with PVB/PEBA. Of the 5 additional patients in the study, only 1 did not receive Adriamycin. The diagnosis for these patients was mediastinal undifferentiated cancer. They did not meet the pathologic criteria for germ cell cancer, and in three of them, neither marker was elevated. The clinical presentation suggested metastatic germ cell tumor, however, although the possibility of primary lung cancer was high. Their median age was slightly older—32 years (range, 22–47 years).

Staging Procedures

Pretreatment evaluation included complete hematologic and biochemical examinations and a determination of the serum levels of α-fetoprotein (AFP) and HCG. To be admitted to the study, patients' cardiac, hepatic, and renal function tests had to be within normal range limits. Radiologic examination included standard chest roentgenography, whole-lung tomography if indicated, and computerized tomography (CT) of the abdomen. Each patient also received a bone scan to evaluate the presence of bone metastases. Patients whose testes appeared normal on palpation underwent testicular ultrasonography before the diagnosis of extragonadal germ cell tumor could be confirmed. Computerized tomography of the chest and intravenous pyelography were performed only if clinically indicated. Computerized tomography of the head was always performed if the tumor was pure choriocarcinoma or if the clinical situation dictated. Pulmonary function tests, including the study of vital capacity and diffusion capacity of carbon monoxide, were scheduled before the beginning of the therapy and before each cycle, or more frequently if indicated. Physical examination, hematologic evaluation, electrocardiogram, liver function tests, renal function tests, marker determination, and chest x-ray were repeated before each cycle of therapy. A complete noninvasive restaging was performed at the end of the chemotherapy and before surgery.

Criteria of Response

A PR after the noninvasive restaging at the end of the remission-induction chemotherapeutic phase was defined as a greater than 50% reduction in the sum of the products of longest perpendicular diameters of the most measurable areas of tumor or a 30% reduction of palpable hepatomegaly lasting in excess of 4 weeks. A CR was defined as a complete disappearance of all clinically evident disease, the return to normal range of all pathologic criteria, and the normalization of all previously abnormal markers for at least 4 weeks. Progressive disease (PD) was defined as an increase of at least 25% in the sum of the products of the longest perpendicular diameters of measurable lesions, an increase in the level of circulating AFP and HCG, or the development of new lesions.

After the surgical restaging, the patient was considered in CR only if the residual mass was fibrosis or completely resectable teratoma. In this situation, no further therapy was administered. If the surgical specimen contained residual viable cancer, even if it was fully resected leaving no microscopic residual disease, the patient was not considered to be in CR, and the additional planned chemotherapy was recommended.

RESULTS

Response to Treatment

The response to this treatment for all patients and for each subgroup is summarized in Table 50–1. Six of the 15 patients (40%) with EGGCC who were treated with four cycles of PVB and surgery achieved a CR (no viable cancer at surgery). Only 1 patient (6%) was in CR at the end of the remission-induction phase, but the other 5 patients were considered in CR after surgery confirmed residual fibrosis in 4 and completely removed residual teratoma from 1. Residual viable cancer was detected in the histologic specimens of 4 more patients who underwent surgery.

Seven of the 13 patients (54%) with EGGCC who were treated with alternating PVB/PEB(A) and surgery achieved a CR. After the initial chemotherapeutic phase, 4 patients (31%) had achieved a clinical CR and 6 a PR. One partial responder with extragonadal seminoma was irradiated in the retroperitoneal region and achieved a durable CR. The 5 other partial responders were operated on; in 2 (40%) only fibrosis or teratoma was found, while 3 still harbored viable cancer.

Five of the 12 patients (42%) with poor-prognosis testicular NSGCT achieved a CR, two (17%) after the initial chemotherapy. Nine were partial responders after chemotherapy; six could undergo surgery, and in three only fibrosis or teratoma remained. Two of the partial responders had unresectable disease, and one died of acute respiratory failure before completing the program. Disease progressed in all five patients with undifferentiated cancer before they completed the chemotherapeutic program.

TABLE 50–1.
Response to Treatment*

| | PVB × 4 Cycles | PVB/PEB(A) × 6 Cycles | | |
	EGGCC	EGGCC	NSGCTT	UC
No. of patients	15	13	12	5
After chemotherapy				
CR	1	4	2	0
PR	9	6	8	0
PD	5	3	1	5
Patients operated on	9	5	6	0
After surgery				
CR (F or T)	5	2	3	—
Viable cancer	4	3	3	—
CR after chemotherapy and surgery	6	7	5	0

*PVB = cisplatin, vincristine, bleomycin; PEB(A) = cisplatin, etoposide, bleomycin, with or without Adriamycin; EGGCC = extragonadal germ cell cancer; NSGCTT, nonseminomatous germ cell tumor of the testis; UC = undifferentiated cancer; CR = complete response; PR = partial response; PD = progressive disease; F = fibrosis; T = teratoma.

Duration of Response

Kaplan-Meier product-limit estimates of overall survival durations for patients with EGGCC are represented in Figure 50–1. In the first group of 15 patients, those treated with PVB and surgery, 3 of the 6 patients who achieved a CR (50%) have remained alive and disease free, 2 have relapsed from CR, and 1 died of surgical complications. Only 1 patient of those whose viable cancer was completely resected was still alive and disease free at 58 months after the beginning of the treatment. In the group of 13 patients who were treated with alternating PVB/PEB(A), none of the 7 who achieved a CR has relapsed after a median follow-up of 36 months (range, 14–48 months). Four of the 5 patients with NSGCT who achieved a CR are continuously disease free after a median follow-up of 20 months. Only one has relapsed after 6 months with brain metastases and increased serum marker levels. All 5 patients with undifferentiated cancer have died a median of 4 months after the beginning of the treatment.

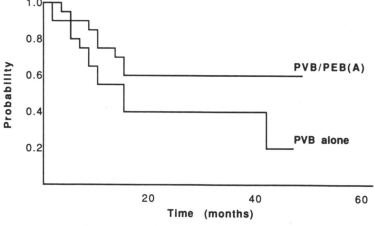

FIG 50–1.
Overall survival duration for patients with extragonadal cancers treated at the Dana-Farber Cancer Institute with either PVB (cisplatin, vinblastine, bleomycin) alone or alternating PVB and PEB(A) (cisplatin, etoposide, bleomycin, with or without doxorubicin (Adriamycin).

Toxicity

The most prominent toxic effect has been myelosuppression (Table 50–2). The severity of myelosuppression frequently mandated a reduction in the dosage of myelosuppressive drugs, but the dosage of cisplatin was never reduced. Toxicities other than hematologic are summarized in Table 50–3. Hospital admissions for infectious complications during the myelosuppression phase have been necessary after 20% of PVB cycles, after 15% of PEB cycles, and after 23% of PEBA cycles. In each case, however, antibiotic and supportive therapy was sufficient to control the infection. Pulmonary function impairment induced by the administration of bleomycin has been observed in 9% of patients treated with PVB alone and in 40% of those treated with PVB/PEB(A). Renal toxic effects were never severe; they were usually completely preventable without mannitol diuresis by administering vigorous saline hydration (3–4 L/day).

Three deaths were due to complications of the therapy. One patient treated with only PVB died of surgical complications, while 2 treated with PVB/PEB(A) died of acute respiratory failure, probably related both to their compromised baseline pulmonary function and to the toxicity of bleomycin.

DISCUSSION

Extragonadal Cancers

The results of using an alternating regimen for patients with EGGCC compare favorably with those of our previous experience using PVB alone followed by surgery. In the alternating series, we obtained a CR (defined as no viable cancer at surgical exploration) in 7 of 13 patients (54%), as compared with 6 of 15 patients (40%) in the previous series. Moreover, 2 patients in the previous series had relapses at 13 and 30 months, whereas no patient in this series has relapsed after a median follow-up of 36 months (range, 14–48 months). However, some important differences between our two series must be taken into consideration. In the first study, 8 patients presented with mediastinal involvement and no patient had a pure seminoma; in the second study, 2 patients had pure seminoma and only 2 patients had mediastinal involvement. This prognostic imbalance in clinical and pathologic characteristics may in effect bias results in favor of the group of patients with EGGCC treated with PVB/PEB(A).

Recently, other researchers have employed aggressive regimens for patients presenting with EGGCC. Logothetis et al. (1985a) report experience at The University of Texas M. D. Anderson Cancer Center treating 49 patients with various chemotherapeutic regimens. They report a disease-free survival in 16 of 19 patients (84%) with extragonadal seminoma, especially good results for those treated with combination chemotherapy that included cisplatin (14 of 14 patients surviving disease free), and disease-free survival overall in 12 of 30 patients (40%) with nonseminomatous EGGCC. When they analyzed the survival results of this latter group as a function of the treatment received, they found that 6 of 9 patients (67%) treated with alternating chemotherapy ($CISCA_{II}/VB_{IV}$, i.e., cisplatin, cyclophosphamide, Adriamycin + vinblastine and bleomycin) were surviving disease free, as compared with 2 of 8 (25%) treated with $CISCA_{II}$ alone or VB + P (vinblastine, bleomycin, cisplatin), a statistically significant difference. After introducing the more aggressive chemotherapeutic program, the authors noted a lack of statistical significance in the differences in response rate between primary abdominal and mediastinal EGGCC.

Bosl et al. (1986) report their experience in treating 19 patients with extragonadal tumors, including 9 with mediastinal disease, with the VAB-6 (vinblastine, dactinomycin (actinomycin

TABLE 50–2.
Hematologic Toxicity*

Component	PVB (% of Patients Affected)	PEB (% of Patients Affected)	PEBA (% of Patients Affected)
	Regimen		
Leukocytes			
<2,000/µl	26	21	9
<1,500/µl	24	26	30
<1,000/µl	14	18	45
Granulocytes			
<1,500/µl	12	9	5
<1,000/µl	32	32	15
<500/µl	34	50	61
Platelets			
<90,000/µl	2	3	5
<70,000/µl	4	21	15
<40,000/µl	4	24	47
Hgb <10 g/100 ml	28	47	48

*PVB = cisplatin, vinblastine, bleomycin; PEB = cisplatin, etoposide, bleomycin; PEBA = PEB + Adriamycin; Hgb = hemoglobin.

TABLE 50–3.
Nonhematologic Toxicity

Toxic Response	PVB Alone (% of Patients Affected)	PVB/PEB(A) (% of Patients Affected)
	Regimen	
Nausea and vomiting	69	73
Mucositis/stomatitis	22	23
Abdominal cramps	19	13
Constipation	30	23
Ileus	9	6
Paresthesias	19	13
Raynaud's phenomenon	13	13
Hypomagnesemia	41	27
Pulmonary abnormalities	9	40
Creatinine level changes from baseline (%):		
25	15	16
25–50	6	16
>50	9	13
Hospital admission for fever	24	60
Treatment-related death	1	2

*PVB = cisplatin, vinblastine, bleomycin; PEB(A) = cisplatin, etoposide, bleomycin, with or without Adriamycin.

D), bleomycin) regimen. They obtained very good results against the extragonadal seminomas—8 of 8 patients alive and disease free; however, only 6 of 11 patients with extragonadal nonseminomatous malignancies (55%) achieved a CR, and 3 of these eventually relapsed, resulting in an ultimate disease-free survival rate of 27% after a median follow-up of 46 months (range, 1–67 months). In a phase II trial alternating etoposide plus cisplatin with VAB-6 for 14 patients with EGGCC, Bosl et al. (1987) obtained a CR in 8 patients (57%) and a disease-free survival in 5 of them (37%) after an unspecified follow-up. They did not find this result statistically different from the response rate obtained in their previous series using VAB-6 alone.

An early report from the Southwest Oncology Group Study (Bokowski et al. 1985) of a trial using four cycles of alternating chemotherapy with PVB/PEBA showed promising results, with 13 of 15 treated patients achieving a CR. It was too early, however, for them to draw conclusions about the curative potential of the regimen. Hainsworth et al. (1982) reported that their results improved when they used sequential chemotherapy—vinblastine, bleomycin, and cisplatin with or without Adriamycin followed by surgical removal of residual abnormalities—for a series of 31 patients with extragonadal tumors, 17 of whom had mediastinal involvement. They obtained CRs in 4 of 6 patients (67%) with extragonadal seminoma and in 17 of 26 (65%) with extragonadal nonseminomatous tumors and a long-term disease-free survival in 18 of 31 patients (58%) after a median follow-up of 30 months (range, 3–52 months). Unfortunately, their exclusion of patients with mediastinal endodermal sinus tumors from this series makes impossible a full comparison with other reported series.

High-Risk Testicular Cancers

Recently, we have identified a subgroup of patients with advanced primary testicular NSGCT whom, we believe, have a very poor prognosis (Garnick et al. 1984). We included patients who presented with bone metastases, brain metastases, a serum HCG titer greater than 2,000 ng/ml, and liver metastases with a concomitant serum HCG titer greater than 2,000 ng/ml. In a subgroup with such a poor prognosis, we have obtained a CR in 5 of 12 patients (42%). Only one patient has relapsed from CR at 6 months. Follow-up is not yet sufficiently long to draw conclusions on the true curative potential of the present alternating regimen. In our previous study (Garnick et al. 1983) using PVB alone followed by surgery, we obtained a CR in 35 of 39 patients (90%) with disseminated germ cell cancer and a long-term disease-free survival in 32 (82%). Most patients in this earlier group, however, did not have as many poor-prognostic risk factors.

Researchers from UT M. D. Anderson Cancer Center (Logothetis et al. 1985b), treating with $CISCA_{II}/VB_{IV}$ 48 patients with disseminated NSGCT, 50% of whom had advanced disease (stage $III-B_4$ and $III-B_5$ by Samuels' staging criteria), obtained a CR in 44 patients (92%). All remain alive and disease-free after a median follow-up of about 35 months (range, 19–57). Researchers from the Memorial Sloan-Kettering Cancer Center (Bosl et al. 1986) evaluated the VAB-6 program for 142 patients with disseminated germ cell tumors of the testis (including 22 patients with seminoma). They reported a CR rate of 79% (112 patients); because 12 (11%) eventually relapsed, the disease-free survival rate was 70% (100 of 142 patients) after a median follow-up of 44 months (range, 1–69 months).

Certainly, the results of our present study are considerably inferior when they are compared to those reported for equivalent aggressive chemotherapeutic programs and even to those we have reported for the PVB combination used in a broader population of patients with advanced primary testicular NSGCT. This fact may truly be the reflection of the poor prognostic group that we have identified among patients with advanced NSGCT. Even an aggressive approach using an alternating regimen like the one we tested in the present study has proved to be insufficient in significantly improving the prognosis of this subset of patients.

Undifferentiated cancers whose clinical syndrome is compatible with a germ cell origin carry a very dismal prognosis. No patient responded to the aggressive PVB/PEB(A) chemotherapeutic program, and the median survival time has been 4 months. Our experience is comparable to that of other groups. Our decision to include patients with mediastinal undifferentiated cancers but no marker elevation may have contributed to the lower response rates.

A CR and no histologic evidence of viable cancer at surgical exploration is the most important goal of the induction chemotherapy program. We detected viable cancer in 4 of the 9 patients with EGGCC treated with PVB alone, and in only 1 of those 4 could we obtain a durable CR after radical resection and intensive additional chemotherapy. Among the 5 patients with EGGCC treated with PVB/PEB(A) who underwent surgery, we identified viable cancer that could not be surgically eradicated in 3. Although 3 of the 6 partial responders with NSGCT could be rendered disease-free after radical resection, all 3 relapsed systemically during the salvage program. Similarly Bosl et al. (1987) report that, in their recent experience, 4 of 5 patients with viable cancer at surgery had an early relapse despite two more courses of alternating chemotherapy, and only 1 of these was still alive. Patients who are found to have viable cancer after the induction chemotherapy phase cannot, in our experience, be considered complete responders, and more effective salvage treatment is needed for them.

Unfortunately, the contribution of Adriamycin to the therapeutic efficacy of this regimen cannot be easily evaluated. Adriamycin has been shown to improve the results when added to etoposide-based salvage regimens for refractory germ cell cancers (Lederman and Garnick 1986), but its role in addition to other active agents in first-line regimens for the poor-prognosis groups has not yet been clearly established; clinical studies are still needed to determine its place.

Toxicity from the alternating regimen seems to be higher than that from PVB alone. The addition of etoposide and Adriamycin has certainly increased myelotoxicity, thereby increasing the need for red blood cell and platelet transfusions. More patients in the second series required hospital admission for fever. However, the incidence of infectious episodes has not been greater after the PEB/PEBA regimens than after PVB chemotherapy. By reducing the total amount of vinblastine administered, we seem to have decreased the incidence of neurotoxic side effects. The only serious and really life-threatening complication has been the pulmonary toxicity from bleomycin, responsible for the two observed treatment-related deaths. Different schedules, including administration of the drug by continuous infusion, have been associated with lower pulmonary toxicity, and this change may be considered for future treatment plans.

CONCLUSION

Clearly, defined areas in the treatment of poor-prognosis germ cell cancers are still open to improvement (Garnick 1985). Although the PVB regimen has proved to be adequate to cure most patients with advanced testicular disease and extragonadal seminoma, future treatment must focus on achieving and maintaining higher cure rates while minimizing both acute and long-term toxicities for patients with nonseminomatous EGGCC or advanced testicular NSGCT with "poor-prognosis" features. More aggressive regimens than the standard PVB are required to provide better results for these patients. However, the superiority of one program over another is difficult to assess without data generated from prospectively randomized trials. Patients who achieve a CR with the initial chemotherapeutic phase have good chances of long disease-free survivals and, ultimately, of cure. For patients who do not achieve a CR and who have residual viable cancer or persistently elevated levels of tumor markers, new intensive salvage strategies are needed. The use of high doses of active drugs such as carboplatin and ifosfamide, along with autologous bone marrow transplantation, may be the next step towards further improving our results in this field.

REFERENCES

1. Bosl GJ, Geller NL, Vogelzang NJ, et al. 1987. Alternating cycles of etoposide plus cisplatin and VAB-6 in the treatment of poor-risk patients with germ cell tumors. *J Clin Oncol* 5:436–440.
2. Bosl GJ, Gluckman R, Geller NL, et al. 1986. VAB-6: An effective chemotherapy regimen for patients with germ-cell tumors. *J Clin Oncol* 4:1493–1499.
4. Bukowski RM, Montie J. 1985. Phase II trial of combination chemotherapy in patients with extragonadal germ cell tumors: Southwest Oncology Group Study (abstract). *Proc Am Assoc Cancer Res* 26:166.
5. Einhorn LH. 1981. Testicular cancer as a model for curable neoplasm: The Richard and Hinda Rosenthal Foundation Award Lecture. *Cancer Res* 41:3275–3280.
6. Einhorn LH, Donohue J. 1977. Cis-diamminedichloroplatinum, vinblastine, and bleomycin combination chemotherapy in disseminated testicular cancer. *Ann Intern Med* 87:293–298.
7. Einhorn LH, Williams SD, Troner M, et al. 1981. The role of maintenance therapy in disseminated testicular cancer. *N Engl J Med* 305:727–731.
8. Garnick MB. 1985. Advanced testicular cancer: Treatment choices in the "land of plenty." *J Clin Oncol* 3:294–297.
9. Garnick MB, Canellos GP, Richie JP. 1983. Treatment and surgical staging of testicular and primary extragonadal germ cell cancer. *JAMA* 250:1733–1741.
10. Garnick MB, Canellos GP, Lederman GS, et al. 1984. Treatment of extragonadal germ cell tumors (letter). *J Clin Oncol* 2:713.
11. Hainsworth JD, Einhorn LH, Williams SD, et al. 1982. Advanced extragonadal germ-cell tumors: Successful treatment with combination chemotherapy. *Ann Intern Med* 97:7–11.
12. Lederman GS, Garnick MB. 1986. Possible benefit of doxorubicin treatment in patients with refractory germ cell cancer. *Cancer* 58:2393–2398.
13. Logothetis CJ, Samuels ML, Selig DE, et al. 1985a. Chemotherapy of extragonadal germ cell tumors. *J Clin Oncol* 3:316–325.
14. Logothetis CJ, Samuels ML, Selig DE, et al. 1985b. Improved survival with cyclic chemotherapy for nonseminomatous germ cell tumors of the testis. *J Clin Oncol* 3:326–335.

Chapter 51

Germ Cell Tumors: Commentary

Christopher J. Logothetis, M.D.

Douglas E. Johnson, M.D.

Andrew C. von Eschenbach, M.D.

Cures of patients with germ cell tumors have been commonplace for more than a decade. Because they were among the first solid tumors to be curable when metastatic, the therapeutic concepts developed for germ cell tumors have served as models for treatments of other solid tumors. Nevertheless, questions remain about the significance of dose intensity in chemotherapy, the duration and amount of chemotherapy required, and the ideal manner of integrating chemotherapy and surgery. In the chapters of this section, the authors have addressed these and other current issues of germ cell tumor therapy.

Since vinblastine-bleomycin–based chemotherapy was introduced in 1970, later supplemented by cisplatin, investigators have learned much about the staging and natural behavior of germ cell tumors that has affected their treatment. Initially, clinical investigators were concerned with developing and refining systemic therapy for patients with advanced metastatic disease. More recently, clinical trials have been directed towards patients with "early stage" disease. This trend has led to the high cure rates with minimal morbidity that this group of patients enjoys.

SEMINOMA

Most investigators agree that seminoma has distinct features that justify its segration from nonseminomatous germ cell tumors and that patients in the seminoma category deserve separate and special consideration. Clinicians treating these patients have recognized their reduced tolerance to the conventional bleomycin-based chemotherapy that is effective against nonseminomatous tumors. The frequency of bleomycin pulmonary complications has since been shown to be high among patients with seminoma (Friedman et al. 1985; Loehrer et al. 1987).

In addition to the increased morbidity of the standard vinblastine-bleomycin-cisplatin combination for patients with seminoma, these patients have been recognized as being more sensitive to alkylating agents (Whitmore et al. 1977; Calman et al. 1979). Accordingly, patients with metastatic seminoma at The University of Texas M. D. Anderson Cancer Center have been treated as a unique subpopulation of patients with germ cell tumors. The choice of regimen has been based on the clinical knowledge of the unique sensitivity of seminomas to alkylating agents. The two-drug combination currently used at our hospital includes a combination of cyclophosphamide and sequential cisplatin (Chong and Logothetis, Chapter 36). A two-drug combination employing etoposide (VP-16-213) and cisplatin, also not incorporating bleomycin (Bosl, Chapter 37), appears in preliminary analysis to be effective.

One can summarize the results of treatment of seminoma easily: seminoma is a disease that is extremely responsive to cisplatin-based chemotherapy. Seminoma appears to be uniquely sensitive to bleomycin-based chemotherapy, and severely myelosuppressive acutely toxic vinblastine-bleomycin combinations are not required. Cisplatin is the essential agent in the treatment of seminoma.

Interpretation of seminoma treatment data requires great caution. The question of combining radiation therapy and chemotherapy has been addressed at both UT M. D. Anderson Cancer Center and the Memorial Sloan-Kettering Cancer Center (Logothetis et al. 1987; Bosl, Chapter 37). Both institutions recognize that persistent discrete masses in the retroperitoneum require further therapy. The arbitrary limit defined at Memorial Sloan-Kettering Cancer Center is a mass 3 cm in diameter. Investigators at Memorial Sloan-Kettering recommend surgical exploration, including an excisional biopsy of this mass; we have recommended definitive radiation as treatment. The correctness of either approach has yet to be established. Because of the overwhelmingly high cure rate among patients treated at both institutions, the difference is likely to be reflected in morbidity of therapy rather than in disease-free survival rate.

A remaining dilemma in treating seminoma is to define which patients with disease confined to the abdomen need radiation therapy only and which require systemic therapy. This dilemma persists because of the lack of a uniform staging system for investigators to use. Arbitrary limits set by different investigators for the staging of these tumors have made it difficult to compare patients reliably. Zagars (Chapter 38) has reviewed the UT M. D. Anderson Cancer Center experience and notes that, for patients with a mass less than 10 cm in maximum diameter, cure with radiotherapy alone has been nearly universal. Patients with a retroperitoneal mass greater than 10 cm need systemic chemotherapy because of the high likelihood of systemic relapse. It is very clear that stringent criteria for measuring retroperitoneal disease are required so that appropriately integrated systemic and local therapy can be defined for these patients.

For patients with a mass measuring less than 10 cm in diameter and confined to the retroperitoneum, the current radiotherapy approach as used in the Princess Margaret Hospital (Thomas, Chapter 39) achieves an overwhelmingly high rate of cure, without the need for irradiation to the mediastinum. Radiotherapists and chemotherapists agree that all patients with disease above the diaphragm need systemic chemotherapy.

NONSEMINOMATOUS GERM CELL TUMORS OF THE TESTIS

Distant Metastatic Disease

The experiences of investigators of the Australasian Germ Cell Study Group, Stanford University and the Northern California Oncology Group (NCOG), Memorial Sloan-Kettering Cancer Center, and M. D. Anderson Cancer Center in treating patients with nonseminomatous germ cell tumors of the testis (NSGCTT) have been presented here for comparison. All investigators agree that vinblastine-bleomycin-platinum–based combination chemotherapy regimens have achieved long-term disease-free survivals. The survival duration is determined by volume of disease, degree of elevation of serum beta-human chorionic gonadotropin (β-HCG), and the sites of metastatic involvement. For patients with low-volume disease, these cure rates are high and durable with vinblastine-bleomycin-cisplatin–based chemotherapy, independent of histology. The activity of etoposide in germ cell tumor therapy has been recognized as equal to that of the drugs originally employed.

The various combination chemotherapy regimens used by the investigators for patients with moderate- and small-volume disease all produce high response rates. At M. D. Anderson Cancer Center and at Stanford University (Lo et al., Chapter 45), a flexible number of courses of chemotherapy, determined by the response of the tumor, are delivered. We administer two chemotherapy courses beyond the development of a complete remission (CR) or stable biomarker-negative mass. We believe that employing this concept has reduced both the relapse rate and the rate of failure to achieve a CR. Most investigators, including those of the Memorial Sloan-Kettering Cancer Center and the Australasian Germ Cell Study Group, administer a fixed number of courses of chemotherapy. All investigators perform equally aggressive surgery following the chemotherapy, and all agree that surgical removal of residual teratoma is necessary.

For patients with advanced metastatic poor-prognostic germ cell tumors, more intense chemotherapy regimens have been proposed. The M. D. Anderson Cancer Center regimen of cisplatin, cyclophosphamide, and Adriamycin alternating with vinblastine and bleomycin (cyclic $CISCA_{II}/VB_{IV}$) has achieved a high and durable CR rate. The results reveal that in excess of 75% of patients with truly advanced disease as defined by the modification of the Samuels' staging system achieved durable CRs. Tondini and Garnick at the Dana-Farber Cancer Institute (Chapter 50) confirm the relative ineffectiveness of vinblastine-bleomycin-cisplatin–based combination chemotherapy regimens for patients with truly advanced disease. Clinicians generally agree that patients with far-advanced disease need very aggressive, intense chemotherapy that may incorporate other active cytotoxic drugs. Dispute persists regarding the relative effectiveness of the more recent aggressive chemotherapy regimens ($CISCA_{II}/VB_{IV}$ vs. POMPACE [cisplatin, vincristine, actinomycin D, methotrexate, chlorambucil, bleomycin, and etoposide]).

Locoregional Disease

Patients with local-regional NSGCTT have been the objects of much interest recently in the literature. The availability of computerized tomography and reliable assays for serum β-HCG and alpha-fetoprotein (AFP) have increased physicians' confidence in their ability to identify true stage I disease.

As a result, investigators have become more willing simply to monitor patients with stage I NSGCTT (Peckham 1985). A number of studies have attempted to refine the clinical staging further. General agreement exists that patients with vascular invasion in the primary testicular tumor have an increased likelihood of developing subsequent metastases. Based on this information, some investigators have proposed that these patients not be incorporated in the stage I surveillance programs. However, the cure rate for all patients with stage I tumors is extremely high, including those with vascular invasion in the primary tumor.

The survival of patients treated with chemotherapy is directly related to the volume of disease at treatment. Although patients with vascular invasion in the primary tumor are at a higher likelihood of relapse, it is not clear that they have a lower chance of achieving an overall cure if they are more closely observed, yet included in surveillance protocols. Furthermore, a portion of such patients, ranging from 30% to 50%, has the opportunity to be cured of any disease with a simple orchiectomy. The fears that delays in delivering systemic chemotherapy will result in a lower cure rate have not been realized. The cure rates reported in the literature from the British experience, from M. D. Anderson Cancer Center (Swanson and Johnson, Chapter 40), and from Memorial Sloan-Kettering Cancer Center (Herr et al., Chapter 41) are uniformly overwhelmingly high. Differences in patient selection notwithstanding, this approach is safe in the hands of these investigators.

It is clear that a surveillance protocol is a therapeutic approach designed to maintain a high cure rate and reduce the morbidity of potentially unnecessary therapy. With the availability of modern chemotherapy and reliable staging criteria, the responsibility lies in the hands of clinician and patient not only to achieve a high rate of cure but also to reduce unnecessary morbidity.

Differences in therapeutic approach for patients in whom NSGCT is confined to the retroperitoneum also exist. The approach of M. D. Anderson Cancer Center is to refine further the treatment of such patients. Our clinical experience has allowed us to identify subgroups that are likely to benefit from primary chemotherapy and subgroups that are more likely to benefit from primary surgery. For those with clinical stage II disease, which includes a higher tumor-volume spectrum than pathologic stage II disease, we believe that the first treatment should be chemotherapy. Chemotherapy is likely to totally eradicate the retroperitoneal metastases of patients with pure embryonal carcinoma, eliminating the need for later surgery. Patients with teratomatous elements in the primary tumor are less likely to achieve total eradication of retroperitoneal metastasis and frequently require postchemotherapy excision of residual teratoma. Therefore, patients with primary embryonal carcinoma benefit by reducing the frequency of double therapy without compromising their ultimate cure. Patients with teratomatous elements in the primary lesion do not have such an obvious benefit, although they continue to have an extremely high survival rate. A more refined therapeutic approach is currently being investigated that should reduce the frequency of double therapy without compromising the long-term survival rate (Logothetis, Chapter 30).

Difficulty in interpreting clinical stage II data, now that therapy for patients with disease confined to the retroperitoneum offers several options, emphasizes the need for a clinical staging system. Requirements are meticulous attention to detail in the pathologic review of the primary tumor and the use of computerized tomography and serum biomarker evaluation to determine the extent of retroperitoneal disease.

EXTRAGONADAL GERM CELL TUMORS

Patients with extragonadal germ cell tumors remain the single most difficult therapeutic challenge. The experiences at the Dana-Farber Cancer Institute (Tondini and Garnick, Chapter 50) and at UT M. D. Anderson Cancer Center (Chong and Logothetis, Chapter 49) confirm the relatively high mortality of this group of patients. Unusual histologic subtypes with relative chemotherapy resistance are disproportionately represented. General agreement currently exists that patients with extragonadal presentations deserve an individualized approach and very intense therapy. Novel therapeutic approaches and increased intensity must be investigated for these patients. Like patients with very advanced NSGCTT, patients with extragonadal germ cell tumors should be the subjects of clinical investigations that incorporate additional cytotoxic drugs at greater intensity.

REFERENCES

1. Calman FMB, Peckham MJ, Hendry WF. 1979. The pattern of spread and treatment of metastases in testicular seminoma. *Br J Urol* 51:154–160.
2. Friedman EL, Garnick MB, Stomper PC, et al. 1985. Therapeutic guidelines and results in advanced seminoma. *J Clin Oncol* 3:1325–1332.
3. Loehrer PJ, Birch R, Williams SD, et al. 1987. Chemotherapy of metastatic seminoma: The Southeastern Cancer Study Group experience. *J Clin Oncol* 5:1212–1220.
4. Logothetis CJ, Samuels ML, Ogden SL, et al. 1987. Cyclophosphamide and sequential cisplatin for advanced seminoma: long-term follow-up in 52 patients. *J Urol* 138:789–794.
5. Peckham MJ. 1985. Orchiectomy for clinical stage I testicular cancer: Progress report of the Royal Marsden Hospital study. *J R Soc Med* 78(suppl):41–42.
6. Whitmore WF Jr, Smith A, Yagoda A, et al. 1977. Chemotherapy of seminoma. W. Vahlensieck (ed): *Recent Results Cancer Res* 60:244–249.

Index